THIRD EDITION

Modern Neuromuscular Techniques

with accompanying DVD-ROM

Leon Chaitow ND DO
Osteopathic Practitioner and Honorary Fellow,
University of Westminster, London, UK

with contributions from

Judith DeLany LMT
(Chapter 10: American neuromuscular therapy)
Director of Neuromuscular Therapy Training Center, St Petersburg, Florida, USA

Dennis J Dowling DO FAAO
(Chapter 11: PINS technique)
Attending Physician and Director of Manipulative Medicine
Physical Medicine and Rehabilitation Department
Nassau University Medical Center
New York, USA
Director of Osteopathic Manipulative Medicine Assessment
The National Board of Osteopathic Medical Examiners Clinical Skills Testing Center
Pennsylvania, USA

Howard Evans MA PgDiP
(Chapter 12: Thai massage and neuromuscular technique)
School of Therapeutic Bodywork, London, UK

Foreword by Professor Cesar Fernandez de las Penaz PT DO MSc PhD
Universidad Rey Juan Carlos, Madrid, Spain

Original Illustrations by **Graeme Chambers** BA (HONS)
Medical Artist

CHURCHILL
LIVINGSTONE

ELSEVIER

Edinburgh London New York Oxford Philadelphia St Louis Sydney Toronto 2011

First edition 1996
Second edition 2003
Third edition 2011

ISBN 9780443069376

British Library Cataloguing in Publication Data
A catalogue record for this book is available from the British Library

Library of Congress Cataloging in Publication Data
A catalog record for this book is available from the Library of Congress

Notices
Knowledge and best practice in this field are constantly changing. As new research and experience broaden our understanding, changes in research methods, professional practices, or medical treatment may become necessary.

Practitioners and researchers must always rely on their own experience and knowledge in evaluating and using any information, methods, compounds, or experiments described herein. In using such information or methods they should be mindful of their own safety and the safety of others, including parties for whom they have a professional responsibility.

With respect to any drug or pharmaceutical products identified, readers are advised to check the most current information provided (i) on procedures featured or (ii) by the manufacturer of each product to be administered, to verify the recommended dose or formula, the method and duration of administration, and contraindications. It is the responsibility of practitioners, relying on their own experience and knowledge of their patients, to make diagnoses, to determine dosages and the best treatment for each individual patient, and to take all appropriate safety precautions.

To the fullest extent of the law, neither the Publisher nor the authors, contributors, or editors, assume any liability for any injury and/or damage to persons or property as a matter of products liability, negligence or otherwise, or from any use or operation of any methods, products, instructions, or ideas contained in the material herein.

£47.99

Modern Neuromuscular Techniques

Publisher: Sarena Wolfaard
Development Editor: Carole McMurray
Project Manager: Kerrie-Anne McKinlay
Designer: Stewart Larking
Illustration Buyer: Merlyn Harvey

Contents

The CD-ROM accompanying this text includes video sequences of all the techniques indicated by the icon. To look at the video for a given technique, click on the relevant icon on the CD-ROM. The CD-ROM is designed to be used in conjunction with the text and not as a stand-alone product.

Abbreviations		vii
Foreword		ix
Preface		xi
Dedication		xiii
1	Soft tissue distress	1
2	Introduction to NMT	35
3	Myofascial trigger points and other reflex phenomena	43
4	The variety of reflex points	75
5	Diagnostic methods	97
6	Basic spinal NMT	123
7	Basic abdominal and pelvic NMT application	141
8	Associated techniques	155
9	NMT in clinical use	203
10	American neuromuscular therapy *Judith DeLany*	221
11	Progressive inhibition of neuromusculoskeletal structures (PINS) technique *Dennis J Dowling*	247
12	Thai massage and neuromuscular technique *Howard Evans*	275
	Appendix – Nimmo, Chiropractic and myofascial pain *Jeffrey Cohen, Russell W. Gibbons, Michael Schneider and Howard Vernon*	291
	Index	315

Abbreviations

ACh	acetylcholine
ASIS	anterior superior iliac spine
ATP	adenosine triphosphate
CFS	chronic fatigue syndrome
CNS	central nervous system
CSF	cerebrospinal fluid
CTM	connective tissue massage
EAV	electroacupuncture according to Voll
EMG	electromyography
FMS	fibromyalgia syndrome
FPR	facilitated positional release
GAS	general adaptation syndrome
HIV	human immunodeficiency virus
HSZ	hyperalgesic skin zone
HVLA	high-velocity low-amplitude
HVT	high-velocity thrust
INIT	integrated neuromuscular inhibition technique
LAS	local adaptation syndrome
MET	muscle energy technique

MI	mechanical interface
MPS	myofascial pain syndrome
MRT	myofascial release technique
NGF	nerve growth factor
NGP	noxious generative point
NMT	neuromuscular technique/therapy (USA)
PINS	progressive inhibition of neuromuscular structures
PIR	post-isometric relaxation
PNF	proprioceptive neuromuscular facilitation
PRT	positional release technique
PSIS	posterior superior iliac spine
RI	reciprocal inhibition
SCM	sternocleidomastoid
SCS	strain/counterstrain
STM	soft tissue manipulation
TCM	traditional Chinese medicine
TFL	tensor fascia lata
TMJ	temporomandibular joint

Foreword

It is my pleasure to write the foreword for the third edition of the textbook Modern Neuromuscular Techniques edited by Leon Chaitow. As always the editor has done excellent work by incorporating the expertise of other authors, in order to improve the quality of this essential textbook, written for manual and physical therapists, osteopaths and chiropractors. Chaitow is an Osteopathic Practitioner and Honorary Fellow at the University of Westminster, London, UK who combines clinical practice, teaching and writing activities. He is also the Editor-in-chief of the Journal of Bodywork and Movement Therapies, one of the most important clinical journals in Europe. Chaitow has written many textbooks, a number of which focus on manual approaches employed in the management of chronic pain and dysfunction. One of these excellent textbooks is the current one.

This textbook provides the most current information relating to the range of modalities known as Neuromuscular Techniques (NMT). The books lead author and contributors have combined both clinical and scientific experience with an in-depth knowledge of the literature, to analyze, integrate, and present useful information and guidelines relevant to the practicing clinician. There are different forms of application of NMT, and most are covered in this edition, from classical European (Lief's) NMT, to the American model of Neuromuscular Therapy (also abbreviated as NMT), as well as a fascinating chapter on the merging of NMT with Thai massage. This is appropriate since European NMT has at least part of its roots in Ayurvedic massage, as explained in the introductory chapters. Another important feature of this edition is the inclusion of an appendix that outlines the work of Raymond Nimmo DC, a contemporary of the early researchers into our understanding of myofascial pain and trigger points. As explained in early chapters, Nimmo's work strongly influenced American NMT, and there remains much to learn from his early chiropractic exploration of the aetiology and treatment of soft-tissue pain and dysfunction.

The clinical usefulness of NMT is acknowledged worldwide as both an assessment and treatment tool for the management of soft tissue disorders. NMT can be used for deactivating trigger points (TrPs) as well as for improving circulation of fascial tissues (Simons et al, 1999). Ibañez-García et al. (2009) demonstrated the effectiveness of NMT for the management of TrPs within the masseter muscle. Other authors have proposed NMT as one key element for the management of headaches (Palomeque-del-Cerro & Fernández-de-las-Peñas, 2010). In fact, in clinical practice NMT methods are commonly combined with other manual local techniques, e.g. ischemic compression, positional release and muscle energy techniques, for inactivating TrPs (Palomeque-del-Cerro & Fernández-de-las-Peñas, 2010). In my own clinical practice, NMT is one key element for the management of soft tissue disorders, in different chronic pain conditions, such as lateral epicondylalgia, tension type headache, carpal tunnel syndrome, fibromyalgia, low back and neck pain.

The editors, authors, publisher, illustrators, and all others involved in the production of this book can be justifiably proud of the final product. I hope you, the reader, will find the important, timely information that it contains, useful in assessing, treating and managing your patients. If both patients and clinicians benefit, then the efforts of people involved in compiling this text will have been well worth it.

César Fernández-de-las-Peñas, PT, DO, MSc, PhD

Departamento de Fisioterapia, Terapia Ocupacional, Rehabilitación y Medicina Física, Universidad Rey Juan Carlos, Madrid, Spain

References

Ibáñez-García J, Alburquerque-Sendín F, Rodríguez-Blanco C, et al: Changes in masseter muscle trigger points following strain-counter/ strain or neuro-muscular technique, *J Bodywork Movement Therapies* 13(1):2–10, 2009.

Simons DG, Travell J, Simons LS: *Myofascial pain and dysfunction: The trigger point manual*, Vol 1, ed 2, Baltimore, 1999, Williams & Wilkins.

Palomeque-del-Cerro L, Fernández-de-las-Peñas C: Neuromuscular approaches? In Fernández-de-las-Peñas C, Arendt-Nielsen L, Gerwin R, editors: *Tension Type and Cervicogenic Headache: pathophysiology, diagnosis and treatment*, Boston, 2010, Jones & Bartlett Publishers, pp. 327–338.

Preface

"What are neuromuscular techniques (NMT)?"

If this subject (NMT) is new to you, that would be a reasonable question to ask.

Simplistically, and literally, the answer would point to NMT comprising methods that involve the nervous system and the musculoskeletal system - which realistically would involve almost all manual therapy techniques and modalities.

However, a more focused and accurate use of the term NMT exists – and this relates to manual treatment of soft tissue dysfunction in general, and mysofascial (trigger point), and other reflexogenically related aspects of dysfunction, in particular.

The roots of NMT, as it evolved in the USA and Europe, are outlined in the opening chapters (particularly chapter 2). There the work of a few key individuals responsible for the body of knowledge that informs what we now term NMT, is described. These include the many years of study, innovation and development, by pioneer British osteopath and naturopath, Stanley Lief, his son Peter Lief ND DC, and his cousin Boris Chaitow ND DO DC. Across the Atlantic Raymond Nimmo DC – an innovative US based chiropractor - as well as the two premier researchers into myofascial pain, Janet Travell MD and David Simons MD added additional clinical and research dimensions.

While these early chapters mirror what was in earlier editions, the content has been updated to take account of recent research

The ways in which the efforts of those named individuals (and others), working separately and sometimes in combination, matured into our current understanding of myofascial pain, and how it can be treated, are therefore detailed in the opening chapters, while novel material regarding Nimmo's concepts, as well as a current review of chiropractic approaches to myofascial pain, is contained in an important appendix.

Understanding how myofascial pain evolves offers the best means for preventing and eliminating it – with chapters 3 and 4 focusing specifically on trigger point and other reflexogenic phenomena.

Following on from that, chapter 5 discusses diagnostic and assessment approaches, followed, in chapters 6 and 7, by details of the methodology of European ('Lief's') NMT, both for the spine and abdomen. A separate chapter (8) details and discusses associated methods, modalities and techniques, while chapter 9 outlines an extremely useful combinations of NMT modalities in trigger point deactivation, as well as other clinical approaches.

In a fully updated chapter 10, American neuromuscular therapy is then reviewed and outlined, with specific examples, by the gifted therapist, author and teacher, Judith Delany. In a chapter on progressive inhibition of neuromuscular structures, (11) osteopathic professor Dennis Dowling describes this innovative pain management approach which has distinctive echoes of NMT.

Howard Evans, in his chapter on Thai massage and NMT (12), skilfully blends these two approaches. Howard obtained his Masters degree in Soft Tissue Manipulation approaches at the University of Westminster, London in the 1990's, and since then has developed ever more subtle variations of NMT and Thai yoga massage.

As mentioned above, the appendix contains expanded material on the Nimmo approach – the pioneer whose work is first introduced in the opening chapters.

This third edition of Modern Neuromuscular Techniques has therefore been conceived as a offering revision updates, as well as new material – emphasising the relevance of NMT to a wide spectrum of professions – many of which contributed to its origins – physical therapy, osteopathy, chiropractic, massage therapy, Thai yoga massage – and more.

Leon Chaitow

Corfu, Greece, April 2010

Dedication

The death of David Simons MD (1922-2010), on April 5th 2010 demands recognition. He was working on a revision of his magisterial trigger point manual until days before he passed away – heading for (as he circulated to family, friends and colleagues) his "next great adventure".

David was also a pioneer of space exploration. On August 19, 1957 he became the first man to travel into outer space in a pressurised gondola travelling to over 100,000 feet as part of the Man High Project. He had volunteered for this 36 hour venture to study the effects of cosmic radiation on living tissue – his own!

David was the last survivor of those whose clinical work, research and writing allowed NMT to evolve. His historically important texts *Myofascial Pain and Dysfunction: The Trigger Point Manual, Volumes 1 and 2* (co-authored with Janet Travell) remain unparalleled in their detailed descriptions and analysis of causes and treatment options, of myofascial pain in general, and trigger points in particular.

This book is dedicated to David, with grateful thanks.

Soft tissue distress

CHAPTER CONTENTS

Somatic dysfunction   2
Identifying sources of pain   2
Coherent and incoherent patterns   3
Reporting stations   3
Effect of contradictory information   4
Contradictory gibberish?   5
Neural 'cross-talk'   5
Mechanisms that alter proprioception   5
Trophic neural influences   6
Neural influences on gene expression   6
Maitland and Butler: 'abnormal neural movement'   8
The role of neuromuscular techniques in management of adaptive overload   9
General adaptation syndrome (GAS) and local adaptation syndrome (LAS), and connective tissue   10
A biomechanical stress response sequence   11
Unsustainable without consequences   12
Causes of soft tissue dysfunction   12
Some major soft tissue stress categories   12
Other models of pain genesis   14
Stoddard's osteopathic perspective   15
Modern pain concepts   15
Sensitization   16
Different responses in postural and phasic muscles   17
Fetal position influences   17
Role of the muscles in low back problems   19
Muscle types   20
Therapeutic choices   20
Postural and phasic muscle lists   21
Fibrositis   22
Fibrositis changes its name to fibromyalgia   22

The fascial network   22
Functional fascial continuities   24
Soft tissue changes – energy and fascial considerations   25
Fascial stress responses and therapeutic opportunities   26
Ligaments and muscle tone   30

Somatic dysfunction

The musculoskeletal system – sometimes referred to as the locomotor system – is the means whereby we act out and express our human existence – 'The primary machinery of life' is what one of osteopathy's greatest researchers, Irwin Korr (1970), called it. While, medically speaking, the musculoskeletal system may lack the glamour and fascination of vital organs and systems, the fact is that the cardiovascular and neuroendocrine and digestive (and other) systems and organs exist only to service this great biomechanical structure through which we live and function. It is by means of our musculoskeletal system (not our kidneys or livers) that we perform tasks, play games, make love, impart treatment, perform on musical instruments, paint and, in these and a multitude of other ways, interact with one another and the planet.

The musculoskeletal system – comprising mainly bones, muscle and connective tissue structures, such as ligaments, gives shape and stability, and allows movement, to the human body, while also protecting the vital organs (Mooar 2007).

The musculoskeletal system is also by far the greatest energy user in the body, as well as being one of our primary sources of pain, discomfort and disability, whether localized or general, referred or reflex, acute or chronic.

The term 'somatic dysfunction' offers an accurate and a comprehensive term to describe all lesions of the musculoskeletal system – osseous and soft tissue (Licciardone 2005).

Somatic dysfunction can be defined as any impairment, or altered function, of related components of the somatic system (body framework), i.e. skeletal, arthrodial and myofascial structures, as well as related vascular, lymphatic and neural elements. This general expression (somatic dysfunction) obviously requires specific definition in any given situation, which should include identification of the particular structure, tissue or area involved.

Sometimes somatic dysfunction is the primary cause of pain, however sometimes it generates reflexive symptoms, or may act as a perpetuating feature. Palpation may provide clues to the true nature of an injury (Stanton 1996). A process of assessment and examinations may help to identify structural factors associated with pain and dysfunction, often associated with repeated injury or cumulative microtrauma involving postural, habitual or occupational ergonomic stresses.

Identifying sources of pain

Different dysfunctional tissues produce different qualities of symptoms (Kuchera 2005). For example: sclerotomal tissues (skeletal, arthrodial, and ligamentous generators) typically relate to dull, aching pain – which may be experienced some distance from the actual source; myotomal (muscle) pain is also poorly localized, possibly also at a distance from the generating site. Trigger point activity in hypertonic tissues might be involved. The pain is typically described as involving stiffness, aching and sometimes having a cramp-like quality. Note: Examples of sclerotomes and myotomes are illustrated in Chapter 5, while the palpatory characteristics (such as tissue texture changes) of dysfunctional tissues that generate pain locally, or at a distance, are to be found in Chapter 3.

The objectives, if not the methods we are discussing, are not new. Carl McConnell, a major force in early 20th century osteopathy, discussed the soft tissues as follows (McConnell 1962):

> A pathological point of prime importance, for example, is that osseous malalignment is sustained by ligamentous rigidity. This rigidity is incepted by way of muscular fascial and tendinous tensions and stresses. Every case portrays a uniqueness in accordance with location, architectural plan and laws, tissue texture, regional and strength ratios, resident properties, environmental settings, resolution of forces etc. Remember I am speaking of the solid biological background of individual pathogenesis, the veritable soil of prediseased conditions. The lack of either sufficient, or efficient, soft-tissue work, is one reason for mediocre technique and recurrence of lesions. The same is evident in the correction of postural defects.

The causes and the results of local and general somatic dysfunction, whether traumatic, functional, postural, pathological or psychological in origin, require a brief overview as we explore different aspects of the issues and the tissues involved, so that some of their possible solutions might become clearer.

Coherent and incoherent patterns

In Chapter 3 we will examine one of the major causes of somatic pain and dysfunction, myofascial trigger points, and the causes of this widespread phenomenon. It will then become clear that, while many forms of (referred) pain follow predictable and neurologically coherent pathways, there also exist patterns of pain and dysfunction that do not.

In this chapter our task is to evaluate a variety of influences on the evolution of soft tissue dysfunction, which follow a chronological sequence – the ways in which what is happening in an acute setting differs from what is taking place in a chronic situation, where an initial alarm state progressively gives way to a degree of organization, adaptation, compensation and (if not prevented) decompensation and dysfunction. It will also be explained just why not all muscles respond to stressors in quite the same way.

Reporting stations

The reporting mechanisms in the soft tissues and joints (Travell & Simons 1983, 1992, Wall & Melzack 1991) may be thought of as providing answers to a number of basic questions that the central nervous system (CNS) requires answering.

These questions were expressed by Keith Buzzell (1970) as follows: 'What is happening in the peripheral machinery with respect to three questions? What is the present position? If there is motion, where is it taking us? And, third, how fast is it taking us there?'

The various neural reporting organs provide a constant information feedback to the CNS and higher centres as to the current state of tone, tension, movement, etc. of the tissues housing them. Such sensory information can be modulated and modified both by the influence of the mind, and by changes in blood chemistry, to which the sympathetic nervous system is sensitive. A variety of inputs of information will give the answers to these important questions so that the body can provide appropriate responses to the demands and adaptations constantly called for by varying situations. Some important structures involved in this internal information highway are summarized in Box 1.1.

There are various ways of 'manipulating' the neural reporting stations to produce physiological modifications in soft tissues – notably of the Golgi tendon organ in muscle energy techniques (METs)

Box 1.1   Reporting stations

Ruffini end-organs
These are found within the joint capsule, around the joint, so that each is responsible for describing what is happening over an angle of approximately 15°, with a degree of overlap between it and the adjacent end-organ. These organs are not easily fatigued, and are recruited progressively as the joint moves, so that movement is smooth and not jerky. The prime concern of Ruffini end-organs is to maintain a steady position. They are also, to some extent, concerned with reporting the direction of movement.

Golgi end-organs
These, too, adapt slowly, and continue to discharge over a lengthy period. They are found in the ligaments associated with the joint. Unlike the Ruffini end-organs, which respond to muscular contraction that alters tension in the joint capsule, Golgi end-organs are not thus affected, and can deliver information independently of the state of muscular contraction. This helps the body to know just where the joint is at any given moment, irrespective of muscular activity.

Pacinian corpuscle
This is found in periarticular connective tissue, and adapts rapidly. It triggers discharges, and then ceases reporting in a very short space of time. These messages occur successively, during motion, and the CNS can therefore be aware of the rate of acceleration of movement taking place in the area. It is sometimes called an acceleration receptor.

There are other end-organs, but these three can be seen to provide information regarding the present position, direction and rate of movement of any joint.

Continued

Box 1.1   Reporting stations—cont'd

Muscle spindle

This receptor is sensitive and complex. It detects, evaluates, reports and adjusts the length of the muscle in which it lies, setting its tone. Acting with the Golgi tendon organ, most of the information as to muscle tone and movement is reported. The spindles lie parallel to the muscle fibres, and are attached either to skeletal muscle or to the tendinous portion of the muscle. Inside the spindle are fibres that may be one of two types. One is described as a 'nuclear bag' fibre, and the other as a chain fibre. In different muscles the ratios of these internal spindle fibres differ. In the centre of the spindle is a receptor called the annulospiral receptor (or primary ending), and on each side of this lies a 'flower spray receptor' (secondary ending). The primary ending discharges rapidly, and this occurs in response to even small changes in muscle length. The secondary ending compensates for this, because it fires messages only when larger changes in muscle length have occurred.

The spindle is a 'length comparator', and may discharge for long periods at a time. Within the spindle there are fine, intrafusal fibres that alter the sensitivity of the spindle. These can be altered without any actual change taking place in the length of the muscle itself, via an independent γ-efferent supply to the intrafusal fibres. This has implications in a variety of acute and chronic problems.

The proprioceptive role of muscles of the suboccipital region is directly related to the number of spindles per gram of muscle. There are an average of 36 spindles per gram in some of the suboccipital muscles, such as rectus capitis posterior minor, and 30.5 spindles per gram in rectus capitis posterior major, compared, for example, with 7.6 spindles per gram in splenius capitis and just 0.8 spindles per gram in gluteus maximus (Peck et al 1984). McPartland & Brodeur (1999) suggest that 'The high density of muscle spindles found in the RCPM muscles suggests a value ... [which] lies not in their motor function, but in their role as "proprioceptive monitors" of the cervical spine and head.'

Buzzell (1970) describes the neural connections with the CNS thus:

The central connections of the spindle receptors are important. The annulospiral fibre has the only known monosynaptic relationship in the body. As the fibre passes to the cord, and through the dorsal horn, it goes without synapse, directly to the anterior horn cells that serve the muscle fibres in the vicinity of the spindle. This is the basis of the so called 'tendon reflex', which actually is not a tendon reflex, but simply a spindle response to a sudden elongation of the muscle.

In contrast, the secondary fibres have various synapses in their central connection which can be traced to higher cortical centres. Conscious activity may, therefore, provide a modifying influence, via these structures, on muscle tone. The activities of the spindle appear to provide information regarding length, velocity of contraction and changes in velocity. How long is the muscle? How quickly is it changing length? And what is happening to this rate of change of length? (Gray 1977).

Golgi tendon receptors

These structures indicate how hard the muscle is working, they reflect the tension of the muscle, rather than its length, as does the spindle. If the tendon organ detects excessive overload it may cause cessation of function of the muscle, to prevent damage. This produces relaxation.

---

and of the spindle in various positional release (PR) techniques, such as strain/counterstrain (SCS) (Jones 1980, Stiles 1984).

Effect of contradictory information

Korr's words regarding the nature of the information that these, and other, reporting stations are providing to the CNS are worth recording (Korr 1976). He reminds us:

The spinal cord is the keyboard on which the brain plays when it calls for activity or for change in activity. But each 'key' in the console sounds, not an individual 'tone', such as the contraction of a particular group of muscle fibres, but a whole 'melody' of activity, even a 'symphony' of motion. In other words, built into the cord is a large repertoire of patterns of activity, each involving the complex, harmonious, delicately balanced orchestration of the contractions and relaxations of many muscles. The brain 'thinks' in terms of whole motions, not individual muscles. It calls selectively, for the preprogrammed patterns in the cord and brain stem, modifying them in countless ways and combining them in an infinite variety of still more complex patterns. Each activity is also subject to further modulation, refinement, and adjustment by the afferent feedback continually streaming in from the participating muscles, tendons, and joints.

This means that the pattern of information fed back to the CNS and brain from neural reporting stations (proprioceptors, mechanoreceptors, nociceptors, etc.) reflects, at any given time, the steady state of joints, the direction as well as speed of alteration in position of joints, together with data on the length of muscle fibres, the degree of load that is being borne, along with the tension this involves. This total input is what occurs, rather than individual pieces of information, as outlined above, from particular reporting stations.

Contradictory gibberish?

But what if any of the mass of information being constantly received should be contradictory, and actually conflict with the other information being received?

Buzzell puts it this way:

It is possible, for example, for the excessive force exerted by external trauma to induce such hyperactivity of the joint and muscle receptors that the reports from that area become gibberish.

Should conflicting reports reach the cord from a variety of sources simultaneously, no discernible pattern may be recognized by the CNS. In such a case no adequate response would be forthcoming, and it is probable that activity would be stopped. Spasm, or splinting, could therefore result.

When somatosensory, vestibular or visual afferent systems provide conflicting information, a variety of symptoms may result. Somatosensory afferent systems depend on coherent input, from the soles of the feet, the neck and lumbar spine (Gagey 1986).

Neural 'cross-talk'

Korr (1976) discussed a variety of insults that could result in increased neural excitability: the triggering of a barrage of supernumerary impulses, to and from the cord, and also what he terms 'cross-talk', in which axons may overload and pass impulses to one another directly; muscle contraction disturbances, vasomotion, pain impulses, reflex mechanisms, disturbances in sympathetic activity, all may result from such activity, due to what might be relatively slight tissue changes, for example in the intervertebral foramina.

In addition, Korr reported that when any tissue is disturbed, whether bone, joint, ligament or muscle, the local stresses feed constant information to the cord, and effectively jam normal patterned transmission from the periphery. These factors, combined with any mechanical alterations in the tissues, are the background to much somatic dysfunction.

He summarized thus (Korr 1976):

These are the somatic insults, the sources of incoherent, and meaningless feedback, that causes the spinal cord to halt normal operations and to freeze the status quo in the offending and offended tissues. It is these phenomena that are detectable at the body surface, and are reflected in disorders of muscle tension, tissue texture, visceral and circulatory function, and even secretory function; the elements that are so much a part of osteopathic diagnosis.

These are the palpable changes that we will be evaluating in later chapters that can allow us the opportunity to 'read' dysfunction, and to potentially choose therapeutic measures – such as neuromuscular technique – to assist in restoration of normal function.

Mechanisms that alter proprioception

(Lederman 1997)

• Ischaemic or inflammatory events at the receptor site may produce diminished proprioceptive sensitivity due to metabolic byproduct build-up stimulating groups III and IV, mainly pain afferents (this also occurs in muscle fatigue).

- Physical trauma can directly affect receptor axons (articular receptors, muscle spindles and their innervations).
- In direct trauma to muscle, spindle damage can lead to denervation and atrophy (e.g. following whiplash) (Hallgren et al 1993).
- Structural changes in parent tissue lead to atrophy and loss of sensitivity in detecting movement, plus altered firing rate (e.g. during stretching).
- Loss of muscle force (and possibly wasting) may result when a reduced afferent pattern leads to central reflexogenic inhibition of motor neurons supplying affected muscle.
- Psychomotor influences (e.g. feeling of insecurity) can alter patterns of muscle recruitment at the local level, and may result in disuse muscle weakness.

Trophic neural influences

Setting aside for the moment the obviously important feature of nerves, and their message-carrying functions, we need to consider the less understood role they play in transporting substances – proteins, phospholipids, glycoproteins, neurotransmitters, enzymes, mitochondria and more (Canals et al 2004).

Transportation takes place, at a rate of anything from 1 mm/24 h to several hundred millimetres per 24 h, depending on what is being transported and the presence, or absence, of interfering factors. Movement occurs in both directions along nerves, with retrograde (returning from the target tissues towards the CNS) transportation seemingly 'a fundamental means of communication between neurons and between neurons and non-neuronal cells' which strongly influences the 'plasticity of the nervous system', according to Korr's research (Korr 1981).

Patterson & Wurster (1997) note that substances known as nerve growth factors (NGFs) are supplied to the neural structures by the target (end) organ to which neurotrophic substances are being transported. 'If the end organ does not

supply the NGF, the synaptic contact is lost.' They continue: 'Complete withdrawal of NGF or of the material delivered by the nerve to its end organ may result in loss of function ... The occurrence of the tissue tensions and fluid flow disturbances often associated with somatic dysfunctions can be factors in altering axoplasmic flows.'

Butler (1991) reports that there are two speeds of delivery of trophic substances via the nerves:

The fast transport moves at approximately 400 mm per day and the substances carried, such as neurotransmitters and transmitter vesicles, are for use in transmission of impulses at the synapse. This transport depends on an uninterrupted supply of energy from the blood. Various toxic substances and deprivation of blood will slow or block the transport.

In the slow antegrade (delivery) transport (1–6 mm per day), cytoskeletal material is carried. The return transportation (retrograde) along the nerve carries recycled transmitter vesicles and extracellular material. Butler suggests that 'It also seems likely that the retrograde flow carries "trophic messages" about the status of the axon, the synapse and the general environment around the synapse including the target tissues.'

Very significantly, Butler states: 'If the retrograde flow is altered by physical constriction, or from loss of blood flow, nerve cell body reactions are induced.'

Korr (1981) demonstrated that red (postural) and white (phasic) muscle fibres, which differ morphologically, functionally, chemically and, as we will discover later in this chapter, in their response to stress, can have all of their characteristic differences reversed if their innervation is 'crossed', so that red muscles receive white muscle innervation and vice versa. 'This means, in effect, that the nerve instructs the muscle what kind of muscle to be, and is an expression of a neurally mediated genetic influence', according to Korr (1981).

Neural influences on gene expression

Korr's research (1981) therefore suggests that it is the nervous system that largely determines which genes in a muscle will be suppressed, and which expressed, and this information is carried in the material being transported along the axons. (See Box 1.2 for additional influences on gene expression.)

When a muscle loses contact with its nerve (as in anterior poliomyelitis, for example) atrophy occurs, not as a result of disuse but because of loss of the integrity of the connection between nerve cells and muscle cells at the myoneural junction, where nutrient exchange occurs irrespective of whether or not impulses are being transmitted.

Korr (1981) also describes just how vulnerable these highways of nutrition are:

Any factor which causes derangement of transport mechanisms in the axon, or that chronically alters the quality or quantity of the axonally transported substances, could cause the trophic influences to become detrimental. This alteration in turn would produce aberrations of structure, function and metabolism, thereby contributing to dysfunction and disease.

What could cause such neurotrophic interference?

Box 1.2   Gene expression

Korr (1981) demonstrated that obstruction of axonal transport modifies gene expression. Additional modulation of gene expression is now known to derive from biomechanical influences, specifically the status of minute structures – integrins – that penetrate the cell surface, acting as a communicating mechanism between the extracellular and intracellular environment.

'Integrin molecules carry tension from the extracellular matrix, across the cell surface to the cytoskeleton which behaves as a tensegrity matrix' (Wang et al 1993).

'Of particular interest are the roles of the integrins in the migration of cells that defend the body against disease and repair injuries' (Horwitz 1997, Hynes 1992).

The precise effects of tense, distorted, contracted, fibrosed or otherwise dysfunctional tissues on the integrins of the cells in these tissues, and subsequent gene expression, are topics for research, as are the potentially beneficial influences of appropriate bodywork designed to normalize such tissues (Oschman 2000).

Moving beyond neural and mechanical influences on gene expression, Martin (2001) interviewed functional medicine expert Jeffrey Bland, who observed:

Functional genomics derived out of the human genome project, in which it was thought that by dissecting the code of life in our 23 pairs of chromosomes, people would be able to understand how they were going to die. They would see locked in

their genes heart disease, cancer, diabetes, arthritis, whatever it might be, and they would tell from these genetic imperfections what day, and what disease, they would finally fall prey to ... Mendelian determinism ... said that locked into our genes, when the sperm met the egg, were these strengths and weaknesses that we call the recessive and dominant characteristics of inheritance, ... [and that] basically if we had the genes for cancer we would die of cancer, [and] if we had the genes for heart disease we would die of heart disease. It turns out that the human genome project has discovered that the genes that we thought were hard-wired to produce these diseases, are not hard-wired at all. Within our genes are multiple messages, and the message that is expressed at any moment – that's in our phenotype – is a consequence of the environmental messages including diet, lifestyle, environment, that wash over our genes to give rise to different expression paths of the genes ... some may be healthy, some may be unhealthy ... what we're really seeing is that the major determinants for the expression of genetic patterns, over decades of living, are the decisions that we make, either consciously or subconsciously, every day. How we exercise, how we work, what our stress patterns are.

A picture emerges that suggests structural features, neural function, stress and emotion, as well as environmental factors including diet, all determine the way in which genetic predispositions are either modified, modulated, contained or expressed.

Korr specifies: 'Deformations of nerves and roots, such as compression, stretching, angulation and torsion', especially, he tells us, 'in their passage over highly mobile joints, through bony canals, intervertebral foramina, fascial layers and tonically contracted muscles'.

Mention by Korr, Butler and others of the changes that can have a negative influence on neurotrophic flow include altered circulatory status as well as hypertonicity. Trigger point activity, as we will see in later chapters, should be capable of directly producing just such changes. Normalization of trigger point activity, and the aetiological factors that produced them, utilizing NMT for example, should therefore be at least one way of assisting more normal neurotrophic function.

More general normalization of somatic dysfunctions, which include not just trigger points but the entire range of shortened, fibrotic, hypertonic, oedematous, inflamed, restricted or otherwise compromised soft and osseous structures, can therefore be seen to offer benefit in restoration of neurotrophic function, and therefore of body functions generally.

Maitland and Butler: 'abnormal neural movement'

Butler & Gifford (1989), building on the original work of Maitland (1986), have shown how what they term 'adverse tension' in the nervous system can impair its mobility and elasticity, and how many painful problems can result from this. Butler and Gifford's detailed analysis of the diagnosis and treatment of such restrictions and tensions is highly recommended to manual therapists. The tissues that surround neural structures are known as the mechanical interface (MI). These adjacent tissues are those that can move independently of the nervous system; for example, supinator muscle is the MI to the radial nerve, as it passes through the radial tunnel.

There is no general agreement as to the terminology that should be used in describing such biomechanical changes in the neural environment. Maitland et al (2001), for example, suggest that 'abnormal neural movement' is a more accurate description than 'neural tension'.

Whatever we term the dysfunctional pattern, Butler and Gifford's focus on those 'adverse mechanical' changes that negatively influence neural function, and that cause a multitude of symptoms, including pain, has been an important contribution to our understanding of some aspects of pain and dysfunction.

Any pathology in the MI can produce abnormalities in nerve movement, resulting in tension on the neural structure with unpredictable ramifications. Examples of MI pathology include nerve impingement by disc protrusion, or osteophyte contact, and carpal tunnel constriction. These problems would be regarded as mechanical in origin as far as the nerve restriction is concerned. Any symptoms resulting from mechanical impingement on neural structures will be more readily provoked in tests that involve movement rather than pure (passive) tension (Alshami & Hodges 2006).

Chemical or inflammatory causes of neural tension can also occur, resulting in 'interneural fibrosis', which leads to reduced elasticity and increased 'tension', and would become obvious with tension testing of these structures.

Pathophysiological changes resulting from inflammation, or from chemical damage (i.e. toxicity), are noted by Butler & Gifford (1989) as commonly leading on to internal mechanical restrictions of neural structures in a different manner to mechanical causes such as those, for example, imposed by a disc lesion.

Korr (1970) states:

To appreciate the vulnerability of the segmental nervous system to somatic insults it must be understood that much of the pathway taken by nerves as they emerge from the cord is actually through skeletal muscle. The great contractile forces of skeletal muscles with the accompanying chemical changes exert profound influences on the metabolism and excitability of neurons. In this environment the neurons are subject to quite considerable mechanical and chemical influences of various kinds, compression and torsion and many others ... slight mechanical stresses may, over a period of time, produce adhesions, constrictions and angulations imposed by protective layers.

Adverse mechanical tension changes do not necessarily affect nerve conduction, according to

Butler and Gifford; however, Korr's research indicates that axonal transport may be affected.

From the perspective of the manual therapist, this knowledge is extremely important.

The dysfunctional tissues and patients being treated by massage therapists, neuromuscular therapists, physiotherapists, Rolfers, Heller Workers, osteopathic and chiropractic practitioners, and those using movement therapies (Pilates, Feldenkrais, etc.), all have the potential to involve the mechanically interfacing structures in which neural tissues lie, and where normal mobility should be present (and often is not).

The role of neuromuscular techniques in management of adaptive overload

This book has, as a primary focus, the use of neuromuscular techniques (NMTs) in assessing and treating somatic dysfunction. The objectives of neuromuscular technique (NMT as practised in Europe) and neuromuscular therapy (NMT as practised in the USA) are summarized in Box 1.3.

To understand the context for application of such approaches, we need to appreciate time-related influences on the evolution of dysfunction: how, over time, a progression occurs that

---

 Box 1.3 NMT: European (Lief's) neuromuscular technique and American neuromuscular therapy (Chaitow & Delaney 2000)

Neuromuscular technique, as the term is used in this book, refers to the manual application of specialized (usually) digital pressure and strokes, most commonly applied by finger or thumb contact. These digital contacts can have either a diagnostic (assessment) or therapeutic objective, and the degree of pressure employed varies considerably between these two modes of application. There are subtle differences between the European and American versions of NMT. Detailed descriptions of Lief's NMT will be found in Chapter 6, while the American NMT version is outlined by Judith DeLany in Chapter 10.

Additional complementary manual methods to NMT (both versions) include massage, muscle energy technique (MET), positional release technique (PRT), myofascial release technique (MRT) and variations of these soft tissue manipulation approaches.

Aims of NMT
Therapeutically, NMT aims to produce modifications in dysfunctional tissue, encouraging a restoration of functional normality, with a particular focus of deactivating focal points of reflexogenic activity, such as myofascial trigger points.

An alternative objective of NMT application is toward normalizing imbalances in hypertonic and/or fibrotic tissues, either as an end in itself or as a precursor to joint mobilization or manipulation.

NMT attempts to:

- offer reflex benefits
- deactivate myofascial trigger points

- prepare for other therapeutic methods such as exercise or manipulation
- relax and normalize tense, fibrotic muscular tissue
- enhance lymphatic and general circulation and drainage
- simultaneously offer the practitioner diagnostic information.

Neuromuscular therapy (USA) utilizes similar manual methods, as well as re-education, rehabilitation and home-care approaches, to those utilized in European methodology.

NMT attempts to address a number of features that are all commonly involved in causing or intensifying pain and dysfunction (Chaitow & DeLany 2000) including, among others:

- *biochemical features* – nutritional imbalances and deficiencies, toxicity (exogenous and endogenous), endocrine imbalances (e.g. thyroid deficiency), ischaemia, inflammation
- *pyschosocial factors* – stress, anxiety, depression, etc.
- *biomechanical factors* – posture, including patterns of use, hyperventilation tendencies, as well as locally dysfunctional states such as hypertonia, trigger points, neural compression or entrapment.

NMT sees its role as attempting to normalize or modulate whichever of these (or additional) influences on musculoskeletal pain and dysfunction can be identified in order to remove or modify as many aetiological and perpetuating influences as possible (Simons et al 1999), without creating further distress or requirement for excessive adaptation.

alters acute responses, as the tissues locally, or the body as a whole, modify, accommodate, compensate and adapt to the demands, stresses and insults of daily life.

General adaptation syndrome (GAS) and local adaptation syndrome (LAS), and connective tissue

Selye (1976) called stress the non-specific element in disease production. In describing the relationship between the general adaptation syndrome (GAS) – i.e. alarm reaction, resistance (adaptation) phase followed by the exhaustion phase (when adaptation finally fails), which affects the organism as a whole – and the local adaptation syndrome (LAS), which affects a specific stressed area of the body, Selye also emphasized the importance of connective tissue. He demonstrated that stress results in a pattern of adaptation, individual to each organism. He further showed that, when an individual is acutely alarmed, stressed or aroused, homeostatic (self-normalizing) mechanisms are activated – this is the alarm reaction of Selye's general (and local) adaptation syndromes.

If the alarm status is prolonged or repetitive, defensive adaptation processes commence and produce long-term – chronic – changes. In assessing (palpating) the patient, these neuromusculoskeletal changes represent a record of the attempts on the part of the body to adapt and adjust to the stresses imposed upon it as time passes. The results of repeated postural and traumatic insults of a lifetime, combined with changes of emotional and psychological origin, will often present a confusing pattern of tense, contracted, bunched, fatigued and ultimately fibrous tissue (Chaitow 1989).

The minutiae of the process are not, for the moment, at issue. What is important is the realization that, due to prolonged stress of a postural, psychic or mechanical type, discrete areas of the body become so altered by the efforts to compensate and adapt that structural and, eventually, pathological changes become apparent. Researchers have shown that the type of stress involved can be entirely physical in nature (Wall & Melzack 1991) (e.g. a single injury or repetitive postural strain) or purely psychic in nature (Latey 1983) (e.g. chronically repressed anger). An example of localized emotional stress influences on muscle tissue is given in Box 1.4. Wider biomechanical

---

Box 1.4   Selective motor unit involvement

The effect of psychological influences on muscles seems to be more complex than a simplistic 'whole' muscle or regional involvement. It has been demonstrated that a small number of motor units in particular muscles may display almost constant, or repeated, activity when influenced psychogenically (Waersted et al 1993). The reaction time taken to perform tasks was evaluated in normal individuals, so creating a 'time pressure' anxiety. Researchers were able to demonstrate low-amplitude levels of activity (using surface EMG in trapezius muscles) even when the muscle was not being employed. It seems that, in spite of low total activity level of the muscle, a small pool of low-threshold motor units may be under considerable load for prolonged periods of time.

Such a recruitment pattern would be in agreement with the 'size principle' first proposed by Henneman (1957), which states that motor units are recruited according to their size. Motor

units with type I (postural) fibres are predominant among the small, low-threshold units. If tension-provoking factors (e.g. anxiety) are frequently present, and the subject repeatedly recruits the same motor units, overload may follow, possibly resulting in a metabolic crisis and the appearance of type I fibres with an abnormally large diameter, or 'ragged-red' fibres, which are interpreted as a sign of mitochondrial overload (Edwards 1988, Larsson et al 1990). The implications of this information are profound, because they suggest that emotional stress can selectively involve postural muscle fibres that have a tendency to shorten over time when stressed (Janda 1983).

The possible 'metabolic crisis' suggested by this research has strong parallels with the evolution of myofascial trigger points as suggested by Simons, a topic that is discussed in greater detail in later chapters (Wolfe & Simons 1992).

responses to emotional stress are discussed later in this chapter.

More often than not a combination of emotional and physical stresses will so alter neuromusculoskeletal structures as to create a series of identifiable physical changes, which will themselves generate further stress, such as pain, joint restriction, general discomfort and fatigue.

As described in this and later chapters, predictable chain reactions of compensating changes will evolve in the soft tissues in most instances of chronic adaptation to biomechanical and psychogenic stress (Lewit 1992). Such adaptation is almost always at the expense of optimal function, as well as being an ongoing source of further physiological embarrassment.

A biomechanical stress response sequence

(Basmajian 1974, Dvorak & Dvorak 1984, Janda 1982, 1983, Korr 1978, Lewit 1999, Travell & Simons 1983, 1992, Liebenson 2006, Key 2007, Vleeming et al 2007)

When the musculoskeletal system is 'stressed', a sequence of events occurs which can be summarized as follows:

- 'Something' (see *Causes of soft tissue dysfunction* below) occurs that leads to increased muscular tone.
- Increased tone, if anything but short-term, leads to a retention of metabolic wastes.
- Increased tone simultaneously leads to a degree of localized oxygen lack (relative to the efforts being demanded of the tissues) – encouraging ischaemia.
- Increased tone might also lead to a degree of oedema.
- These factors (retention of wastes, ischaemia, oedema) result in discomfort or pain.
- Discomfort or pain leads to increased or maintained hypertonicity.
- Inflammation, or at least chronic irritation, may be a result.
- Neurological reporting stations in hypertonic tissues will feed the CNS with information regarding their status, leading to a degree of

sensitization of neural structures, and the evolution of facilitation – hyperreactivity (see Ch. 2).
- Macrophages are activated, as is increased vascularity and fibroblastic activity.
- Connective tissue production increases, with cross-linkage, leading to shortened fascia.
- As all fascia/connective tissue is continuous throughout the body, any distortions that develop in one region can potentially create distortions elsewhere, so having a negative influence on structures that are supported by, or attached to, the fascia, including nerves, muscles, lymph structures and blood vessels.
- Changes occur in the elastic (muscle) tissues, leading to chronic hypertonicity and, ultimately, to fibrotic changes.
- Hypertonicity in a muscle will produce inhibition of its antagonist muscles.
- Chain reactions evolve in which some muscles (postural – type I) shorten, while others (phasic – type II) lengthen.
- Because of sustained increased muscle tension, ischaemia in tendinous structures occurs, as it does in localized areas of muscles, and periosteal pain areas develop.
- Abnormal biomechanical effects occur, involving malcoordination of movement – with antagonist muscle groups becoming hypertonic (e.g. erector spinae) or inhibited (e.g. the rectus abdominis group).
- The firing sequences of antagonistic and synergistic muscles alter.
- Joint restrictions and/or imbalances as well as fascial shortenings develop.
- Progressive evolution of localized areas of hyperreactivity of neural structures occurs (facilitated areas) in paraspinal regions or within muscles (trigger points).
- The degree of energy wastage due to unnecessarily maintained hypertonicity leads to generalized fatigue.
- More widespread functional changes develop – for example affecting respiratory function – with repercussions on the total economy of the body.

Unsustainable without consequences

In the presence of a constant neurological feedback of impulses to the CNS/brain from neural reporting stations indicating heightened arousal (a hypertonic muscle status is the alarm reaction of the flight/fight alarm response), there will be increased levels of psychological arousal and an inability to relax adequately with consequent increase in hypertonicity. Functional *patterns of use*, of a biologically unsustainable nature, will emerge, commonly involving chronic musculoskeletal problems and pain.

At this stage, restoration of normal function requires therapeutic input which addresses the multiple changes that have occurred as well as the need to re-educate the individual as to how to use their body – to breathe, to carry and to use themselves – in less stressful ways.

The chronic adaptive changes that develop in such a scenario lead to the increased likelihood of future acute exacerbations, as the progressively chronic, less supple and resilient, biomechanical structures attempt to cope with new stress factors resulting from the normal demands of modern living.

Causes of soft tissue dysfunction

The many elements that can contribute to the 'stress' sequence, leading to musculoskeletal pain include:
1. Congenital factors (short or long leg, small hemipelvis, fascial, cranial and other distortions, hypermobility tendencies) (Gofton & Trueman 1971, Schamberger 2002)
2. Acquired malalignment, asymmetry, resulting from overuse, misuse and abuse (and disuse) factors (such as injury or inappropriate patterns of use involved in work, sport or regular activities) (Schamberger 2002)
3. Postural stresses (Key 2007, Vleeming et al 2007)
4. Chronic negative emotional states (anxiety, etc.) – see Box 1.4 (Bendtsen et al 1996)
5. Reflexive factors (trigger points, facilitated spinal regions) (Simons, Travell & Simons 1999)
6. Pathology (arthritis, etc.).

As a result of the processes described above – most of which affect each and every one of us to some degree – acute and painful problems, overlaid on chronic soft tissue changes, become the norm – the raw material on which bodywork therapies focus.

Some major soft tissue stress categories

Physiological factors

These might involve an overall increase of muscle hypertonicity/tension or localized soft tissue changes due to habitual patterns of use or from patterns of overuse. Occupational, sporting, leisure and general activities are all potential producers of such repetitive or constant stress involving the soft tissues (Janda 1982, 1988).

Emotional factors

All emotional changes are mirrored in muscular changes. Emotional attitudes such as anger or fear, as well as moods such as excitement, anxiety or depression, are known to produce altered muscular postures and patterns. There is a close relationship between habitual tension patterns and posture, and psychological attitudes and conflicts. The use of the body as a metaphor for emotional feelings ('pain in the neck') is well documented (Boadella 1978).

Reich's 'Armouring'

Reich (1949) outlined his understanding of the postures and defensive armouring produced by neurotic patients. He believed that such individuals often behaved as though they were 'half-dead' and that their normal functioning, on all levels, was diminished and restricted. He described an all too frequently seen pattern: 'They were disturbed sexually, they were disturbed in their work function, their bodily processes lacked rhythm, their breathing was uncoordinated' (Boadella 1978).

Reich and his followers demonstrated how emotions can 'mobilize' or 'paralyse' the body, with continued and repeated stress producing 'blockages' and restrictions which, if unreleased, become self-perpetuating and are themselves the source of pain and further stress. The ability to relax is lost, and the drain on nervous energy is profound in such situations. The bioenergetic answer to this problem is to aid in the release of these tensions by a complex set of exercises, including facial expressions and body positions, accompanied by breathing techniques.

Behavioural factors

All movement requires muscular activity. Certain patterns of use establish themselves. Often, individual awareness of the pattern of use is diminished, and habitual, repetitive actions leading to muscular hypertonicity developing (Feldenkrais 1977). Reforming habitual use patterns is far more difficult than altering the resultant soft tissue changes, in the short term. Breathing patterns that are habitual, such as hyperventilation, should be included in this category of stress factors impacting the musculoskeletal system (Chaitow et al 2002, Timmons 1994).

Structural factors

Over and above inborn features, such as a short leg, acquired structural changes make further demands on the adaptive capacity of the body. Depending upon the mechanical and structural loads it bears and responds to, muscle tissue will change in texture, chemistry, tone, etc., and will also modify and alter the framework of the body, warping and cramping its potential for normal use. It's worth remembering that bone also remodels when loaded. Wolff's law states: *'bone in a healthy person or animal will adapt to the loads it is placed under'*.

In other words the body will be bent and distorted to meet the stresses imposed from without and within. Barlow (1959), whose work follows that of Alexander (1957), suggested that there is a self-regulating tendency in the way muscles behave in response to stress.

Function in this example can be seen to remodel structure. This is the mirror opposite of the response of the body to structural modification – which leads inevitably to functional changes.

These 'laws' reflect a basic rule, usefully summarized by the acronym SAID – specific adaptation to imposed demand ... and of course this is used as the basis for many rehabilitation programmes.

Mobilization before rehabilitation?

Rehabilitation of normal pain-free function, following soft tissue changes such as those described above – whether from behavioural, emotional or structural causes – requires an appropriate sequence, so that functionality can be restored.

In other words, before an individual can learn to breathe more normally, or stand upright, or walk more normally, there is a need to modify the soft tissue and joint changes that have occurred.

Dommerholt (2000), points out:

In general, assessment and treatment of individual muscles must precede restoration of normal posture and normal patterns of movement. Claims that muscle imbalances would dissolve, following lessons in the Alexander technique are not substantiated in the scientific literature (Rosenthal 1987). Instead muscle imbalances must be corrected through very specific strengthening and flexibility exercises, since generic exercise programs tend to perpetuate the compensatory muscle patterns. Myofascial trigger points must be inactivated using either invasive or non-invasive treatment techniques. Associated joint dysfunction, especially of the cervical and thoracic spine must be corrected with joint mobilizations. Once the musculoskeletal conditions for 'good posture' have been met, postural retraining [Alexander or other methods], can proceed.

Hypermobility

Clearly hypermobility tendencies may be inborn; however, acquired hypermobility may result from trauma, or over-zealous manipulation of particular joints (Protopapas & Cymet 2002).

Kappler (1997) cautions: 'A normal physiological reaction to a painful hypermobile joint is for muscles surrounding the joint to splint the joint, and protect it from excess motion. Physical examination reveals restriction of motion. Underneath the protective muscle splinting is the unstable joint.'

It may be useful to reflect that one way in which the body might maintain excess tone in a muscle offering such protective support would be for it to evolve trigger point activity. These distressed supporting muscles (and their associated trigger points) might best be left untreated until underlying use patterns can be modified. Kappler (1997) suggests: 'Management [of hypermobile structures] involves modifying patient activity that contributes to instability, mobilizing adjacent hypomobile joints, and prescribing active rehabilitation exercises.'

Understanding pain

Research into the mechanisms involved in muscular pain has evolved rapidly over the past 50 years.

Barlow's (1959) suggestions that in the absence of other pathology muscular pain results from one of the following:

- The muscle itself, through noxious metabolic product, such as 'factor P' (Lewis 1942), or an interference in blood circulation due to spasm, resulting in relative ischaemia. Butler & Mosely (2003) note that when pain sensors (nociceptors), which are scattered throughout the body, are sufficiently stimulated they transmit messages towards the spinal cord that produce a release of excitatory chemicals into the synapse. When the synapse is sufficiently stimulated the pain message is sent to the brain.
- Acidic build-up within muscles (Issberner et al 1996) and inflammatory responses, involving what Butler & Mosely (2003) call *'inflammatory soup'*, add to the irritation of nociceptors – but of course are part of the internal repair system that allows healing to take place. See more on this topic below, under the sub-heading 'Medical acupuncture model'.
- Muscular insertions into the periosteum, may be just such sites of nociceptor irritation, due to excessive or repetitive, muscular activity leading, for example, to 'tennis elbow' and periosteal pain points – as described in Chapter 3 (Lewit 1992).
- Joints, which can become restricted and over-approximated may also be sources of muscular pain. In advanced cases, osteoarthritic changes can result from the regular microtrauma of repeated muscular

misuse. Over-approximation of joint surfaces, due to soft tissue shortening, can also lead to uneven wear and tear, as, for example, when the tensor fascia lata structure shortens and crowds both the hip and lateral knee joint structures.

- Neural irritation, which can be produced spinally or along the course of the nerve as a result of chronic muscular contractions may produce pain. These can involve disc and general spinal mechanical faults (Korr 1976), as well as altered neural status in which there is abnormal tension between nerves and the mechanical interface they have with their surrounding nerve sheaths (Butler & Gifford 1991, Maitland et al 2001).
- Variations in pain threshold, largely to do with perception, but also with gender, with fibromyalgia occurring in a female:male ratio of approximately 4:1 (Mense & Simons 2001) as well as ethnicity, modify the interpretation of pain messages in the brain – making them more or less significant (Wall & Melzack 1991). The brain processes pain messages and ascribes value to these based on whether danger is perceived, and this perception of danger has cultural and personal belief aspects (Butler & Mosely 2003).
- Gender differences relate largely to 'a higher sensitivity of the pain system in females'.

Other models of pain genesis

Medical acupuncture model and trigger points

Baldry (1993) described the progression from muscle in a normal state, to muscle in painful chronic distress, as commonly involving initial or repetitive trauma (strain or excessive use), resulting in the release of chemical substances such as bradykinin, prostaglandins, histamine, serotonin and potassium ions. Sensitization of A-*d* and C (group IV) sensory nerve fibres may follow, with involvement of the brain (limbic system and the frontal lobe).

Trigger points (see Ch. 3), which evolve from such a progression, themselves become the source of new problems in their own locality, as well as at distant sites, as their sarcoplasmic reticulum is damaged and free calcium ions are released, leading to the formation of localized taut bands of tissue (involving the actin–myosin contractile mechanisms in the muscle sarcomeres).

If free calcium and energy-producing adenosine triphosphate (ATP) is present, this becomes a self-perpetuating feature, compounded by the relative (compared with surrounding tissues) ischaemia that has been identified in such chronically contracted tissues (Simons 1987). Local myofascial changes are considered in Chapter 3.

Much of this description by Baldry has been confirmed by research which assessed the chemicals in the tissues surrounding trigger points (Shah et al 2008a).

Shah & Gilliams (2008b) report:

Painful MTrPs activate muscle nociceptors that, upon sustained noxious stimulation, initiate motor and sensory changes in the peripheral and central nervous systems, [resulting in] sensitisation. In order to investigate the peripheral factors that influence the sensitisation process, a microdialysis technique was developed to quantitatively measure the biochemical milieu of skeletal muscle. Differences were found between active and latent MTrPs,, as well as in comparison with healthy muscle tissue.

Note: Where pain has been produced by repetitive habits, postural and otherwise, with emotional and psychological overtones, the task of the therapist is complex because hypertonicity can often be only partially released or relaxed without resolving the underlying pattern of use. If repeated recurrence of painful episodes is to be minimized, a state of relative equilibrium of body structure and function is needed, which calls for treatment of structural restrictions as well as re-education regarding posture and use.

Stoddard's osteopathic perspective

Stoddard (1969), in discussing contracted musculature, describes its 'stringy' feel, resulting from the continuous contraction of some muscle fibres, and ascribes the cause to the underlying joint dysfunction. The resulting ache and pain, he believes, is usually a result of circulatory embarrassment as metabolic wastes build up due to sustained muscular contraction. Muscular guarding is always seen to indicate deeper pathological changes (e.g. tuberculosis of the spine, osteomyelitis, disc herniation).

Stoddard sees the metabolic wastes, which may result from a degree of stasis, as causing a vicious cycle in perpetuating muscular contraction, leading eventually to fibrous changes. There is no indication that Stoddard considers such changes to be of primary importance in his treatment programme. He does stress the importance of exercises (to strengthen muscle groups) and of correct posture, but does not indicate any great interest in treatment of the soft tissues themselves.

While release of muscular restrictions and shortening could be considered a desirable step in the restoration of normality, it is worth emphasizing that once adaptive fibrotic changes have taken place in the soft tissues (whether in response to emotional stress or anything else) these changes are no longer under purely neurological control and therefore cannot simply be 'released' (by exercises or anything else): they require a physical input that alters, stretches and effectively breaks down concretions such as fibrotic tissue.

Modern pain concepts

The complexity of muscular pain mechanisms becomes clearer as the diligent research and reporting of Mense & Simons (2001) is examined. Interestingly, many of the ideas promoted half a century ago, by Barlow and others, are confirmed by modern research, although far more detail is now available with regard to pain mechanisms.

A brief summary of the key elements described by Mense and Simons is offered below; however, this captures no more than a superficial glimpse of the material in their book.

Common subgroups of muscular pain are identified:

- *myofascial pain* resulting from trigger points (often also used to describe regional pain syndromes)
- *fibromyalgia* (also used to describe myoglossis, muscular induration, non-articular rheumatism and tendomyopathy)
- *muscular pain* related to articular dysfunction.

Mense and Simons consider that most other terms used to describe muscular pain can be subsumed into these three terms.

Sensitization

Sensitization of nociceptors by vasoneuroreactive substances (such as bradykinin and prostaglandins) leads to long-lasting tenderness of trigger points (Fig. 1.1). This is discussed further in Chapter 3.

The process of sensitization involves local oedema, release of neuropeptides such as substance P, subsequent compression of venous vessels, venous congestion (which reduces blood supply) and therefore local ischaemia. Ischaemic conditions lead to the release of more bradykinin, ensuring a vicious cycle, which engenders sensitization of pain receptors.

In skeletal muscle, ischaemia results in interference with normal energy (ATP) production, which leads to disturbance of normal calcium pump activity, preventing actin and myosin filaments from releasing their contractured state. This is the hypothesized cause of 'taut bands', which are a key feature of myofascial trigger points (see Ch. 3).

Mense & Simons (2001) suggest that when inflammation occurs in muscle for a period as short as 12 days, the concentration of thin nerve fibres containing neuropeptides increases markedly, leading to a greater reporting of pain sensations (Reinert & Mense 1993).

The widely held belief that a pain–spasm–pain cycle exists is questioned by Mense & Simons (2001). Their arguments are too complex to summarize without losing accuracy, but the following remarks offer a glimpse:

> The [pain–spasm–pain] cycle is assumed to start with a muscle lesion that excites nociceptors. The small-diameter group III and IV muscle afferent fibers from the muscle nociceptors excite interneurons in the dorsal horn, which in turn activate α-motor neurons. Via their efferent fibers (α-motor axons) these motor neurons activate the neuromuscular endplate and cause spasm of the muscle. A longer-lasting spasm is painful and further activates muscle nociceptors.

Mense and Simons argue that although excitation of dorsal horn neurons by muscle nociceptors is established there is no proof that homonymous [alpha]-motor neurons are similarly activated: 'An acute noxious stimulus to a muscle is likely to inhibit rather than excite homonymous motor neurons if the muscle is an extensor.'

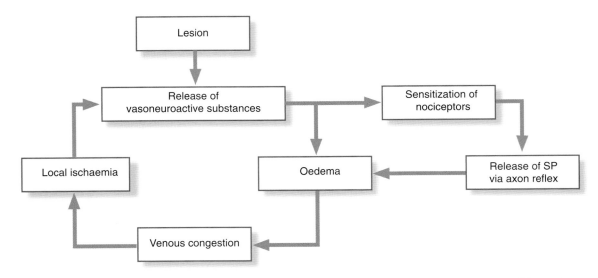

Figure 1.1   Schematic diagram showing hypothesized mechanism for sustained tenderness in trigger points. (SP = substance P) Redrawn from Mense S & Simons D, Muscle pain, Williams & Wilkins, 2001, with permission.

They believe that because flexor muscle motor neurons display only short-lasting excitation (if any), and painful muscles frequently show little or no electrical activity when at rest, 'the postulated [pain–spasm–pain] reflex is not functional in every muscle and cannot explain long-lasting spasm.'

Apart from the idea that spasm results via reflex arcs, as outlined above, a variety of other working hypotheses exists to explain the phenomenon of spasm, none of which is proven. These include the possibility that joint nociceptors act as initiators resulting in reflex stabilization via chronic muscle spasm.

Mense and Simons reject this, saying it cannot be universally valid, because 'in many cases of painful joint lesions ... neighbouring muscles are reflexly inhibited.'

Neuroplastic sensitization involves a process in which nociceptive input to the cord or brainstem leads to synaptic sensitization in the dorsal horn neurons. 'Following such an input, the neurons are thought to increase their excitability and exhibit enhanced responses to both pathologic and normal afferent inflow.'

Central sensitization is then thought to perpetuate nociceptive activity.

This is a concept close to facilitation mechanisms, as hypothesized by osteopathic medicine, and discussed in Chapter 3.

There may be a malfunctioning of the descending antinociceptive system, in which central damping down of pain messages fails to be effective. Mense and Simons state: 'It is conceivable that a malfunction of the descending antinociceptive system, which might occur spontaneously, or following a central or peripheral lesion, leads to chronic pain sensations from deep tissues, even in the absence of a peripheral lesion.'

Fibromyalgic pain may result from such a process.

Psychological factors modulate pain perception; however, controversially, Mense & Simons (2001) contend that whilst 'psychological stress can be a potent aggravating factor ... as we learn more about the pathophysiology concerning the origin of muscle pain, the less psychogenic and more somatic it becomes.'

A variety of mechanical (e.g. poor posture, asymmetry) and systemic (e.g. anaemia, low thyroid function, vitamin B deficiency) factors may interact to aggravate and perpetuate painful conditions.

Mense and Simons insist that it is essential to be aware of, and able to distinguish between, pain and tenderness that is local, projected (caused by peripheral nerve irritation), referred and of central origin – and of overlaps between these.

Additional insights from Mense and Simons will be introduced in later chapters.

At this stage it is useful to observe that pain is complex, confusing and demanding. The task of uncovering the mechanisms involved in any given patient's painful muscular condition calls for the ability to evaluate muscular and articular status, and neurological features, as well as identification of myofascial trigger points and fibromyalgia characteristics.

One requirement for such a process is the ability to distinguish between different muscular responses to stress: overuse, misuse, disuse and abuse.

Different responses in postural and phasic muscles

It is not within the scope of this book to provide detailed physiological analysis; however, it is vital that the ways in which different muscle fibre types respond to stress are understood. To be sure there are several models in which different muscle groups are designated according to their main functions and characteristics, and an attempt is made in Box 1.5 to summarize these.

In this book the categorizations *'postural'* and *'phasic'* (Janda 1982, 1996, Lewit 1992, Liebenson 2006) are used, as these have been found by the principal author to be the most useful in clinical practice. What has been demonstrated is that, when stressed (overuse, misuse, abuse, disuse, etc.), postural muscles have a propensity to shorten, whereas phasic muscles undergoing similar 'stress' are inhibited, become weaker, and possibly lengthen (although localized contractures may be present).

Fetal position influences

Kolar (1999) reports that the muscles that tend to hypertonicity and shortening (i.e. 'postural'

Box 1.5   Categorization of muscles

Postural and phasic muscles (sometimes called type I and type II)

Muscles have a mixture of fibre types, although there is usually a predominance of one type or another. There are those that contract slowly ('slow twitch fibres' or 'slow white fibres'), which are classified as type I. These have very low stores of energy-supplying glycogen but carry high concentrations of myoglobulin and mitochondria. These fibres fatigue slowly and are mainly involved in postural and stabilizing tasks (Engel et al 1986, Woo et al 1987).

There are also several phasic/active type II fibre forms, notably:

- Type IIa fibres ('fast twitch' or 'fast red' fibres), which contract more speedily than type I and are moderately resistant to fatigue, with relatively high concentrations of mitochondria and myoglobulin.
- Type IIb fibres ('fast twitch/glycolytic fibres' or 'fast white fibres'), which are less fatigue-resistant and depend more on glycolytic sources of energy, with low levels of mitochondria and myoglobulin.
- Type IIm ('superfast' fibres), found mainly in the jaw muscles, which depend on a unique myosin structure which, along with a high glycogen content, differentiates this from the other type II fibres (Rowlerson 1981).

The implications of the effects of prolonged stress on these different muscle types cannot be emphasized too strongly, because long-term stress involving type I muscles indicates that they will shorten, whereas type II fibres undergoing similar stress will weaken without shortening over their whole length (they may, however, develop shortened areas within the muscle). It is important to emphasize that shortness or tightness of a postural muscle does not imply strength. Such muscles may test as strong or weak. However, a weak phasic muscle will not shorten overall and will always test as weak (Janda 1982).

Fibre type is not totally fixed, in that evidence exists as to the potential for adaptability of muscles, so that committed muscle fibres can be transformed from slow-twitch to fast-twitch and vice versa (Lin et al 1994).

An example of this potential, which is of profound clinical significance, involves the scalene muscles, which Lewit (1999) confirms can be classified as either postural or phasic. If the largely phasic scalene muscles, which are dedicated to movement, have postural functions thrust upon them (as in an asthmatic condition in which they will attempt to maintain the upper ribs in elevation to enhance lung capacity) and if, owing to the laboured breathing of such an individual, they are thoroughly and regularly stressed, their fibre type will alter and they will shorten, becoming postural muscles (Lin et al 1994). A list of postural and phasic muscles is given later in this chapter.

Stabilizers and mobilizers

Norris (1995a, b, c, d, e, 1998) designates muscles according to their major functions, i.e. as 'stabilizers' or 'mobilizers'. According to Norris, research has shown that muscles that are inhibited or weak may lengthen, adding to the instability of the region in which they operate. It is the 'stabilizer' muscles that have this tendency: if they are inhibited because of deconditioning they become unable adequately to perform the role of stabilizing joints in their 'neutral posture'.

'Stabilizer' muscles, which are more deeply situated, slow twitch, and have a tendency to weaken and lengthen if deconditioned, include: transverse abdominis, multifidus, internal obliques, medial fibres of external oblique, quadratus lumborum, deep neck flexors, serratus anterior, lower trapezius, gluteus maximus and medius. These muscles can be correlated to a large extent (apart from quadratus lumborum) with muscles designated by Lewit (1999) and Janda (1982, 1983) as 'phasic'.

The more superficial, fast-twitch muscles which have a tendency to shortening (i.e. 'mobilizers' in Norris's terminology) include: suboccipital group, sternocleidomastoid, upper trapezius, levator scapulae, iliopsoas and hamstrings. These fall into the category of 'postural' muscles as described by Lewit (1992), Janda (1982) and Liebenson (1996).

Norris calls these 'mobilizers' because they cross more than one joint. This redefining of 'postural' as 'mobilizer' appears to be confusing, and many prefer to refer to these muscles simply as 'having a tendency to shortening' (Liebenson 1999).

Examples of patterns of imbalance that emerge as some muscles weaken and lengthen and their synergists become overworked, while their antagonists shorten, can be summarized as follows:

Continued

Box 1.5   Categorization of muscles—cont'd

Underactive stabilizer	Overactive synergist	Shortened antagonist
Gluteus medius	Tensor fascia lata, quadratus lumborum, piriformis	Thigh adductors
Gluteus maximus	Iliocostalis lumborum, hamstrings	Iliopsoas, rectus femoris
Transversus abdominis	Rectus abdominis	Iliocostalis lumborum
Lower trapezius	Levator scapulae, upper trapezius	Pectoralis major
Deep neck flexors	Sternocleidomastoid	Suboccipitals
Serratus anterior	Pectoralis major/minor	Rhomboids
Diaphragm		Scalenes, pectoralis major

Multijoint or monoarticular muscles

Richardson et al (1999, 2000) have argued for the use of the terms multijoint muscles (also described as 'global' or 'deep' – slow twitch) and monoarticular muscles (also described as 'local' or 'superficial' – fast twitch). Richardson (2000) states:

> For many years traditional exercise therapy was mainly focussed on building strength or endurance of whole muscle groups e.g. rotators of the trunk, extensors of the knee, internal rotators of the shoulder. Those involved in rehabilitative exercise gradually realized that people with injury not only needed general strength and endurance of whole muscle groups to perform an activity e.g. lifting a load, but also needed more specifically directed exercise.
> More specifically exercise regimes were necessary to take into account that some individual muscles of a synergistic group:
> (1) have distinct and different individual functions
> (2) react in different ways to injury of the associated joint (reflex inhibition and excitation)
> (3) react in different ways to lack of use or lack of gravitational load
> (4) react in different ways to specific patterns of use (e.g. ballistic, repetitive activity)

> In each of the above it can be easily predicted that individual muscles would fall consistently into basically two groups:
> Group A
> [Note: These are the 'phasic', stabilizer', multijoint (deep, global) muscles.]
> (1) more linked with joint stabilization
> (2) more likely to undergo reflex inhibition with injury to associated joint
> (3) more likely to atrophy quickly due to lack of use or lack of gravitational load
> (4) more likely to decrease activity and change their function when exposed to ballistic repetitive exercise
> Group B
> [Note: These are the 'postural', 'mobilizer', monoarticular (superficial/local) muscles.]
> (1) more linked with efficient movement of joints
> (2) more likely to undergo reflex excitation with injury to associated joint
> (3) not prone to atrophy quickly due to lack of use or lack of gravitational load
> (4) more likely to become more active (and tighten) when exposed to ballistic repetitive exercise.

To minimize confusion, this book will follow the Janda/Lewit/Liebenson categorizations of *postural* and *phasic* muscles.

muscles) include most muscles shortened in the fetal position. These include finger, hand and wrist flexors; shoulder internal rotators and adductors; shoulder girdle elevators, as well as ankle plantar flexors and inverters; hip flexors, internal rotators and adductors.

The antagonists to these tend to become reciprocally inhibited (i.e. 'phasic' muscles). Janda (1996) suggests that these are the muscles whose neurodevelopment brings about the upright posture.

Role of the muscles in low back problems

If we examine the role of the muscular component of musculoskeletal structures, we find strong evidence for its involvement in many acute and chronic conditions.

Jokl (1984) tells us that disuse muscular atrophy, following back injury, is a major factor in the progression from an acute back problem to a chronic one. Changes take place that are observable, histologically and biochemically, in the muscle fibres, and that are translated into functional changes. The effects of these changes involve decreased endurance and weakened muscles, as well as spasm. We should remind ourselves of the basic anatomy of the low back, which includes the division of the musculature into:

1. The *deep muscles*, connecting the adjacent spinous processes (interspinales), adjacent transverse processes (intertransversari) and the rotatores, connecting the transverse process below to the laminae above.
2. The *intermediate muscles* include multifidus, which connects the transverse processes to the spinous processes of the vertebra above.
3. The *superficial* group includes iliocostalis, longissimus and spinalis (erector spinae). The origin of this is on the ischium, and the insertion on the sixth and 12th ribs. Together with the psoas (major and minor) and the quadratus, these greatly influence spinal stability.
4. The *prevertebral* muscles, which further stabilize and support the spine, are those that encircle the abdomen, such as the internal and external oblique, and rectus abdominus muscles.

Muscle types (see Box 1.5)

Any, or all, of these muscles can have a major influence on the onset of low back problems and pain. The division of muscles with regard to their different postural and phasic (volitional movement) types is worthy of re-emphasis. As mentioned earlier, muscle fibres may be differentiated into types by virtue of their role, as well as their main energy source.

- For example, type I muscles require stamina, rather than speed of action, and derive their energy via oxidative phosphorylation.

- This is in contrast to type II muscles, which produce power and speed, and derive energy from carbohydrate sources via glycolytic breakdown.

The muscles that support the spine are mainly type I, endurance and stamina muscles. Their activities are in the main related to static, antigravity efforts, which require prolonged contraction, and these muscles are far more susceptible to disuse atrophy and shortening. The strength of such muscles may not indicate much change, even after a period of disuse, but the endurance factor could be greatly affected. This necessitates a certain degree of caution when interpreting muscle strength tests involving the paravertebral musculature.

Jokl (1984) points out that electromyographic (EMG) studies indicate that paraspinal muscles show marked fatigue in individuals with low back pain. This fatigue factor may play a major part in worsening, or accentuating, an already demonstrable degree of dysfunction in this region. When such a situation exists (pain and easy fatigue of supporting musculature), it may be assumed that an increasing number of muscle fibres has been recruited in order to maintain spinal stability, which in turn results in increased muscular pressure. Jokl tells us that normal muscle can work for long periods without any EMG evidence of fatigue. As muscles become weaker, they work at an increased percentage of their maximum voluntary contraction. Ultimately this leads to muscle spasm, which allows ischaemia to develop, and pain to result.

The cycle of increased effort, local spasm and ischaemia, leading to pain, may ultimately result in paraspinal spasm and splinting.

Therapeutic choices

The use of both neuromuscular technique (NMT) and muscle energy technique (MET), are indicated in such a situation, as a means of disrupting the cycle and, initially, relaxing the contracted muscles. NMT methods have a combined effect, both relaxing the tissues as well as increasing the vascularity and mobility of these structures. They become more 'extensible', to use Grieve's phrase (Grieve 1985). He enlarges on this aspect thus:

There is new evidence to support the view that suppleness and flexibility of muscle and connective tissue, are of prime importance. Long and continued occupational and postural stress, asymmetrically imposed upon the soft tissues, tends to cause fibroblasts to multiply more rapidly and produce more collagen. Besides occupying more space within the connective tissue element of the muscle, the extra fibres encroach on the space normally occupied by nerves and vessels. Because of this trespass, the tissue loses elasticity and may become painful when the muscle is required to do work in coordination with others. In the long term collagen would replace the active fibres of the muscle and since collagen is fairly resistant to enzyme breakdown these changes tend to be irreversible.

The explanations of Jokl, Korr, Patterson and Grieve, as discussed above, help us to gain a clearer picture of the structural changes that take place as stress factors, operating over a period of time, impact on the soft tissues.

Postural and phasic muscle lists

Type I postural muscles are prone to loss of endurance capabilities when disused or subject to pathological influences and become shortened or tighter, whereas type II phasic muscles, when abused or disused, become weak (Janda 1982, Lewit 1992, Liebenson 2006).

Postural muscles that become hypertonic and shorten in response to dysfunction include (Fig. 1.2):

- Trapezius (upper), sternocleidomastoid, levator scapulae and upper aspects of pectoralis major, in the upper trunk; and the flexors of the arms. Quadratus lumborum, erector spinae, oblique abdominals and iliopsoas, in the lower trunk. Tensor fascia lata, rectus femoris, biceps femoris, adductors (longus brevis and magnus) piriformis, hamstrings, semitendinosus.

Phasic muscles, which weaken (i.e. are inhibited), and may lengthen, in response to dysfunction, include:

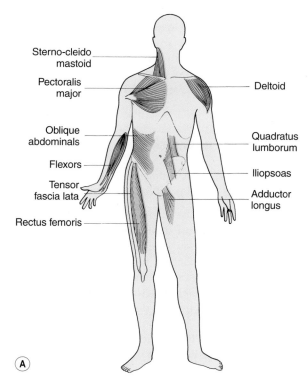

Figure 1.2A   Major postural muscles of the anterior aspects of the body.

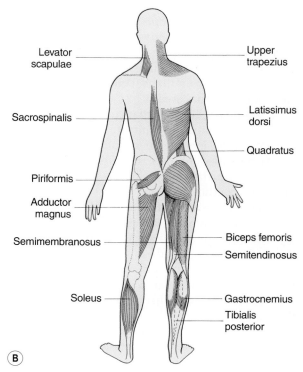

Figure 1.2B   Major postural muscles of the posterior aspects of the body.

- The paravertebral muscles (not erector spinae) and scaleni, the extensors of the upper extremity (flexors are primarily postural), the abdominal aspects of pectoralis major; middle and inferior aspects of trapezius; the rhomboids, serratus anterior, rectus abdominus; the internal and external obliques, gluteals, the peroneal muscles and the extensors of the arms.

Muscle groups such as the scaleni are equivocal: they start out as phasic muscles but can end up as postural.

Note: Lewit (1999) does not subscribe to the theory that phasic and postural muscles can be differentiated by virtue of their fibre type, as do Grieve and Jokl, but certainly subscribes to their differences in all other regards.

Fibrositis

Having evolved from 'muscular rheumatism', via fibrositis, to the currently favoured term 'fibromyalgia', generalized muscular pain is a manifestation of multiple causative influences. The great British orthopaedic physician and writer James Cyriax (1962) believed, like Stoddard, that all primary 'fibrositic' conditions were a result of articular lesions (dysfunctions).

A secondary librotic change could result, he stated, from traumatic injury to soft tissues (e.g. capsular adhesion at the shoulder after injury) which he called fibrosis, not fibrositis. He saw fibrosis as scar tissue formation. Other secondary fibrositic conditions were said to result from rheumatoid disease, infection (such as epidemic myalgia) and parasitic infection (*Trichinella spiralis*). All other muscular and soft tissue dysfunctions, Cyriax regarded as one result of joint dysfunction, which then produced muscular protective spasm, muscular wasting, pain, etc., and which could be normalized only by correction of the joint lesion.

NMT theory and practice holds an almost precisely opposing view to that held by Cyriax – maintaining that appropriate normalization of the soft tissues can, more often than not, achieve joint normalization, when restriction exists, without active manipulation of the joint, since most joint problems appear to be the direct result of myofascial dysfunction (Cantu & Grodin 1992, Janda 1988, Stiles 1984).

Cyriax did point out that fibrous tissue is capable of maintaining inflammation, originally traumatic, almost as a matter of habit. In such cases he opted for hydrocortisone injections as the appropriate measure to 'break' this habit. Such treatment can work, but such an approach all too often fails if underlying fibrotic changes have not been normalized or habits of use modified.

Fibrositis changes its name to fibromyalgia

In Chapter 3, in which the phenomenon of local soft tissue dysfunction, most notably myofascial trigger point activity, is analysed in detail, the evolution of thinking regarding 'fibrositis' is also examined. Fibromyalgia (the new incarnation of fibrositis), with its causes, associated conditions and diagnostic criteria, requires discussion in that context because of the confusion that currently exists regarding the overlap between fibromyalgia syndrome (FMS), myofascial pain syndrome (MPS) and chronic fatigue syndrome (CFS). The fascia of the body has profound influence, and it is to this focus that we now turn.

The fascial network

(DiGiovanna 1991, Frankel 1980, Ingber 2008, Myers 2001, Schelip 2006)

Of major significance in understanding musculoskeletal function and dysfunction is the fact that the fascia comprises one connected network – from the fascia attached to the inner aspects of the skull to the fascia in the soles of the feet, there exists just one fascial structure.

If any part of this is deformed or distorted, negative stresses may be imposed on distant aspects, and on the structures that it divides, envelops, enmeshes and supports, and with which it connects. There is ample evidence that Wolff's law applies, in that fascia accommodates to chronic stress patterns and deforms itself –

something that often precedes deformity of osseous and cartilaginous structures in chronic diseases.

Note: Wolff's law states that biological systems (including soft and hard tissues) deform in relation to the lines of force imposed on them.

The musculoskeletal system, the mechanical component of the human machine, comprising as it does 60% of the mass of the body, exists in a state of structural and functional continuity between all of its hard and soft tissues, and fascia is the ubiquitous elastic–plastic, gluey, component that invests, supports and separates, connects and divides, wraps and gives cohesion to the rest of the body – the fascial, connective tissue network. It is the connective tissues/fascia that provide most of that continuity. Any tendency to think of a local 'lesion' as existing in isolation should be discouraged as we try to visualize a complex, interrelated, symbiotically functioning assortment of tissues, comprising skin, muscles, ligaments, tendons and bones, as well as the neural structures, blood and lymph channels, and vessels that bisect and invest these tissues – all given shape, cohesion and functional ability by the fascia (connective tissue).

One of the major researchers into the role of connective tissue in the economy of the body is Donald Ingber. He has summarized aspects of this work, that are pertinent to manual therapists, by saying:

> [The study of] mechanotransduction has revealed that molecules, cells, tissues, organs, and our entire bodies use "tensegrity" architecture to mechanically stabilize their shape, and to seamlessly integrate structure and function at all size scales. Through use of this tension-dependent building system, mechanical forces applied at the macroscale produce changes in biochemistry and gene expression within individual living cells. This structure-based system provides a mechanistic basis to explain how application of physical therapies might influence cell and tissue physiology (Ingber 2008).

Apart from its immense role in the support, structural organization and motion of the body, fascia is involved in numerous complex biochemical activities:

- Connective tissue provides a supporting matrix for more highly organized structures and attaches extensively to muscles, offering support and strength (Huijing & Baan 2007).
- Individual muscle fibres are enveloped by endomysium, which is connected to the stronger perimysium which surrounds the fasciculi. The perimysium's fibres attach to the even stronger epimysium, which surrounds the muscle as a whole and attaches to fascial tissues nearby.
- Because it contains mesenchymal cells of an embryonic type, connective tissue provides a generalized tissue capable of giving rise, under certain circumstances, to more specialized elements.
- It provides, by its fascial planes, pathways for nerves, blood and lymphatic vessels, and structures.
- Many of the neural structures in fascia are sensory in nature.
- It supplies restraining mechanisms by the differentiation of retention bands, fibrous pulleys and check ligaments, as well as assisting in the harmonious production and control of movement.
- Where connective tissue is loose in texture, it allows movement between adjacent structures and, by the formation of bursal sacs, reduces the effects of pressure and friction.
- Deep fascia ensheathes and preserves the characteristic contour of the limbs, and promotes the circulation in the veins and lymphatic vessels.
- The superficial fascia, which forms the panniculus adiposus, allows for the storage of fat and also provides a surface covering which aids in the conservation of body heat.
- By virtue of its fibroblastic activity, connective tissue aids in the repair of injuries by the deposition of collagenous fibres (scar tissue).
- The ensheathing layer of deep fascia, as well as intermuscular septa and interosseous membranes, provides vast surface areas for muscular attachment.
- The meshes of loose connective tissue contain the 'tissue fluid' and provide an essential medium through which the cellular elements of other tissues are brought into functional relation with blood and lymph. Connective

tissue has a nutritive function and houses nearly a quarter of all body fluids (Dicke 1978).

- The histiocytes of connective tissue comprise part of an important defence mechanism against bacterial invasion by their phagocytic activity. They also play a part as scavengers in removing cell debris and foreign material.
- Connective tissue represents an important 'neutralizer' or detoxicator to both endogenous toxins (those produced under physiological conditions) and exogenous toxins (those introduced from outside the organism). The mechanical barrier presented by connective tissue has important defensive functions in cases of infection and toxaemia.
- Recent research has shown evidence of the presence in connective tissue of contractile smooth muscle cells, indicating the potential for fascial tone to be actively modified (Schleip et al 2006).

Fascia, then, is not just a background structure with little function apart from its obvious supporting role, but is a ubiquitous, tenacious, connective tissue that is involved deeply in almost all of the fundamental processes of the body's structure, function and metabolism.

In therapeutic terms there can be little logic in trying to consider muscle as a separate structure from fascia, because they are so intimately related. Remove connective tissue from the scene and any muscle left would be a jelly-like structure without form or functional ability.

See Box 1.6 for definitions relating to the characteristic features of connective tissue/fascia.

Functional fascial continuities

Myers (2001) has created a model in which myofascial linkages are described in terms of railway junctions and tracks, which he has termed 'myofascial meridians'. While the interconnectedness of fascia throughout the body has long been understood, Myers' descriptions highlight specific linkages. The myofascial chains, which he describes as 'long functional continuities', are of important clinical value when attempting to identify functional connections between anatomically distant structures, for example the plantar fascia and fascia of the scalp, attaching to the brow ridge, as described in his *superficial back line* (Fig. 1.3), or

---

Box 1.6   Biomechanical terms relating to fascia

Creep
Continued deformation (increasing strain) of a viscoelastic material with time under constant load (traction, compression, twist). 'Creep' can occur during the process of myofascial release or in response to postural or functional patterns of use.

Hysteresis
Process of energy loss due to friction when tissues are loaded and unloaded, which may occur during treatment using stretching or other manual methods.

Load
The degree of force (stress) applied to an area.

Strain
Change in shape as a result of stress.

Stress
Force (load) normalized over the area on which it acts (all tissues exhibit stress–strain responses).

Thixotropy
A quality of colloids in which the more rapidly force is applied (load), the more rigid the tissue response, highlighting the need for sustained and slowly applied force when attempting to modify fascial status.

Viscoelastic
The potential to deform elastically when load is applied, and to return to the original non-deformed state when load is removed.

Viscoplastic
A permanent deformation resulting from the elastic potential having been exceeded, or pressure forces sustained.

Figure 1.3   Myers' superficial back line. Redrawn from *Journal of Bodywork and Movement Therapies* 1997; 1(2):95, with permission.

the anterior compartment of the periosteum of the tibia and the sternocleidomastoid attachment to the temporal bone, as described in his *superficial front line* (Fig. 1.4). These fascial bridges are also of potential clinical importance in application of the progressive inhibition of neuromuscular structures (PINS) method, described by Dennis Dowling in Chapter 11 of this book.

Soft tissue changes – energy and fascial considerations

Taylor (1958) has postulated that tissue changes, apparent to the trained palpating hand, often result from changes in thermodynamic equilibrium. He states that the body is a thermodynamic system and, as such, alterations in the extracellular fluids, viscosity, pH, electrophoretic changes, colloidal osmotic pressure, etc., are subject to thermodynamic laws. One of these laws states that the total energy of such a system and its surroundings must remain constant,

although the energy may be changed from one form to another as a result of alterations of the stresses imposed.

For example, through postural stress and gravitational effects, particular changes in the fascia involved would result in energy loss and therefore stasis and stagnation. One of the characteristics of thermodynamics is that of thixotropy, in which gels become more solid with energy loss and more fluid with energy input. Such changes are certainly palpable in soft tissues, before and after neuromuscular and other forms of manual treatment (Mikova et al 2008).

- Taylor (1958) has stated that manipulative pressure and stretching are the most effective ways of modifying energy potentials of abnormal soft tissues.
- Little (1969) believes that an additional beneficial effect results from the interaction of the bioenergy mechanism of the practitioner with the bioenergy field of the patient.

Figure 1.4   Myers' superficial front line. Redrawn from *Journal of Bodywork and Movement Therapies* 1997; 1(2):97, with permission.

Over and above the important factors of posture, functional ability and pain, the musculoskeletal component of the body plays a vital role in the conservation – wastage – of energy and in the attainment, or otherwise, of a truly relaxed mind. Whilst the origins of musculoskeletal dysfunction can be either psychic or physical, the constant interaction of the soma with the mind ensures a degree of psychic stress occurring as a feedback from physically caused chronic muscular tensions.

Rolf (1962) suggests that the human organism, as an energy mass, is subject to gravitational law. As a plastic medium, capable of change, Rolfing attempts to reorganize and balance the body in relation to gravitational forces. This is done by using pressure and stretch techniques on the fascial tissues in a precise sequence of body areas. The beneficial effects are claimed to be physical, emotional, postural and behavioural.

Rolf (1962) states:

Our ignorance of the role and significance of fascia is profound. Therefore even in theory it is easy to overlook the possibility that far-reaching changes may be made not only in structural contour, but also in functional manifestation, through better organisation of the layer of superficial fascia which enwraps the body. Experiments demonstrate that drastic (beneficial) changes may be made in the body, solely by stretching, separating and relaxing superficial fascia in an appropriate manner.

Osteopaths have observed and recorded the extent to which all degenerative change in the body – whether muscular, nervous, circulatory or organic – reflects in the superficial fascia. Any degree of degeneration, however minor, changes the bulk of the fascia, modifies its thickness and draws it into ridges in areas overlying deeper tensions and rigidities. Conversely, as this elastic envelope is stretched, manipulative mechanical energy is added to it, and the fascial colloid becomes more 'sol' and less 'gel' (Greenman 1989). Without minimizing the clinical importance of the structural and biomechanical aspects of the connective tissues, Oschman (2000) has examined and evaluated research, which suggests that far more may be taking place during manual treatment than current understanding can fully explain. See Box 1.7 for a brief summary of aspects of these concepts.

Fascial stress responses and therapeutic opportunities

Changes in the fascia can result from passive congestion, which results in fibrous infiltration and a more 'sol'-like consistency than is the norm. Under healthy conditions a 'gel'-like ground substance follows the laws of fluid mechanics. Clearly, the more resistive drag there is in a colloidal substance, the greater will be the difficulty in normalizing this.

Scariati (1991) points out that colloids are not rigid: they conform to the shape of their container, and respond to pressure even though they are not compressible. The amount of resistance they offer increases proportionally to the velocity of motion applied to them, which makes a gentle touch a fundamental requirement if viscous drag and resistance are to be avoided when attempting to produce a release.

Box 1.7   Oschman's energy concepts: connective tissue, crystallinity and continuity

Peters (2001) discusses Oschman's research into energy phenomena as this relates to health enhancement. He reports that Oschman (2000) makes the point that the intricate traffic of biochemical, structural and electrical information is modulated not only through an electromagnetic flux, and 'clouds' of neuroreceptor traffic, but also as mechanical and rhythmic impulses of sound, heat, gravity, elasticity and pressure.

Oschman (2000) describes the processes:

What we refer to as health is when all the systems, both known and unknown, are functioning collectively, co-operatively ... The solid state, electronic, photonic and vibratory properties, of this living matrix continuum, play key roles in the integration of function, including injury repair and defence against disease. A debate about whether there is such a thing as 'healing energy' or 'life energy' has been replaced with study of the interaction between biological energy fields, structures and functions ... There are now instruments sensitive enough to detect the bio-magnetic fields produced by the different organs ... photometers and thermographs of parallel sensitivity allow us to detect almost infinitesimal variations in light and heat emanating from the body. Previous images of the organism – as being built up of parts – have concealed the most significant attribute of living matter – its continuity.

Oschman (2000) goes on:

The major structural and functional domains of the body are the connective tissues, the cells within them, and the cytoskeletons, nuclei and genetic material within the cells ... [this] assembly is best described by a single word, continuum ... Structural and functional continuity has now been confirmed and appreciated by science.
Continuity in living systems is simultaneously mechanical, structural, regulatory, and energetic. A second key to the emerging concepts has come about from recognition of the crystalline properties

of living tissues ... Crystals have important vibratory characteristics that arise as collective properties of the whole system. When a crystal is broken into its constituents, these unique vibratory phenomena disappear. This is why collective properties such as functional organization and consciousness have been elusive for those who study the system's components piece-by-piece. Molecular arrays or crystals are the dominant structural feature of living matter. Crystallographic techniques such as X-ray diffraction have been essential for determining the structure of nerves, muscles, cell membranes, and connective tissues. From the biophysical perspective, molecular arrays or crystals cannot be described in terms of their constituents alone. (See Fig. 1.5.)

British biophysicist Mae-Wan Ho has developed an elegant quantum theory which describes the organism as a vibrant sentient whole (Ho 1993). Key to Ho's theory (Ho 1997) is the role of the connective tissue as a liquid crystalline material constituting a noiseless excitable vibratory continuum for rapid intercommunication and energy flow, permeating the entire organism and enabling it to function and perceive as a coherent whole.

Oschman (2000) attempts to describe a unitary concept:

The quantum coherence phenomenon, described by biophysicists, may be the origin of Sheldrake's morphogenetic field (Sheldrake 1995). Quantum coherence is a source of measurable light emissions from living systems (Popp et al 1992). Quantum coherence in the living matrix provides a basis for a unitary theory. Water and vibrations of the crystalline molecular lattices play key roles in energy and information storage, transfer, and release.

The conclusion reached by Oschman (2000) is that, almost irrespective of the mode of treatment, a primary interaction occurs between the therapist and the patient, which may involve communication between their energy fields.

When stressful forces (undesirable or therapeutic) are applied to fascia, there is a first reaction in which a degree of slack is allowed to be taken up, followed by what is colloquially referred to as 'creep' – a variable degree of resistance (depending on the state of the tissues).

Creep is an honest term that accurately describes the slow, delayed yet continuous, stretch that occurs in response to a continuously applied load, as long as this is gentle enough to not provoke the resistance of colloidal 'drag'.

As the fascia comprises a single structure, the implications for body-wide repercussions

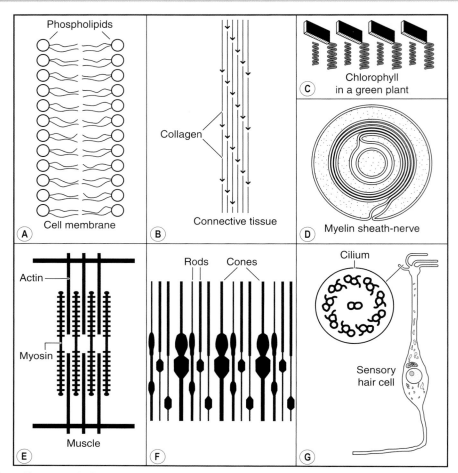

Figure 1.5   Crystalline arrays in living systems. Crystalline arrangements are the rule and not the exception in living systems. (A) Arrays of phospholipid molecules from cell membranes. (B) Collagen arrays form connective tissue. (C) Arrays of chlorophyll molecules in the leaf. (D) The myelin sheath of nerves. (E) The contractile array in muscle is composed of actin and myosin molecules organized around one another. (F) The array of sensory endings in the retina. (G) Arrays of microtubules, microfilaments and other fibrous components of the cytoskeleton occur in nerves and other kinds of cells. The example shown here is the cilia of sensory organs such as those responsible for detecting odours and sound. Reproduced from Oschman (2000) (illustration (D) is reproduced with permission of Arnold).

of distortions in that structure are clear (Fig. 1.6). An example of one possible negative influence of this sort is to be found in the fascial divisions within the cranium, the tentorium cerebelli and falx cerebri, which are commonly warped during birthing difficulties (too long or too short a time in the birth canal, forceps delivery, etc.) and which are noted in craniosacral therapy as affecting total body mechanics via their influence on fascia (and therefore the musculature) throughout the body (Brookes 1984).

Cantu & Grodin (1992) describe what they see as the 'unique' feature of connective tissue as its 'deformation characteristics'. This refers to a combined viscous (permanent) deformation characteristic as well as an elastic (temporary) deformation characteristic. This leads to the clinically important manner in which connective tissue responds to applied mechanical force by first changing in length, followed by some of this change being lost while some remains. The implications of this phenomenon can be seen in the application of stretching techniques to such

Figure 1.6 Balanced posture (A) compared with two patterns of musculoskeletal imbalance that involve fascial, and general, tissue and joint adaptations.

tissues, as well as in the way they respond to postural and other repetitive insults.

Such changes are not, however, permanent, because collagen (the raw material of fascia/connective tissue) has a limited (300–500 days) half-life and, just as bone adapts to stresses imposed upon it, so does fascia. Therefore, if negative stresses (posture, use, etc.) are modified for the better and/or positive 'stresses' are imposed (e.g. manipulation and/or exercise), dysfunctional connective tissue can usually be improved over time (Neuberger et al 1953).

Cantu & Grodin (1992), in their evaluation of the myofascial complex, concluded that therapeutic approaches that sequence their treatment protocols to involve the superficial tissues (involving autonomic responses) as well as deeper tissues (influencing the mechanical components of the musculoskeletal system), and which also address the factor of mobility (movement), are in tune with the requirements of the body when dysfunctional. NMT, as it will be presented here, does take this comprehensive approach, and much that it offers seems to be similar to the

myofascial release methods currently receiving so much attention in the USA.

Cathie (1974) maintains that the contractile phase of fascial activity supersedes all its other qualities. The attachments of fascia, he states, have a tendency to shorten after periods of marked activity that are followed by periods of inactivity, and the ligaments become tighter and thicker with advancing age. The properties of fascia (connective tissue) that he regards as being important to therapeutic consideration are:

1. It is richly endowed with nerve endings.
2. It has the ability to contract and to stretch elastically.
3. It gives extensive muscular attachment.
4. It supports and stabilizes, thus enhancing the postural balance of the body.
5. It is vitally involved in all aspects of motion.
6. It aids in circulatory economy, especially of venous and lymphatic fluids.
7. Fascial change will precede many chronic degenerative diseases.
8. Fascial changes predispose towards chronic tissue congestion.
9. Such chronic passive congestion precedes the formation of fibrous tissue, which then proceeds to an increase in hydrogen ion concentration of articular and periarticular structures.
10. Fascial specializations produce definite stress bands.
11. Sudden stress (trauma) on fascial tissue will often result in a burning type of pain.
12. Fascia is a major arena of inflammatory processes.
13. Fluids and infectious processes often travel along fascial planes.
14. The CNS is surrounded by fascial tissue (dura mater) that, in the skull, attaches to bone, so that dysfunction in these tissues can have profound and widespread effects.

Greenman (1989) describes how fascia responds to loads and stress in both a plastic and an elastic manner, its response depending upon the type, duration and amount of the load. The responses to either acute injury or repetitive microtrauma (e.g. resulting from a short leg imbalance) are, according to Greenman, likely to follow a sequence of inflammation which subsequently leads to absorption of inflammatory fluids into the superficial fascia, as well as into tight compartmentalized areas in the deep fascia – with this latter event being both palpable and detrimental.

Another variable (apart from the nature of the stress load) that influences the way in which fascia responds to stress, and what the individual feels of the process, relates to the number of collagen and elastic fibres contained in any given region.

Neural receptors within the fascia report to the CNS as part of any adaptation process, with the Pacinian corpuscles being particularly important in terms of their involvement in reflex responses.

Ligaments and muscle tone

Other neural input into the pool of activity, and responses to biomechanical stress, involve specialized fascial structures such as tendons and ligaments that contain highly specialized and sensitive mechanoreceptors and proprioceptive reporting stations.

Solomonow (2009) summarizes the role of ligaments as follows:

> As joints go through their range of motion, with or without external load, the ligaments ensure that the bones associated with the joint travel in their prescribed anatomical tracks, keep full and even contact pressure of the articular surfaces, prevent separation of the bones from each other by increasing their tension, as may be necessary, and ensuring stable motion. Joint stability, therefore, is the general role of ligaments without which the joint may subluxate, cause damage to the capsule, cartilage, tendons, nearby nerves and blood vessels, discs (if considering spinal joints) and to the ligaments themselves. Such injury may debilitate the individual by preventing or limiting his/her use of the joint and the loss of function. Unstable joints are also known to drastically modify the intra-articular pressure

> and the muscular activity pattern about the joint, resulting in early onset of osteoarthritis, pain, disability and eventually the need for joint replacement surgery.

Solomonow adds some important information regarding the link between muscle behaviour and ligamentous function:

> Ligaments are also sensory organs and have significant input to sensation and reflexive/synergistic activation of muscles. The muscles associated with any given joint, therefore, also have a significant role as restraints.
>
> For example muscular activity associated with the reflex from the ACL acts to prevent distraction of the joint, while simultaneously reducing the strain in the ACL. Evidence also supports the possibility that ligamento-muscular reflexes may also have inhibitory effects on muscles associated with that joint – inhibiting muscles that destabilize the joint or increasing antagonist co-activation to stabilize the joint.

A strong clue relative to the potential therapeutic use of ligament behaviour, in for example positional release methodology (see Ch. 8), can be gained from Solomonow's (2009) observation that:

> Ligaments are functional (effective) under tension, or when stretched, and completely non-functional in compression or when shortened below their resting length.

Having briefly scanned the influences of stress, both short and long term, on the musculoskeletal system, and of the varying ways in which the soft tissues respond – acutely, chronically and with variations based on their structure – and before looking more closely at reflex phenomena a brief introduction to neuromuscular technique (see Ch. 2) will provide an indication of its potential for dealing with soft tissue distress.

References

Alexander FM: *The use of the self*, London, 1957, Educational Publications.

Alshami CM, Hodges A: An experimental pain model to investigate the specificity of the neurodynamic test for the median nerve in the differential diagnosis of hand symptoms, *Arch Phys Med Rehabil* 87(10):1412–1417, 2006.

Baldry P: *Acupuncture, trigger points and musculoskeletal pain*, Edinburgh, 1993, Churchill Livingstone.

Barlow W: Anxiety and muscle tension pain, *Br J Clin Prac* 3(5):339–350, 1959.

Basmajian J: *Muscles alive*, Baltimore, 1974, Williams & Wilkins.

Bendtsen L, Jensen R, Olesen J: Qualitatively altered nociception in chronic myofascial pain, *Pain* 65: 259–264, 1996.

Boadella D: The language of the body in bioenergetic therapy, *Journal of the Research Society for Natural Therapeutics*, 1978.

Brookes D: *Cranial osteopathy*, London, 1984, Thorsons.

Butler D: *Mobilisation of the nervous system*, Edinburgh, 1991, Churchill Livingstone.

Butler D, Gifford L: Adverse mechanical tensions in the nervous system, *Physiotherapy* 75:622–629, 1989.

Buzzell K: *The physiological basis of osteopathic medicine*, New York, 1970, Postgraduate Institute of Osteopathic Medicine and Surgery.

Canals J, Pineda J, Torres-Peraza J, et al: Brain-derived neurotrophic factor regulates the onset and severity of motor dysfunction associated with enkephalinergic neuronal degeneration in Huntington's disease, *J Neurosci* 24:7727–7739, 2004.

Cantu R, Grodin A: *Myofascial manipulation*, Gaithersburg, Maryland, 1992, Aspen Publications.

Cathie A: *Selected writings. Academy of Applied Osteopathy Yearbook 1974*, Colorado Springs, 1974, Academy of Applied Osteopathy.

Chaitow L: *Soft tissue manipulation*, London, 1989, Thorsons.

Chaitow L, DeLany J: *Clinical applications of neuromuscular technique*, Edinburgh, 2000, Churchill Livingstone.

Chaitow L, Bradley D, Gilbert C: *Interdisciplinary approaches to breathing pattern disorders*, Edinburgh, 2002, Churchill Livingstone.

Cyriax J: *Textbook of orthopaedic medicine*, London, 1962, Cassell.

Dicke E: *A manual of reflexive therapy*, Scarsdale, New York, 1978, Sydney Simons.

DiGiovanna E: *An osteopathic approach to diagnosis and treatment*, London, 1991, Lippincott.

Dommerholt J: Posture. In Tubiana R, Camadio P, editors: *Medical problems of the instrumentalist musician*, London, 2000, Martin Dunitz.

Dvorak J, Dvorak V: *Manual medicine – diagnostics*, Stuttgart, 1984, Georg Thiem.

Edwards R: Hypotheses of peripheral and central mechanisms underlying occupational muscle pain and injury, *Eur J Appl Physiol* 57:275–281, 1988.

Feldenkrais M: *Awareness through movement*, New York, 1977, Harper & Row.

Frankel V: *Basic biomechanics of the skeletal system*, Philadelphia, 1980, Lea & Febiger.

Gagey PM: Postural disorders among workers in building sites. In Bles W, Brandt T, editors: *Disorders of posture and gait*, New York, 1986, Elsevier.

Gofton J, Trueman G: Studies in osteoarthritis of the hip: Part II. Osteoarthritis of the hip and leg-length disparity, *CMA Journal* 104:791–799, 1971.

Gray H: *Gray's anatomy*, ed 35, Edinburgh, 1977, Churchill Livingstone.

Greenman P: *Principles of manual medicine*, Baltimore, 1989, Williams & Wilkins.

Grieve G: *Mobilisation of the spine*, Edinburgh, 1985, Churchill Livingstone.

Hallgren R, Greenman P, Rechtien J: MRI of normal and atrophic muscles of the upper cervical spine, *J Clin Eng* 18(5):433–439, 1993.

Henneman E: Relation between size of neurons and their susceptibility to discharge, *Science* 126:1345–1347, 1957.

Ho MW: *The rainbow and the worm. The physics of organisms*, Singapore, 1993, World Scientific.

Ho MW: Quantum coherence and conscious experience, *Kybernetes* 26:265–276, 1997.

Horwitz A: Integrins and health, *Sci Am* 276:68–75, 1997.

Huijing P, Baan: Epimuscular myofascial force transmission between antagonistic and synergistic muscles can explain movement limitation in spastic paresis, *J Electromyogr Kinesiol* (6):708–724, 2007.

Hynes R: Integrins: versatility, modulation and signalling, *Cell* 69:11–26, 1992.

Ingber D: Tensegrity and mechanotransduction, *Jnl Bodywork and Movement Therapies* 12(3):198–200, 2008.

Issberner U, Reeh P, Steen K: Pain due to tissue acidosis: a mechanism for inflammatory and ischemic myalgia? *Neurosci Lett* 208(3):191–194, 1996.

Janda V: Introduction to functional pathology of the motor system, Proceedings of the VIIth Commonwealth and International Conference on Sport. *Physiotherapy in Sport* 3:39, 1982.

Janda V: *Muscle function testing*, London, 1983, Butterworths.

Janda V: Grant R, editor: *Physical therapy of the cervical and thoracic spine*, Edinburgh, 1988, Churchill Livingstone.

Janda V: Evaluation of muscle imbalances. In Liebenson C, editor: *Rehabilitation of the spine*, Baltimore, 1996, Williams & Wilkins.

Jokl P: Muscle and low back pain, *J Am Osteopath Assoc* 84(1):64–65, 1984.

Jones L: *Strain and counterstrain*, Colorado Springs, 1980, Academy of Applied Osteopathy.

Kappler R: Thrust techniques. In Ward R, editor: *Foundations for Osteopathic Medicine*, Baltimore, 1997, Williams & Wilkins.

Key J, et al: A model of movement dysfunction provides a classification system guiding diagnosis and therapeutic care in spinal pain and related musculoskeletal syndromes: a paradigm shift. Part 2, *Journal of Bodywork & Movement Therapies* 12(2):105–120; 2007.

Kolar P: Sensomotor nature of postural functions, *J Orthop Med* 212:40–45, 1999.

Korr I: *The physiological basis of osteopathic medicine*, New York, 1970, Postgraduate Institute of Osteopathic Medicine.

Korr I: *Spinal cord as organiser of disease process*, Colorado Springs, 1976, Academy of Applied Osteopathy Yearbook.

Korr I: *Neurologic mechanisms in manipulative therapy*, New York, 1978, Plenum Press.

Korr I: Axonal transport and neurotrophic functions in spinal cord as organiser of disease processes (part 4), *Academy of Applied Osteopathy* 451–458, 1981.

Kuchera M: Osteopathic Manipulative Medicine Considerations in Patients With Chronic Pain, *J Am Osteopath Assoc* 4(105):29–36, 2005.

Larsson SE, Bodegard L, Henriksson KG, et al: Chronic trapezius myalgia. Morphology and blood flow studied in 17 patients, *Acta Orthop Scand* 61:394–398, 1990.

Latey P: *Muscular manifesto*, London, 1983, P Latey.

Lederman E: *Fundamentals of manual therapy*, Edinburgh, 1997, Churchill Livingstone.

Lewis Sir T: *Pain*, New York, 1942, Macmillan.

Lewit K: *Manipulation in rehabilitation of the locomotor system*, ed 2, London, 1992, Butterworths.

Lewit K: *Manipulation in rehabilitation of the locomotor system*, ed 3, London, 1999, Butterworths.

Licciardone, et al: Osteopathic manipulative treatment for low back pain: a systematic review and meta-analysis of randomized controlled trials, *BMC Musculoskelet Disord* 6:43, 2005.

Liebenson C, editor: *Rehabilitation of the spine*, Baltimore, 1996, Williams & Wilkins.

Liebenson C: *Rehabilitation of the spine*, ed 2, Baltimore, 2006, Williams & Wilkins.

Liebenson C: *Muscular imbalance – an update. Dynamic Chiropractic*, 1999, Online. Available: http://www.chiroweb.com/dynamic.

Lin JP, Brown JK, Walsh EG: Physiological maturation of muscles in childhood, *Lancet* 343:1386–1389, 1994.

Little KE: Toward more effective manipulative management of chronic myofascial strain and stress syndromes, *J Am Osteopath Assoc* 68:675–685, 1969.

McConnell C: *Osteopathic Institute of Applied Technique Yearbook 1962*, London, 1962.

McPartland J, Brodeur R: Rectus capitis posterior minor, *Journal of Bodywork and Movement Therapies* 3(1):30–35, 1999.

Maitland G: *Vertebral manipulation*, London, 1986, Butterworths.

Maitland G, Hengeveld E, Banks K, et al: *Maitland's vertebral manipulation*, ed 6, London, 2001, Butterworth Heinemann.

Martin S: Interview with Jeff Bland: lessons from the genome, *CAM Magazine* November 2001.

Mense S, Simons D: *Muscle pain*, Philadelphia, 2001, Williams & Wilkins.

Miková M, Krobot A, Janura M, et al: Viscoelastic properties of fibrous connective tissue and manual treatment, *Rehabilitace a Fyzikalni Lekarstvi* 15(1):3–10, 2008.

Mooar P: Introduction. Merck Manual, 2007, http://www.merck.com/mmhe/sec05/ch058/ch058a.html Retrieved 2008-11-12.

Myers T: *Anatomy trains*, Edinburgh, 2001, Churchill Livingstone.

Neuberger A, et al: Metabolism of collagen, *Biochem. J.* 53:47–52, 1953.

Norris CM: Spinal stabilisation. 1. Active lumbar stabilisation – concepts, *Physiotherapy* 81(2):61–64, 1995a.

Norris CM: Spinal stabilisation. 2. Limiting factors to end-range motion in the lumbar spine, *Physiotherapy* 81(2):64–72, 1995b.

Norris CM: Spinal stabilisation. 3. Stabilisation mechanisms of the lumbar spine, *Physiotherapy* 81(2):72–79, 1995c.

Norris CM: Spinal stabilisation. 4. Muscle imbalance and the low back, *Physiotherapy* 81(3):127–138, 1995d.

Norris CM: Spinal stabilisation. 5. An exercise program to enhance lumbar stabilisation, *Physiotherapy* 81(3):138–146, 1995e.

Norris CM: *Sports injuries, diagnosis and management*, ed 2, London, 1998, Butterworths.

Oschman J: *Energy medicine*, Edinburgh, 2000, Churchill Livingstone.

Patterson M, Wurster R: Neurophysiologic system: integration and disintegration. In Ward R, editor: *Foundations for osteopathic medicine*, Baltimore, 1997, Williams & Wilkins.

Peck D, Buxton D, Nitz A: A comparison of spindle concentrations in large and small muscles acting in parallel combinations, *J Morphol* 180:243–252, 1984.

Peters D: Vitalism revisited, *Journal of Bodywork and Movement Therapies* 5(3):198–204, 2001.

Popp FA, Li KH, Gu Q: *Recent advances in biophoton research*, Singapore, 1992, World Scientific.

Protopapas M, Cymet T: Joint cracking and popping: Understanding noises that accompany articular release, *J Am Osteopath Assoc* 102(5):283–287, 2002.

Reich W: Character analysis, 1949, Vision Press.

Reinert A, Mense S: Inflammatory influence on the density of CGRP- and SP-immunoreactive nerve endings in rat skeletal muscle, *Neuropeptides* 24:204–205, 1993.

Richardson C: The muscle designation debate, *Journal of Bodywork and Movement Therapies* 4(4):235–236, 2000.

Richardson C, Jull G, Hodges P, et al: *Therapeutic exercise for spinal segment stabilisation in low back pain*, Edinburgh, 1999, Churchill Livingstone.

Rolf I: *Structural dynamics. British Academy of Applied Osteopathy Yearbook 1962*, New York, 1962, BAAO.

Rosenthal E: The Alexander technique and how it works, *Medical Problems in the Performing Arts* 2:53–57, 1987.

Rowlerson A: A novel myosin, *J Muscle Res Cell Motil* 2:415–438, 1981.

Scariati P: DiGiovanna E, editor: *An osteopathic approach to diagnosis and treatment*, London, 1991, Lippincott.

Schamberger W: *The malalignment syndrome*, Edinburgh, 2002, Churchill Livingstone.

Schleip R, Naylor I, Ursu D, et al: Passive muscle stiffness may be influenced by active contractility of intramuscular connective tissue, *Med Hypotheses* 66(1):71, 2006.

Selye H: *The stress of life*, Philadelphia, 1976, McGraw Hill.

Shah J, Danoff J, Desai M, et al: Biochemicals associated with pain and inflammation are elevated in sites near to and remote from active myofascial trigger points, *Arch Phys Med Rehabil* 89:16–23, 2008a.

Shah J, Gilliams E: Uncovering the biochemical milieu of myofascial trigger points using in vivo microdialysis: An application of muscle pain concepts to myofascial pain syndrome, *Journal of Bodywork and Movement Therapies* 12(4):371–384, 2008b.

Sheldrake R: *A new science of life,* The hypothesis of morphic resonance, Rochester, Vermont, 1995, Park Street Press.

Simons D: *Myofascial pain due to trigger points. International Rehabilitation Medicine Association Monograph (Series 1),* Ohio, 1987, Rademaker.

Simons D, Travell J, Simons L: *Myofascial pain and dysfunction: the trigger point manual. vol. 1: Upper half of body,* ed 2, Baltimore, 1999, Williams & Wilkins.

Solomonow M: Ligaments: A source of musculoskeletal disorders, *Journal Bodywork and Movement Therapies* 13(2):136–154, 2009.

Stanton DF, Dutes JC: Chronic pain and the chronic pain syndrome: the usefulness of manipulation and behavioural interventions, *Phys Med Rehabil Clin North Am* 7:863–875, 1996.

Stiles E: *Patient Care* 15 May:16–97 & 15 August:117–164, 1984.

Stoddard A: *Manual of osteopathic practice,* London, 1969, Hutchinson.

Taylor RB: *Bioenergetics of man. Academy of Applied Osteopathic Yearbook 1958,* California, 1958, Carmel.

Timmons B: *Behavioral and psychological approaches to breathing disorders,* New York, 1994, Plenum Press.

Travell J, Simons D: *Myofascial pain and dysfunction: the trigger point manual,* vol. 1, Philadelphia, 1983, Williams & Wilkins.

Travell J, Simons D: *Myofascial pain and dysfunction: the trigger point manual,* vol. 2, Philadelphia, 1992, Williams & Wilkins.

Vleeming A, Mooney V, Stoeckart R, editors: *Movement stability & lumbopelvic pain - Integration of research and therapy,* ed 2, Edinburgh, 2007, Churchill Livingstone.

Waersted M, Eken T, Westgaard R: Psychogenic motor unit activity – a possible muscle injury mechanism studied in a healthy subject, *Journal of Musculoskeletal Pain* 1(3/4): 185–190, 1993.

Wall P, Melzack R: *Textbook of pain,* Edinburgh, 1991, Churchill Livingstone.

Wang N, Butler JP, Ingbes DE, et al: Mechanotransduction across the cell surface and through the cytoskeleton, *Science* 260:1124–1127, 1993.

Wolfe F, Simons D: Fibromyalgia and myofascial pain syndromes, *J Rheumatol* 19(6):944–995, 1992.

Woo SL-Y, et al: *Injury and repair of musculoskeletal soft tissues,* Savannah, Georgia, 1987, American Academy of Orthopedic Surgeons Symposium.

2

Introduction to NMT

CHAPTER CONTENTS

NMT: A brief historical overview   **35**
Stanley Lief   35
Associated approaches   36
Assessment is key   36
A brief history of NMT   37
Peter Lief   38
Tissues involved in NMT   **38**
Site of application   38
Chemical structure   39
A function of circulation   39
Stressor stimulus   40
Judith DeLany's overview of NMT in the USA   40
Various chiropractic perspectives on Nimmo's work   41

NMT: A brief historical overview

Imagine a palpation technique that becomes a means of therapeutic intervention by virtue of the addition of increased pressure.

Imagine also a palpation technique that, in a non-invasive manner, meets and matches the tone of the tissues it is addressing and sequentially seeks out changes from the norm in almost all accessible (to finger or thumb) areas of the soft tissues.

Imagine this approach as systematically providing information regarding tissue tone, induration, fibrosity, oedema, discrete localized soft tissue changes, areas of altered structure, adhesions or pain – and being able to switch from a painless and pleasant assessment mode to a treatment focus that starts the process of normalizing the changes it uncovers.

This is neuromuscular technique (NMT).

Stanley Lief

The developer of European NMT was Stanley Lief, who was born in Lutzen in the Baltic state of Latvia in the early 1890s. He was one of the five children of Isaac and Riva Lief (Riva was the author's grandfather's eldest sister, i.e. her maiden surname was Chaitow). The family emigrated to South Africa in the 1890s where Stanley was given a basic primary school education before starting work in his father's trading store in Roodeport, Transvaal.

Lief's poor health led to an interest in physical culture, one source of which was found in popular health magazines published in the USA.

Eventually Lief worked his passage to the USA in order to train under the legendary 'physical culturist' Bernard Macfadden. He qualified in chiropractic and naturopathy before World War I, and was in Britain at its outbreak. After serving in the army he returned to England and worked in institutional 'Nature Cure' (naturopathic) resorts until 1925, when he established his own clinic, Champneys, at Tring in Hertfordshire.

At this world-famous healing resort he established his reputation as a daring and pioneering healer. By using the dietetic, fasting, hydrotherapeutic and physical education and manual methods by which naturopathy aims to restore normality to the sick body, he developed a huge following. It was during his most successful years, before World War II, that he evolved the technique that this book attempts to describe.

Stanley Lief, together with his cousin Boris Chaitow, who worked as his assistant at Champneys before and during World War II, developed and refined the uses of NMT. Boris Chaitow was also born in Latvia and grew up in South Africa in the small mining town of Pilgrim's Rest, now a 'museum town', where the Chaitow trading store-cum-home still stands. He later qualified as an attorney, and was in practice with my father when he became inspired by Stanley Lief's example and, with Lief's help, trained as a chiropractor at National College, Chicago, before joining the staff at Champneys in 1937.

Associated approaches

In this book, Lief's basic NMT applications, together with a variety of specialized associated soft tissue manipulation techniques, will be presented. There will also be discussion of various reflex systems that fall within the scope of soft tissue treatment in general, and NMT in particular.

For example, detailed reference to, and illustrations of, the neurolymphatic reflexes of Chapman, together with illustrations of other reflex patterns such as myofascial trigger points, have been included.

Another of Lief's assistants at Champneys, Tom Moule, continued the development of NMT in health care, and his son, Terry Moule, has contributed his thoughts in Chapter 9, in which his particular focus, the use of NMT in treatment of sports injuries, is briefly outlined. Another evolution of an NMT-like approach, known as Progressive Inhibition of Neuromuscular Structures (PINS), is described by its developer, Denis Dowling, in Chapter 11.

In Chapter 12 a description is given of Thai yoga massage – or rather a Western modification, which explains some of the overlaps between this ancient system, and NMT. That there is a similarity should not be surprising, since aspects of modern NMT derive from Ayurvedic techniques, as will become clear later in this chapter.

In the appendix the work and influence of Raymond Nimmo are evaluated. The lead author of this book had the opportunity to attend a course conducted by Nimmo in the 1960s in London, and was struck then by the similarity his concepts and methods had, as compared with those of Stanley Lief, the primary developer of NMT in Europe. Brief evaluations of Nimmo's work are given later in this chapter.

As a modality, NMT complements and may be incorporated into any system of physical medicine. It may – and indeed often should – be used as a means of treatment on its own, or it may accompany (preceding for preference) manipulative and other physical modalities. Its main use up to the present has been in the hands (literally) of the osteopathic profession; however, many physiotherapists, chiropractors, massage therapists and doctors of physical medicine who have studied and used NMT have found it complementary to their own methods of practice.

As it offers a simultaneous diagnostic and therapeutic capability, NMT is time-saving, energy-saving and, above all, efficient.

Other soft tissue manipulative methods such as muscle energy technique (MET) and functional positional release approaches (strain/counterstrain, for example) are commonly used as part of NMT treatment. These are briefly explained in Chapter 8: Associated Techniques.

Assessment is key

The key to the successful use of NMT is an ability to sense accurately what it is that the hands are feeling while at the same time having a clear picture of what the particular movement or technique being employed is aimed at achieving. If the practitioner can learn to 'see', with the hands, and by using them let the patient's body 'tell its own tale', then the intelligent application of the methods described has much to offer towards the recovery of normal function.

Holistic methods of healing demand that, in order to create the situation for the maintenance or the restoration of health, the individual must be seen as a totality.

It is necessary, therefore, to attempt to recognize the various factors affecting both the internal and external environment of the individual, because these are part of the complex interacting totality that can influence the individual for good or ill. In the end, the body is self-healing, self-repairing and self-maintaining, if the prerequisites for health are present. Emotional stability, nutritional balance and hygienic considerations all play their part, as do structural and mechanical integrity.

A brief history of NMT

In Europe neuromuscular technique has evolved over the past 60 years from the original work of Stanley Lief. In the mid-1930s he was seeking improved means for preparing soft tissue structures for subsequent manipulation. The development of NMT (neuromuscular therapy) in the USA is described at the end of this chapter.

Lief had studied the work of Rabagliatti, whose book Initis influenced his interest in connective tissue problems.

Lief also became aware of (and studied) the work of Dr Dewanchand Varma, a practitioner of Ayurvedic manipulation (Varma called his method 'pranotherapy') who was practising in Paris. In Varma's book The Human Machine and Its Forces (Varma 1935), he states:

We have discovered that the circulation of the nervous currents, slows down occasionally because of the obstruction caused by adhesions; the muscular fibres harden and the nervous currents can no longer pass through them. We have demonstrated effective and positive methods designed to restore nervous equilibrium which promotes the healthy circulation of blood, so that

new tissues begin to be built up again. Our method of treatment, by the removal of all obstacles to the flow of nervous current, allows energy to proceed unimpeded.

Lief found various of Varma's techniques clinically useful, and from these ideas and methods developed his own soft tissue approach – NMT. Lief's cousin, Boris Chaitow, describes this early development of NMT as follows (B. Chaitow, personal communication, 1983):

In the middle of the 1930s Stanley Lief realised that the integrity of a joint was to a great extent related to the character of the tissues surrounding the joint, related to muscle, tendons, ligaments, blood and nerve supply etc. He felt that in order the better to achieve effective mobility and integrity of function of joints – particularly in the spine but also in all bony articular relationships – it was advisable to normalise, as best one could, the adjacent soft tissues by removing any function-interfering factors, such as tensions, contractions, adhesions, spasms, fibrositic contractures etc., with appropriate application of fingers and hands to those tissues. To this end the neuromuscular technique was evolved to cover every possible type of lesion in whatever part of the body (articular, soft tissue, abdominal, glandular, nervous, vascular etc).

It so happened that at that particular time Stanley Lief had heard of a well-known Indian practitioner named Varma operating in Paris, who was applying an unusual but very effective soft-tissue technique on patients with remarkable benefits. Lief decided to arrange to have a series of treatments on himself from Varma, and finally persuaded the latter to teach him this specialised technique. Much as he appreciated the method used by Varma, he felt it could be improved, and began to develop and subsequently practised the method for which he devised the name of 'Neuromuscular Technique'. This name was an accurate definition of the purpose of the method he evolved from the cruder technique used by Varma. NMT involved an application of hands and fingers to the appropriate areas of soft tissue related to the affected bony articulations, as well as all other areas of soft tissue which his sensitive fingers found to be abnormal in texture.

This enables adverse factors in such tissue to be corrected to allow the full function of muscles and nerves to be re-established. In doing so the double benefits are achieved in improving nerve and blood circulation, improving texture of muscle tissue and in being better able to get effective results in manipulating the bony articulations involved, and assuring lasting integrity of their normal function.

Stanley Lief also maintained that joint lesions were not the only factors in the interference in nerve force integrity, but that tensions, contractions, adhesions, muscle spasms and fibrositic contractures in soft tissues could in themselves constitute primary factors in disease (symptom) causation by reducing effective nerve and blood circulation. To this end he developed his diagnostic sensitivity with his fingers so that in a few seconds of palpation over any area of the body, he was able to assess abnormalities present in relation to tensions, adhesions and spasms.

The body's integrity, and its functional efficiency, depends not only on its chemistry influenced by the nature of the food and drink we consume, but also on the effective nerve and blood circulation free of mechanical and functional obstructions. To this second vital purpose there is no formula devised by the osteopathic or chiropractic professions that will more effectively achieve the optimum result than the philosophy and technique devised by Stanley Lief. There is no single part of the body that he was not able to apply his method to to achieve remarkable physiological responses.

Peter Lief

Stanley Lief's son, Peter (also a naturopath, chiropractor and osteopath), has described (Lief 1963) the 'neuromuscular' lesion as being associated with:

1. Congestion of the local connective tissues
2. Disturbance of the acid–base balance of the connective tissues
3. Fibrous infiltration (adhesions)
4. Chronic muscular contractions, or hypertrophic or hypotrophic (tone) changes.

The aetiology of the neuromuscular lesion, according to Stanley and Peter Lief, includes a number of causative factors, giving rise to neuromuscular lesions, which may include:

- fatigue, exhaustion, bad posture
- local trauma
- systemic toxaemia
- lack of exercise and oxygen (ischaemia)
- dietetic deficiencies
- psychosomatic causes bringing about muscular tensions.

The presence of a 'lesion' (current terminology would define this as an area of somatic dysfunction) is always revealed by an area of hypersensitivity to pressure. It is remarkable to note just how close Lief came to defining the causes and characteristics of myofascial trigger points, although working many years before the trigger point research of Travell and Simons (Simons et al 1999, Travell, Simons & Travell 1999) (see Ch. 3).

Tissues involved in NMT

Boris Chaitow and Peter Lief have both taken part in the development and evolution of the theory and application of NMT as first described by Stanley Lief, as has Brian Youngs.

At the time of writing (2009) Youngs remains (in his ninth decade) a leading naturopathic/osteopathic practitioner in the UK. He was a colleague of both Stanley and Peter Lief, and was for many years, from the 1950s, a leading tutor at the British College of Naturopathy and Osteopathy – now the British College of Osteopathic Medicine, founded by Lief.

Youngs (1962) has given the following descriptive overview of the tissues involved in NMT.

Site of application

As the technique (NMT) operates primarily on connective tissue it will usually be concentrated at those areas where such tissue is most dense, e.g. muscular origins and insertions, especially the broad aponeurotic insertions. The most frequent sites are the superior curved line of the occiput, the numerous insertions and origins of the large, medium and small muscles which attach to the vertebral column; the iliac-crest insertions; the intercostal insertions and abdominal-muscle insertions. Nevertheless, the technique can of course be applied to any area which requires it – head, face, wrists, etc. Connective tissue is, after all, ubiquitous.

To understand the therapeutic effect of the technique one must have some knowledge of the pathophysiology of the tissue upon which it operates. Connective tissue consists of a matrix containing cells and fibres. It was largely ignored until recently, but has now been made the subject of close study – and even international conferences – in regard to its structure and functions. Dr Rabagliatti, 45 years ago (note: Youngs was writing in the mid-1960s) was so interested and far-seeing that his book, Initis, contained concepts the general truth of which is being proved today. He was, however, a lone voice and because he held unorthodox ideas he was, typically, ignored.

The ubiquity of connective tissue caused Dr Rabagliatti to analogize it to the ether – as the medium for, as he termed it, 'the zoodynamic life force'. (See Box 1.7 for current thinking along these lines.)

Through the connective tissues' planes run the trunks and plexuses of veins, arteries, nerves, and lymphatics. Connective tissue is the support for the structural and, therefore, functional relationships of these systems.

Chemical structure

Briefly, the matrix consists of a jelly-like ground substance in which the fibres, cells, vessels, etc., lie. This ground substance is the 'physical expression of the milieu interieure' intervening everywhere between the blood and lymph vessels and the metabolizing cells; it plays a major role in the transport, storage and exchange of water and electrolytes. The chemical structure is essentially polysaccharide, hyaluronic acid, chondroitin sulphuric acid, chondroitin sulphate and chondroitin itself, together with proteins which contain a considerable amount of the amino acid tyrosine, which forms the majority of the thyroxine molecule.

The fibres are white fibrous (collagen), yellow (elastin), and reticulin. The collagen fibres are also protein and polysaccharide in composition and are stabilized chemically by the presence of the ground substance constituents. The presence of chondroitin sulphate, for example, renders the enzymatic breakdown of collagen much more difficult. The importance of this point will become clearer later. The formation of fibres appears to be due to a precipitation of fibre constituents by serum glycoproteins under the influence of adrenocorticotrophic hormone.

Reticulin contains more polysaccharide than collagen, and some lipid also. Elastin is also protein and polysaccharide in composition. Sulphur is a constituent of all three. Cells include fibroblasts, mast cells, macrophages and others.

A function of circulation

The nature and composition of connective tissue is a function of circulation. Circulatory efficiency in any area will determine (1) the influx of materials to the area, and (2) the drainage of the area.

Incoming blood leads to the production of lymph and this fluid permeates the ground substance, bringing all the constituents of the blood except the proteins to the connective tissue. Some of these constituents are hormones. Thyroxine, adrenoglucocorticoids and adrenomineralocorticoids are only three of these. Oestrogen and androgens are two more. All these have known effects upon the structure of connective tissue. Thus, a diminution of thyroxine leads to an increase of water retention in most cells and an increase in the quantity of ground substance. The sex hormones also do this, but of most interest to us here are the opposing groups of the adrenocortical hormones. Selye divides these into anti- and pro-inflammatory hormones (A-Cs and P-Cs). These are produced in response to stress situations and they exert both a general and a local effect. By regulating the balance between these two the body can control the ability of the tissues to produce an inflammatory response. But when the A-Cs and the P-Cs are both present in the blood the A-Cs always win *the contest, i.e., there is an anti-inflammatory response.*

Stressor stimulus

The A-Cs are produced in response to a stimulus – the stressor. The stressor in neuromuscular technique is pain. Effective technique appears to be accompanied by pain in all such conditions (and also in the condition without treatment). Pain is probably due to two factors. A much reduced threshold in the area due to circulatory inhibition enabling a build up to just below the threshold level of Lewis pain substance or, alternatively, a disturbance of electrolyte level (e.g., increase of hydrogen ions or disturbance in the calcium/sodium/potassium balance due to the same circumstances). Consequently pain will be produced by even slight stimulus, let alone the heavier movements of neuromuscular technique. Also, pressure and tension proprioceptors may be overstimulated and pain can result from an over application of any ordinary stimulus.

The A-Cs liberated will produce both general effects (general adaptation syndrome) and local effects (local adaptation syndrome) and their effect is anti-inflammatory, both generally and locally, at the area of application of the stressor, i.e., at the areas of technique application. Consequently, there is a breakdown of collagen fibres and a general decrease in water retention in the ground substance; the congested area is decongested.

What Youngs has described tallies closely with what is now known about the biochemical status of tissues under stress, and particularly of the trigger point entity, which will be evaluated in following chapters.

Stanley Lief, albeit inadvertently, provided for the generation of practitioners who were to follow him a tool with which to deal with this pain-producing adaptive end-result of the multiple stresses faced by the modern musculoskeletal system.

In the latter part of the lives of Stanley Lief (d. 1963) and Boris Chaitow (d. 1996), awareness grew as to other applications of use for NMT, most notably its potential to identify and commence elimination of myofascial trigger points.

The principal author has, over the past 40 years, since working as assistant to Boris Chaitow in the early 1960s, helped to promote knowledge of NMT – particularly in its diagnostic mode – so that it stands today as a major therapeutic instrument for use by manipulative and massage therapists worldwide. The use of NMT as a broadly applicable sequential assessment and treatment tool was enhanced by exposure to the work of Raymond Nimmo in the late 1960s. Nimmo and his 'receptor-tonus' work seems to be a common link between 'European' NMT and American NMT. Descriptions of Nimmo's work will be found in the Appendix, however a brief perspective on his influence, from one of the USA's leading NMT teachers, Judith DeLany, is given below.

Judith DeLany's overview of NMT in the USA

What has today become neuromuscular therapy in the USA, was spawned in the late 1970s from receptor-tonus method (the work of the late Dr Raymond Nimmo). Nimmo, a 1926 graduate of Palmer College of Chiropractic, states in his writings that he questioned many of the philosophical and theoretical teachings of his profession (Nimmo 1959). He studied many aspects of classical chiropractic even though he was convinced that adjustment of the spine was not enough to ensure the health of the individual. He also sought out information as to the role that soft tissues play in pain and dysfunction in an attempt to explain the syndromes he was confronted with in his work.

As Nimmo developed his skill in palpating muscles, he noted particular points within the muscles which, when pressed, referred pain to various distant areas. He called these 'noxious generative points' (NGPs). In 1952 Nimmo purchased Connective Tissue: Transactions of the Second Conference *(Travell 1952), in which Janet Travell discussed her theories of trigger points. Nimmo found illustrations of referred pain patterns in Travell's work that coincided precisely with his own discoveries. He began working obsessively to develop a sensible treatment plan and states that, as time went by, he learned from others, but it is estimated that 80–90% of the techniques he taught were his own work.*

Nimmo's constant striving to prove the physiological basis of his work, complete with integration of neurological laws that gave validity and substance to his principles of practice, derived not only from being in the forefront of a newly emerging profession, but also from the fact that his interest in the soft tissue component of the body placed him at the fringes of the teachings of that profession.

He faced peers at a time when they were attempting to validate the principles of chiropractic and asked them to question the very basis of their beliefs. His work endured and many healthcare practitioners who studied with him carried the work forward, under a variety of names (see below).

In 1979, Paul St John, who had studied receptor-tonus methodology with Nimmo, published course manuals relating to similar techniques, which he called neuromuscular therapy (NMT). His concepts were influenced by not only Nimmo (Vannerson & Nimmo 1971), but also Travell & Simons (1983), Mariano Racabado, Leon Chaitow, Rene Cailliet (1977), Aaron Mattes, John Barnes, John Upledger and others, through their writings and seminars.

Judith (Walker) Delany's professional association with St John in 1984–1989 led to revisions of previous concepts, with significant changes in treatment techniques and teaching materials, which came to include the influence of posture and craniosacral methods.

During this phase, the work of Janet Travell and David Simons had enormous influence. Their book Myofascial Pain and Dysfunction: The Trigger Point Manual, Volume 1: The Upper Body *(Travell & Simons 1983), and numerous articles by them, began to explain in greater detail the background to what Nimmo had taught. In 1989, St John and Delany separated their work and both continue to teach neuromuscular therapy. The approaches they have taken, although still containing elements of Nimmo's original work, have now diverged, with the St John Method focusing on structural homeostasis of the body and cranium by applying the*

law of cause and effect, and Delany's NMT American Version *incorporating a systematic approach towards pain relief which addresses six physiological factors: ischaemia, trigger points, nerve compression/entrapment, postural distortion (biomechanics), nutritional components and emotional well-being (stress reduction).*

Judith Delany provides a detailed overview of *NMT American Version* in its current stage of evolution in Chapter 10.

Various chiropractic perspectives on Nimmo's work

Cohen & Gibbons (1998) have detailed the chiropractic perspective on the work of Nimmo. They point out that, in a survey carried out in 1993 of procedures currently employed by chiropractors in the USA, fully 40% were using Nimmo's receptor tonus methodology, which closely approximates NMT (National Board of Chiropractic Examiners 1993).

Gatterman & Lee (1995) summarize Nimmo's approach:

> *Nimmo found noxious generative points [trigger points] in muscles that referred pain in characteristic patterns. Viewing these hypersensitive areas, the trigger points of Travell, as abnormal reflex arcs he developed a manual technique designed to reduce the irritable loci. He referred to the inter-relationship of muscle tonus and the central nervous system as 'reverberating circuits', whereby stimulus was self-perpetuating until the cycle was broken ... This procedure referred to by Travell as ischemic compression offers a noninvasive chiropractic technique instead of the common medical practice of injection of the painful trigger points.*

To reach a point where his belief in soft tissue origin of much musculoskeletal pain was widely accepted by his own profession, Nimmo had to contend with, and overcome, the prevailing chiropractic model of 'bone on nerve' concepts. He was certainly an original thinker and his trigger point research was contemporary with, and in some ways ahead of, that of Janet Travell, the major medical researcher into this field. At the very least, Cohen & Gibbons (1998) suggest:

'The similarities are striking and suggest one concept developed concurrently by two outstanding independent researchers.'

There were, nevertheless, distinct differences between the early treatment approaches advocated by Travell, compared with those suggested by Nimmo, in the developmental years of their research into the pain generated by trigger points.

Cohen & Gibbons (1998) explain:

Travell advocated injections to the trigger points and later spray and stretch and 'ischemic compression' to relax the involved muscle. On the other hand Nimmo stated, 'I have found that a proper degree of pressure, sequentially applied, causes the nervous system to release a hypertonic muscle'. Nimmo did not see the trigger points as an object to be injected, stretched, massaged or dissolved by ultrasound.

We should recall that Nimmo's concepts were evolving in the 1950s and that, at that stage of her work, Travell was advocating injection as the primary tool for trigger point deactivation. Over the years, direct compression ('ischaemic') – now called 'trigger point release' – has become the preferred method of trigger point treatment, along with stretching (restoring the muscle housing the trigger point to its normal resting length; see Ch. 3).

Nimmo's insistence that trigger points had a neurological origin has not been validated, however, as evaluation of the latest findings of Simons et al (1999) will show (see Ch. 3). This in no way detracts from the enormous contribution made by Nimmo to this area of study. See the Appendix for more information on Nimmo's work.

References

Cailliet R: *Soft tissue pain and disability*, Philadelphia, 1977, FA Davis.

Cohen J, Gibbons R: Raymond L Nimmo and the evolution of trigger point therapy 1929–1986, *J Manipulative Physiol Ther* 21(3):167–172, 1998.

Gatterman M, Lee H: Chiropractic adjusting techniques. In Peterson D, Weise G, editors: *Chiropractic: an illustrated history*, Chicago, 1995, Mosby, pp 240–261.

Lief P: British Naturopathic, *British Naturopathic Journal* 5(10):304–324, 1963.

National Board of Chiropractic Examiners: *Job analysis of chiropractic*, Colorado, 1993, Greely.

Nimmo R: Factor X. The Receptor (1) 4. Reprinted in Schneider M, Cohen J, Laws S, editors: 2001 *The collected writings of Nimmo and Vannerson, pioneers of chiropractic trigger point therapy*, Pittsburgh, 1959, Self-published.

Simons D, Travell J, Simons L: *Myofascial pain and dysfunction: the trigger point manual*, vol. 1, Upper half of body, ed 2, Baltimore, 1999, Williams & Wilkins.

Travell J: *Connective tissue: transactions of the second conference*, New York, 1952, The Josiah Macy Jr Foundation.

Travell J, Simons D: *Myofascial pain and dysfunction: the trigger point manual*, vol. 1, The upper body. Baltimore, 1983, Williams & Wilkins.

Vannerson J, Nimmo R: Specificity and the law of facilitation in the nervous system, The Receptor 2(1). Reprinted in Schneider M, Cohen J, Laws S, editors: 2001, *The collected writings of Nimmo and Vannerson, pioneers of chiropractic trigger point therapy*, Pittsburgh, 1971, Self-published.

Varma D: *The human machine and its forces*, London, 1935, Health for All.

Youngs B: Physiological background of neuro-muscular technique, *British Naturopathic Journal* 5(6):176–190, 1962.

Myofascial trigger points and other reflex phenomena

3

CHAPTER CONTENTS

Pain patterns   **43**

Difference between referred phenomena and   43
radicular pain

Historical perspectives on non-radicular patterns of   44
referred pain

Other reflexogenic models   46

Central sensitization   50

Understanding facilitation   **51**

Tension headache as an example of facilitation   52

Viscerosomatic reflexes   53

Palpating facilitated spinal tissues   54

Causes of local facilitation   55

Trigger points   **56**

STAR or TART   59

Trigger points: symptoms other than pain   61

Production of trigger points   62

Identifying trigger points   62

Trigger point features   63

Trigger point deactivation   64

Other views on trigger points   67

The stress burden and trigger points   68

Hyperventilation: an example of compound   **69**
stress influences

Pathophysiology of fibromyalgia/fibrositis/   **69**
myodysneuria

Conclusion and hypothesis   **72**

Pain patterns

The radiating and/or referred symptoms deriving from myofascial trigger points are a major cause of sustained pain and dysfunction, according to Wall & Melzack (1989), the leading researchers into pain. Trigger points are indeed stated by them to be a part of all chronic pain conditions, often the major part. To be sure there are many other descriptions and classifications of reflex pain patterns – many of which are outlined in the following chapters – and these demand a brief review of the possible mechanisms involved.

A priority involves the need to differentiate between pain and referred symptoms that are of a spinal, nerve root, origin and those that have different aetiologies.

Difference between referred phenomena and radicular pain

Pain and other root syndrome effects, deriving from damaged or dysfunctional vertebral or intervertebral structures, need to be differentiated from the non-radicular pain and symptoms that derive from reflexogenic activity, such as myofascial trigger points.

The key characteristics of radicular dysfunction from, for example, a herniated disc, will include (Lavelle et al 2008, Fairbank 2008, Dvorak & Dvorak 1984):

- pain located in the regions supplied by the nerve roots from the segment(s) involved
- a loss of sensitivity in the appropriate dermatomes related to the segment(s) involved

- a loss of motor power – possibly to the point of paralysis – of the muscle innervated by the nerve roots involved, and possible atrophy
- disturbances of the deep tendon reflexes in the related areas. Diagnosis of the presence of such dysfunction requires expert neurological assessment; however, practitioners and therapists should be aware of these key signs, which alert them to the possibility that nerve root syndromes may be a feature of the patient's problem.

Historical perspectives on non-radicular patterns of referred pain

Before looking at current explanations for the evolution of chronic pain, it may be useful to look at the perspectives offered by clinicians and researchers during the middle and later 20th century. These insights are valuable in understanding where modalities such as neuromuscular technique fit into the therapetic spectrum.

Five variations

Dvorak & Dvorak (1984) have described five variations on the theme of referred symptomatology, different ways of seeing the same phenomena, aside from nerve root syndromes. These are:

1. Referred pain – which includes the findings described by researchers such as Lewis (1938), Kellgren (1938), Hockaday & Whitty (1967), who demonstrated that mechanical and chemical stimulation to various spinal structures produces referred pain. This is discussed further in this chapter.
2. Myofascial trigger points, which are discussed extensively in this chapter, and which form the major focus of neuromuscular technique application in North America.
3. Pseudoradicular syndromes, which Brugger (1962) describes as being quite distinct from root syndromes and which derive from a 'nociceptive somatomotoric blocking effect' occurring in tissues such as joint capsules, tendon origins and other local (to joint) tissues. These painful reflex effects are noted in muscles and their tendinous junctions as well as the skin – which Brugger calls 'tendomyosis' – defined as, 'the reflexogenic

functional change in the muscle in the presence of concurrent functionally dependent muscle pain'. Dvorak & Dvorak (1984) include in this category of referred pain and symptoms the phenomena of viscerosomatic and somatovisceral influences, in which, for example, organ dysfunction is said to produce tendomyotic changes (Korr 1975). Some aspects of these phenomena form part of the discussion of facilitation in this chapter.

4. Tender points, as described by Jones (1981), which Dvorak & Dvorak equate with the tender points described by Kellgren (1938) (see Ch. 4 for more on Jones' work), are seen to be spontaneously arising areas of tenderness related to acute or chronic strains, usually located in those soft tissues shortened at the time of the strain. These seem to equate with so-called 'Ah shi' points in traditional Chinese acupuncture methodology (i.e. points not necessarily present on acupuncture meridian maps, but occurring spontaneously in association with strain in the region).
5. Spondylogenic reflexes, knowledge of which Dvorak & Dvorak describe as being based on empirical clinical observation that demonstrates relationships between the axial skeleton and the peripheral soft tissues which 'are not easily explained on the basis of radicular, vascular or humoral reasoning'. The effects of these reflexes include 'demonstrable zones of irritation . . . which are painful swellings, tender upon pressure, located in the musculofascial tissue in topographically well-defined sites' (Sutter 1975).

Dvorak & Dvorak (1984) suggest that these different classifications and descriptions are focusing on the same phenomena, with terminology and interpretations being the variables, rather than there being a host of different physiological patterns of response to stress and trauma.

In this context, earlier research into referred pain is worth re-evaluating, because it highlights basic issues – of which many have lost sight.

Speransky

Speransky, in his classic book *A Basis for the Theory of Medicine* (Speransky 1943), demonstrated clearly that 'From any nerve point it is easy to bring into action nerve mechanisms, the functioning of which terminates at the periphery, in changes of a bio-physico-chemical character.' And further: 'Justification exists for the thesis that any nerve point, not excluding peripheral nerve structures, can become the originator of neurodystrophic processes, serving as the temporary nerve centre of these processes.'

Speransky continued: 'It is obvious from this [evidence] that the irritation of any point of the complex network of the nervous system, can evoke changes, not only in the adjacent parts, but also in remote regions of the organism.'

 Kellgren

Following on from the pioneering work of Sir Thomas Lewis, the researcher J. H. Kellgren performed a series of studies in the late 1930s which deserve our attention since he clearly identified the character and nature of what became known as 'myofascial trigger points' (Kellgren 1938, 1939, Lewis 1938).

Kellgren (1938) effectively showed (using himself and volunteers) that by irritating fascia and muscle he could produce referred sensations in other structures. For example, among his early findings was evidence that a saline injection into the occipital muscles would produce a headache, while similar irritation to the masseter muscle produced a toothache.

Kellgren (1939) concluded that such distribution of pain usually followed segmental pathways, although he modified this position when he applied his studies to clinical work, at which time he not only identified localized, exquisitely painful spots that referred painful symptoms to distant areas, but also noted that the distribution of pain from such spots did not in fact always follow peripheral neural pathways. He also showed that a local anaesthetic injection into such spots could obliterate the referred pain sensations.

Kellgren (1939) stated:

Superficial fascia (of the back) and supraspinous ligaments induce local pain when stimulated, while stimulation of the superficial portions of the interspinous ligaments and superficial muscles results in diffuse pain. Deep muscles,

ligaments and periostium of the apophyseal joints as well as the joints themselves can cause referred pain according to segmental innervation when stimulated [saline solution or mechanical stimulus].

Additional research at that time (1940s) indicated that there was not always a predictable pattern of pain distribution from such experiments (Feinstein et al 1954) (Fig. 3.1).

Research by many others in the 1940s, continuing up to the present, has further investigated referred patterns of pain that do not seem to follow neurological pathways, or even known patterns of viscerally caused pain – or, for that matter, the common acupuncture pathways as described in traditional Chinese medicine – myofascial trigger points.

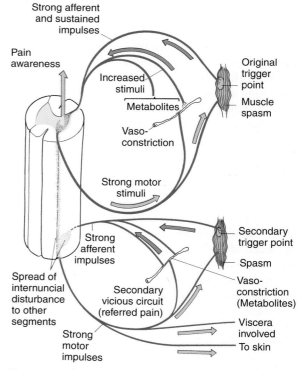

Figure 3.1 Schematic representation of the secondary spread of neurologically induced influences deriving from acute or chronic soft tissue dysfunction and involving trigger point activity and/or spasm.

Evans

Evans, in discussing reflex pain, describes the mechanism as follows:

A prolonged bombardment of pain impulses sets up a vicious circle of reflexes spreading through a pool of many neuron connections upward, downward and even across the spinal cord and perhaps reaching as high as the thalamus itself. Depending upon the extent of the pool (internuncial pool), we detect the phenomena of pain and sympathetic disturbances a long distance from the injured (trigger) area of the body and occasionally even spread to the contralateral side.

Dittrich

Dittrich (1954) has shown a constant pattern of fibrosis of subfascial tissue, with adhesions between this and the overlying muscle fascia, in a number of distinctive and common pain patterns. For example, in what he calls the 'mid-sacral syndrome' which develops from sacral lesions, referred pain is almost always present in the buttock and sometimes in the thigh, leg or foot. Referred tenderness is elicited in the lower part of the buttock. The fibrous adhesions (trigger area) are found at the level of the 3rd sacral vertebra, near the spine.

In the 'mid-lumbar syndrome', Dittrich showed that there is referred pain and tenderness in the lower lumbar, upper sacral and sacroiliac regions. The trigger point is found over the lateral third of the sacrospinalis muscle at the level of the upper margin of the iliac crest.

The 'latissimus dorsi syndrome' could result from irritation of the aponeurosis of this muscle at either of the sites of injury, sacral or lumbar, mentioned above. Referred pain would develop in the sclerotonic distributions of the 6th, 7th and 8th cervical nerves.

Dittrich pointed out that pathological changes at the two sites had been discovered by operative findings. His technique was to remove these triggers surgically or to obliterate the triggers by injection of local anaesthetic. (No concern is expressed as to the mechanical, postural or other reasons that may have produced them, nor any mention made of more conservative manipulative methods of normalization.)

The presence of 'fibrosed subfascial tissue' supports the theories of Stanley Lief and Boris Chaitow, and their use of NMT in treating such problems (see Ch. 2). The locale of these, close to bony insertions, further supports the rationale behind neuromuscular technique application.

It seems that soft tissue lesions, characterized by fibrosis of subfascial tissue (fat, etc.) with fibrous connections between the structure and the overlying fascia, can initiate sensory irritation that produces referred pain and tenderness. In addition, autonomic nervous involvement may be activated to produce vasomotor, trophic, visceral or metabolic changes. Symptoms will disappear when the offending lesion is normalized, by whatever method. However, a system that both corrects the offending trigger and attempts to prevent its recurrence would seem to offer greater clinical benefits. Before surveying some of the other reflex patterns that are pertinent to this text, a brief summary of current thinking on the aetiology of muscle pain, as described by Mense & Simons (2001) is provided in Box 3.1.

Other reflexogenic models

Gutstein

Gutstein (1956) showed that conditions such as ametropia may result from changes in the neuromuscular component of the craniocervical area, as well as from more distant conditions involving the pelvis or shoulder girdle. He states:

Myopia is the long-term effect of pressure of extraocular muscles in the convergence effort of accommodation involving spasm of the ciliary muscles, with resultant elongation of the eyeball. A sequential relationship has been shown between such a condition and muscular spasm of the neck.

Normalization of these muscles by manipulation relieves eye symptoms as well as fascial, dorsolumbar and abdominal tenderness. Gutstein terms these reflexes 'myodysneuria' and suggests that the reference phenomena of such spots or triggers would include pain, modifications of pain, itching, hypersensitivity to physiological stimuli, spasm, twitching, weakness and trembling of striated muscles; hypertonus or hypotonus of smooth muscle of blood vessels, and of internal organs; hypersecretion or hyposecretion of visceral,

Box 3.1   Mense & Simons perspective on muscle pain

In Chapter 1 a brief overview (see 'Modern pain concepts') was provided of how muscle pain evolves, as described by Mense & Simons (2001). In this section some of the major causes of muscle pain are outlined, based on the same researchers' descriptions and discussions.

Local muscular pain

Local muscular pain is defined as deriving from local pain receptors, in the muscle, rather than via neural or central neurons. These free nerve endings (nociceptors) may be sensitized by mechanical (blows, repetitive or single strain injuries, rupture of fibres, etc.) and chemical (e.g. bradykinin) influences that either irritate or increase nociceptor sensitivity, leading to tenderness and soreness (such as occurs following unaccustomed exercise). Non-steroidal anti-inflammatory drugs decrease the degree of such sensitization. The types of situation that bring about such sensitization include trauma, inflammation and ischaemic circulatory deficit (such as that resulting from intermittent claudication or prolonged voluntary contraction, especially if this involves an already ischaemic muscle).

Local muscle pain involving inflammation may additionally lead to feelings of weakness and dysaesthesia. Local muscle pain may also be caused by the influence of a trigger point within the painful muscle, or referring to it from a distant muscle.

Metabolic causes of local muscle pain include enzyme deficiencies and hypothyroid status that 'compromise oxidative metabolism in the muscle mitochondria' (Mense & Simons 2001). Inflammatory process may result from injury or infection (e.g. *Staphylococcus aureus*) or infestation (e.g. trichinosis caused by *Trichinella spiralis* deriving from undercooked meat such as pork).

Local muscle pain resulting from compartment syndrome may result from development of a haematoma, oedema or infection in a muscle surrounded by a fascial envelope (such as flexor digitorum longus muscle in the deep posterior compartment). Surgical intervention may be called for to relieve the pressure before irreparable tissue damage occurs. A similar scenario may result from a plaster cast applied too tightly. Rarely toxicity-induced myalgic pain may derive from contaminated tryptophan, a sleep-inducing and pain-relieving amino acid, useful in the treatment of fibromyalgia. As pure tryptophan is no longer available because of contamination in the manufacturing process following a Japanese attempt to modify genetically the bacteria used in its production, tryptophan is now available in a plant-derived form, free of contaminants, as 5-hydroxytryptophan (Chaitow 2000).

Nerve lesion or dysfunction

Neuropathic muscle pain derived from a nerve lesion or dysfunction in the cranial (spinal) or dorsal root nerves. Causes may be mechanical (trauma) or entrapment (see notes on Maitland, Butler and Gifford in Ch. 1), or as a result of the development of a neuroma, which can lead to phantom pain. Pain from a herniated disc is an example of radicular pain. Peripheral neuropathies may occur in conditions such as diabetes. The causes of widespread pain conditions, which also involve autonomic symptoms, such as complex regional pain syndrome (previously called reflex sympathetic dystrophy), are thought to involve the sympathetic nervous system in an as-yet unknown way.

Referred pain

Pain that is referred to and from muscles can be confusing. Mense & Simons (2001) use the term 'mislocalization of pain', in which 'the muscle in which the pain is felt serves only as a starting point for finding the source of pain, which is really what requires treatment'. The mechanisms are not clear, although the phenomenon is at the very heart of the pain often found to derive from distant trigger point activity. Mense & Simons indicate that there are confusing influences from trigger points when they reflexly influence other structures: 'Why trigger points cause reflex spasm in one situation and reflex inhibition in another is not at all clear. One possibility is that the distinction between muscles prone to tightness (postural – see Ch. 1) and muscles prone to weakness (phasic – see Ch. 1) may be of fundamental physiologic significance.' What is known is that specific dermatome and myotome distribution of sensations is not constant in relation to the symptoms produced by an active trigger point. Discussion in this chapter on the phenomena of local and segmental facilitation, and also of viscerosomatic reflex activity, covers aspects of this form of reflexogenic and referred pain.

Continued

Box 3.1   Mense & Simons perspective on muscle pain—cont'd

Muscular tension
Pain deriving from muscular tension may involve biomechanical rather than neural influences. Factors such as the viscoelastic tone and the colloidal nature of soft tissues involving thixotropic qualities, as well as non-neurologically mediated contractures, may be present (see notes on fascia in Ch. 1).

This topic is complex and the reader is referred to Mense & Simons (2001, Ch. 5) for greater detail.

Aspects of the influence on muscular pain deriving from organ dysfunction, postural imbalances, the presence of active trigger points, and conditions such as fibromyalgia are all discussed in this and later chapters.

---

sebaceous and sudatory glands. Somatic manifestations may also occur in response to visceral stimuli of corresponding spinal levels (Gutstein 1944).

Many such trigger areas are dormant and asymptomatic. Gutstein's method of treatment was the injection of an anaesthetic solution into the trigger area. He indicated, however, that, where accessible (e.g. muscular insertions in the cervical area), the chilling of these areas combined with pressure yielded good results. This is in line with Mennell's work (1975), and fits into the field of NMT.

Amongst the patterns of vasomotor sebaceous, sudatory and gastrointestinal dysfunction mentioned by Gutstein (1944a) are the following, all of which relate to reflex trigger points or 'myo-dysneuria' (fibrositis/fibromyalgia):

1. Various patterns of vasomotor abnormality such as coldness, pallor, redness, cyanosis, etc. These variations in response to stimulation relate to the fact that most organs respond to weak stimuli by an increase in activity and to very strong stimuli by inhibiting activity. Menopausal hot flushes are one example, and these seem often to be linked to musculoskeletal pain. Gutstein found that obliteration of overt and silent triggers in the occipital, cervical, interscapular, sternal and epigastric regions was accompanied by years of alleviation of premenopausal, menopausal and late menopausal symptoms. Proponents of NMT have long emphasized the importance of normalizing these very structures.
2. Gutstein maintains that normalization of skin secretion, and therefore of hair and skin

texture and appearance, may be altered for the better by the removal of active trigger areas in the cervical and interscapular areas.
3. The conditions of hyperhidrosis, hypohidrosis and anhidrosis may accompany vasomotor and sebaceous dysfunction. Gutstein noted that abolition of excessive perspiration as well as anhidrosis followed adequate treatment.
4. Gutstein quoted a number of practitioners who have achieved success in treating gastrointestinal dysfunctions by treating trigger areas. Some of these were treated by procaine injection, others by pressure techniques and massage. The abdominal wall lends itself to the latter procedure, as evidenced by the work of Cornelius (1909), whose treatment was not dissimilar to Lief's NMT.

Among the conditions that have responded to such treatment are pylorospasm, bad breath, heartburn, regurgitation, nausea, abdominal distension, constipation and nervous diarrhoea. Gutstein (1944b) called localized functional sensory and/or motor abnormalities of musculoskeletal tissue (comprising muscle, fascia, tendon, bone and joint) *myodysneuria* (now known as fibromyalgia; formerly known as 'fibrositis' and 'muscular rheumatism').

He viewed the causes of such changes as multiple; among them are:

1. Acute and chronic infections which, it is postulated, stimulate sympathetic nerve activity via their toxins.
2. Excessive heat or cold, changes in atmospheric pressure, and draughts.

3. Mechanical injuries, both major and repeated minor microtraumas. Postural strain, unaccustomed exercises, etc., which may predispose towards future changes by lowering the threshold for future stimuli (facilitation).
4. Allergic and endocrine factors, which can cause imbalance in the autonomic nervous system.
5. Inherited factors that make adjustment to environmental factors difficult.
6. Arthritic changes – because muscles are the active components of the musculoskeletal system it is logical to assume that their circulatory state has influence over bones and joints. Spasm in muscle may contribute towards osteoarthritic changes, and such changes may produce further neuromuscular changes, which themselves produce new symptoms.
7. Visceral diseases may intensify and precipitate somatic symptoms in the distribution of their spinal and adjacent segments.

In these examples of Gutstein's concept, we can see strong echoes of the facilitation hypothesis in osteopathic medicine, and it seems likely that they are describing the same set of circumstances leading to hyperreactive responses – and all that this leads to in terms of pain and dysfunction.

Diagnosis of myodysneuria was made according to some of the following criteria:

• A varying degree of muscular tension and contraction is usually present, although sometimes adjacent, apparently unaffected, tissue is more painful.
• Sensitivity to pressure or palpation of affected muscles and their adjuncts.
• Marked hypertonicity may require the application of deep pressure to demonstrate tenderness.

Travell and Bigelow

Travell & Bigelow (1947) produced evidence to support much of what Gutstein had reported. They indicated that high-intensity stimuli from active trigger areas produced, by reflex, prolonged vasoconstriction with partial ischaemia in localized areas of the brain, spinal cord or peripheral nerve structures (Fig. 3.2). A wide pattern of dysfunction might result, affecting almost any organ of the body. The phenomenon of hysteria, with symptoms as varied as disordered vision, respiration, motor power and cutaneous sensation,

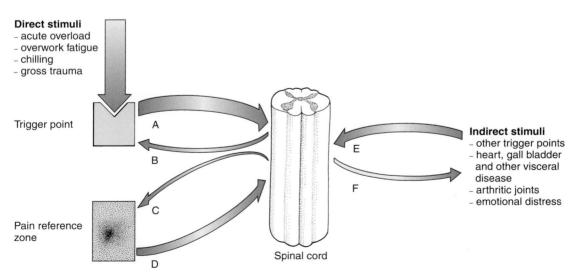

Figure 3.2 Direct stress influence can affect the hyperreactive neural structure of a myofascial trigger point, leading to increased activity (A–B) as well as referring sensations (pain, paraesthesia, increased sympathetic activity) to a target area (C–D) that feed back into the cord to increase the background stress load. Other stimuli reach the cord from distant trigger points and additional dysfunctional areas (E–F).

was often mediated by afferent neural impulses from trigger areas in skeletal muscle. These triggers, when similarly located, produced the same pattern of clinical effects, whether activated in one patient by psychogenic factors or in another by different factors (e.g. mechanical or traumatic).

It is worth noting that Travell (1981) has shown that the effect of a trigger point on the muscle housing it is to produce weakness of contraction without atrophy, and that this is often accompanied by a decreased range of movement in associated joints.

Dowling

Dowling (2000) has described a variation on the use of inhibitory pressure (see Box 3.5), which allies itself closely with the methods of NMT and other soft tissue approaches utilizing the effects of compression in a physiologically useful manner. Using two points of contact, progressive, sequential pressure applications are used to

inhibit pain and modify function. Dowling's work fits well with other approaches (acupressure, strain/counterstrain, use of neurolymphatic reflexes, etc.) that depend on the underlying mechanisms that allow manual input to modify neuromuscular function and pain. See Chapter 11 for a full explanation of progressive neuromuscular inhibition technique (PINS).

Central sensitization (see Fig. 3.3)

All these historical perspectives are describing, in one way or another, what is now known as peripheral and central sensitization. In osteopathic medicine the evolution over time of hypersensitivity and reactivity in neural structures, is known as facilitation, and this is described later in this chapter (Korr 1970).

In brief, sensitization involves what happens when a simple stimulus, that is repeated, becomes irritable, and eventually painful.

Figure 3.3   Diagram showing possible aetiological pathways to somatic dysfunction and sensitization. Modified from Fryer G, Fossum C. Possible etiology of somatic dysfunction. In: Physical Therapy for tension type and cerviocogenic headache. Fernández de las Peñas C., Arendt-Nielsen L., Gerwin R. (Eds): Jones & Bartlett, Boston, 2009.

A demonstration of this process can be seen in the example of a repetitively pressed, or rubbed, or knocked area of the body. This stimulation might initially feel warm, uncomfortable and eventually painful. The pain would be the result of the progressively amplified synaptic response of the peripheral nerves producing an alarm message that the repetitive stimulation is potentially harmful. Neural structures peripherally, or in the cord, or the brain may be involved in different variations of this process.

Sensitization may underlie both adaptive as well as maladaptive learning processes for the organism. This process is also known as long-term potentiation, and involves complex biochemical changes in the tissues involved (Ji et al 2003, McEachern et al 1999).

Just how manual therapy can modify this process is another matter, and this will be explored in other chapters.

Understanding facilitation

If we are to make sense of the phenomenon of myofascial trigger points there is a need to grasp the processes that lead to hyperirritability and hyperreactivity of specific neural structures – facilitation (aka sensitization). Trigger points are localized areas of soft tissue dysfunction that negatively influence distant target areas, and that evolve in a manner similar to that observed when spinal segments become facilitated as a result of stress of one sort or another.

To understand trigger points, we need to understand spinal facilitation first. Facilitation occurs in both spinal and paraspinal tissues (segmental facilitation) as well as in discrete local areas of muscles, mainly near their origins and insertions but also close to their bellies and in areas where fascial stress occurs due to external influences and forces (myofascial trigger points). Understanding facilitation helps us to see how the different classification systems, all describing variations on the same phenomenon of referred pain – listed by Dvorak & Dvorak (1984) and described earlier in this chapter – are held together aetiologically.

Patterson (1976) explains segmental (spinal) facilitation as follows:

The concept of the facilitated segment states that because of abnormal afferent or sensory inputs to a particular area of the spinal cord, that area is kept in a state of constant increased excitation. This facilitation allows normally ineffectual or subliminal stimuli to become effective in producing efferent output from the facilitated segment, causing both skeletal and visceral organs innervated by the affected segment to be maintained in a state of overactivity. It is probable that the 'osteopathic lesion', or somatic dysfunction with which a facilitated segment is associated, is the direct result of the abnormal segmental activity as well as being partially responsible for the facilitation.

A facilitated segment therefore emerges from a prolonged period during which abnormal or altered inputs from a single source (or more than one source) of irritation, impinging on the spinal cord, keep the interneurons or motor neurons of that spinal segment in a constant state of excitement, thus allowing normally ineffectual inputs to produce outputs to all organs receiving innervation from the excited area. This concept implies that the spinal cord is a relatively passive mediator of the influences imposed on it and that the neural paths act as communicators of that activity (Denslow et al 1949).

Research on spinal functions seems to indicate, however, that the spinal cord, besides being the determiner of where abnormal activity is sent, by virtue of predetermined pathways, may participate actively in either controlling abnormal or unusually intense inputs, or amplifying and retaining such inputs in certain circumstances (Korr 1986).

Initially, only intensities of afferent input above a certain level would result in increased sensitivity of the spinal pathway. Inputs of lower intensity would either produce no alterations, or would cause an actual decrease in sensitivity as a protective mechanism against undue changes in homeostatic processes. It is apparent that the potential for sensitization by different types of afferent inputs may differ widely. Thus, inputs from pain receptors may sensitize the pathway at low levels because of the properties of the initial synapses between pain afferent fibres and interneurons. In this event an initially protective increase in response might occur, followed eventually by detrimental facilitation of a segment. On the other hand, inputs from joint receptors seem to have a less dramatic effect at similar input levels (Dowling 1991).

It is now known that emotional arousal would also affect the susceptibility of the pathways to sensitization (Baldry 1993). The increase in descending influences from the emotionally aroused subject would result in an increase in toxic excitement in the pathways and allow all additional inputs to produce sensitization at low intensities. Thus, highly emotional people, or those in a highly emotional situation, would be expected to show a higher incidence of facilitation of spinal pathways.

As the higher brain centres influence the tonic levels of the spinal paths, it might also be expected that physical training and mental attitudes would tend to alter the tonic excitability, reducing the person's susceptibility to sensitization from everyday stress. Thus the athlete would be expected to withstand a comparatively high level of afferent input before experiencing the self-perpetuating results of sensitization.

A further corollary of the hypothesis is that slowly developing conditions, or slowly increasing inputs, would result in less sensitization at high levels than sudden inputs. A process known as 'wind-up' can be part of sensitization, with the rate of stimulus, as well as the size of stimuli, determining how rapidly the process evolves. If noxious stimuli occur rapidly, the degree of stimulus required to produce symptoms (pain mainly) decreases (Codere et al 1993, Li 1999).

Windup is just such a mechanism that is thought to operate in fibromyalgia where relatively minor stimuli can produce symptoms that appear to be proportionately excessive (Staud 2006).

The slow development of a chronic source of increased sensory input initially causes habituation, resulting in resistance to sensitization until the input level is abnormally high. On the other hand, sudden increases in input, such as a sudden mechanical stress, would be expected to rapidly produce sensitization of the neural pathways.

Korr

The premier researcher into facilitation over the past half-century has been Irwin Korr (Korr 1970, 1976). In early studies he demonstrated, for example, that if readings were taken of resistance to electricity in the paraspinal skin of an individual there were often marked differences, with one side showing normal resistance and the other showing reduced resistance (facilitated area).

When 'stress' was applied elsewhere in the body and the two areas of the spine were monitored, it was the area of facilitation, where electrical resistance was reduced, that showed a dramatic rise in electrical (i.e. neurological) activity. In one experiment, volunteers had pins inserted into one calf muscle in order to gauge the effect in the paraspinal areas under investigation – with the spinal areas being monitored for electrical activity. Almost no increase occurred in the normal region, but the facilitated area showed enormously enhanced neurological activity after 60 seconds (Korr 1977) (Fig. 3.4).

The implications of this and hundreds of similar studies are that any form of stress impacting the individual, be it climatic, chemical, emotional, physical or anything else, would produce just such a rise in neurological output from facilitated areas.

In many instances involving spinal segmental facilitation there is a chronic degree of neurological bombardment resulting from internal organ dysfunction. For example, it is almost always possible to predict that cardiovascular disease is present (or will soon be present) when two or more segments of the spine in the region of T2, T3 and T4 display tense, rigid, 'board-like' characteristics on palpation, especially if these tissues do not respond to normal efforts to reduce their hypertonicity (Beal 1983).

Tension headache as an example of facilitation

Danish research (Bendtsen 2000) suggests that there exists:

> ... a pathophysiological model for tension-type headache [resulting from] central sensitization

Figure 3.4   Pain stimuli produce a marked reaction in the facilitated area (red line) and little reaction in the normal area (black line).

[facilitation] at the level of the spinal dorsal horn/trigeminal nucleus due to prolonged nociceptive inputs from pericranial myofascial tissues. The increased nociceptive input to supraspinal structures may in turn result in supraspinal sensitization. The central neuroplastic changes may affect the regulation of peripheral mechanisms and thereby lead to, for example, increased pericranial muscle activity, or sensitization may be maintained even after the initial eliciting factors have been normalized, resulting in conversion of episodic into chronic tension-type headache.

This research demonstrates the need to understand how, over time, a reversible problem may become entrenched and chronic. It is knowledge of facilitation and sensitization that also explains how multiple stress elements affecting the person as a whole (climatic, emotional, postural, nutritional, etc.) might feed into the sensitized structures, exacerbating symptoms, despite apparently not directly impacting the involved structures.

Viscerosomatic reflexes

Many of the various systems involving reflexively active points described in this and the next chapter, such as connective tissue zones, Chapman's reflexes and Bennett's reflexes, as well as trigger points, may involve viscerosomatic reflex activity.

Beal

Myron Beal (1985) has described this phenomenon as resulting from afferent stimuli, arising from dysfunction of a visceral nature. The reflex is initiated by afferent impulses arising from visceral receptors, which are transmitted to the dorsal horn of the spinal cord, where they synapse with interconnecting neurons. The stimuli are then conveyed to sympathetic and motor efferents, resulting in changes in the somatic tissues, such as skeletal muscle, skin and blood vessels.

Abnormal stimulation of the visceral efferent neurons may result in hyperaesthesia of the skin, and associated vasomotor, pilomotor and sudomotor changes. Similar stimuli of the ventral horn cells may result in reflex rigidity of the somatic musculature. Pain may result from such changes.

The degree of stimulus required, in any given case, to produce such changes will differ, because factors such as prior facilitation of the particular segment, as well as the response of higher centres, will differ from person to person.

In many cases it is suggested, by Korr and others, that viscerosomatic reflex activity may be noted before any symptoms of visceral change are evident, and that this phenomenon is therefore of potential diagnostic and prognostic value.

The first signs of viscerosomatic reflexive influences are vasomotor reactions (increased skin temperature), sudomotor (increased moisture of the skin), skin textural changes (e.g. thickening), increased subcutaneous fluid and increased contraction of muscle. The value of light skin palpation in identifying areas of facilitation cannot be too strongly emphasized (Lewit 1992).

These signs disappear if the visceral cause improves. When such changes become chronic, however, trophic alterations are noted, with increased thickening of the skin and subcutaneous tissue, and localized muscular contraction. Deep musculature may become hard, tense and hypersensitive. This may result in deep splinting contractions, involving two or more segments of the spine, with associated restriction of spinal motion. The costotransverse articulations may be significantly involved in such changes.

Patterns of somatic response will be found to differ from person to person, and to be unique, in terms of location, the number of segments involved, and whether or not the pattern is unilateral or bilateral. The degree of intensity will also differ, and is related to the degree of acuteness of the visceral condition (Hix 1976). Research involving animals, as well as observations in humans, using regional nerve blocks, has helped to define site locations of response, in various forms of visceral dysfunction. Beal (1985) notes that, when the voluminous research into segmental associations with organ dysfunction is compounded, three distinct groups of visceral involvement are found in respect of particular sites:

1. T1–T5: heart and lungs
2. T5–T10: oesophagus, stomach, small intestine, liver, gall bladder, spleen, pancreas and adrenal cortex

3. T10–L2: large bowel, appendix, kidney, ureter, adrenal medulla, testes, ovaries, urinary bladder, prostate gland, uterus.

There appears to be a consensus as to sidedness being apparent, in reflexes of unpaired organs. Thus, left-sidedness is noted in conditions involving the small intestine and heart, and right-sidedness for gall bladder disease and appendix. The stomach may produce reflex activity on either, or both, sides. Many studies have been concerned with the identification of viscerosomatic reflexes. One 5-year study involved more than 5000 hospitalized patients (Beal 1985), and concluded that most visceral disease appeared to influence more than one spinal region, and that the number of spinal segments involved seemed to be related to the duration of the disease. Kelso noted in this study that there was an increase in the number of palpatory findings in the cervical region, related to patients with sinusitis, tonsillitis, diseases of the oesophagus and liver complaints. Soft tissue changes were noted in patients with gastritis, duodenal ulceration, pyelonephritis, chronic appendicitis and cholecystitis, in the region of T5–T12.

Palpating facilitated spinal tissues

Somatic dysfunction is usually assessed by means of palpatory investigation, and Beal (1983) insists that investigation should pay attention to the various soft tissue layers:

The skin for changes in texture, temperature and moisture; the subcutaneous tissue for changes in consistency and fluid; the superficial and deep musculature for tone, irritability, consistency, viscoelastic properties, and fluid content; and the deep fascial layers for textural changes.

He advises that 'Special attention [should] be given to the examination of the costotransverse area, where it is felt that autonomic nerve effects are predominant', and notes that tests for the quality and range of joints have not been found to differentiate between visceral reflexes and somatic changes, which confirms the importance of the soft tissue assessment in order to elicit such information.

Beal (1983) notes that the supine position is ideal for assessment of paraspinal tissues – the

Figure 3.5 Beal's 'springing' assessment for paraspinal facilitation rigidity associated with segmental facilitation.

hand being gently inserted under the region, and pressure, or springing techniques applied (Fig. 3.5). He has not investigated the use of patient examination in the prone position, as he suggests that this position is precluded in acutely ill patients.

Nevertheless, since Beal notes the difficulty of applying diagnostic measures with the patient supine when the mid to lower thoracic area is under review, a prone position is suggested, unless the patient cannot manage this. The availability of a couch with a split head-piece would make this more comfortable. As we will see, the methods employed by those using connective tissue massage involve the patient being seated. This helps in assessing skin and superficial tissue status, but is not really suitable for deeper penetration.

Beal suggests that the diagnosis of a paraspinal viscerosomatic reflex be based on two or more adjacent spinal segments showing evidence of somatic dysfunction, and being located within the specific autonomic reflex area. There should be deep confluent spinal muscle splinting, and resistance to segmental joint motion. Skin and subcutaneous tissue changes that are consistent with the acuteness or chronicity of the reflex should be noted.

Specific identification of the origin of the reflex is, he suggests, difficult.

The usefulness of understanding the nature of such reflexes often involves clinical frustration when, for instance, localized soft tissue dysfunction fails to respond to treatment. Suspicion may then be alerted to possible visceral activity maintaining the muscular or joint dysfunction.

According to Beal, treatment of the acute stage should be aimed primarily at breaking into the reflex arc. In cases of serious illness the treatment may consist of gentle digital pressure, of short duration, to effect a local change in superficial tissues. When relaxation has been accomplished in the subcutaneous and superficial paraspinal musculature, the deep muscle contraction can be addressed. The duration of treatment is dependent upon the patient's condition and perceived energy level. Beal suggests that acute conditions that are not life threatening may be addressed in a more aggressive manner (asthma is given as an example).

It is suggested that NMT is also an ideal method of addressing soft tissue manifestations of such reflex activity, because it offers a diagnostic as well as a therapeutic opportunity to address both superficial and deep tissues. Viscerosomatic reflex changes are just one of the many reasons for altered tissue findings, which may be noted in the general NMT assessment. Awareness of the possibility that what is being noted is of reflex origin adds to the potential for accurate diagnosis. In Chapter 4 a variety of other reflex systems are evaluated.

Causes of local facilitation

Melzack & Wall (1989), in their exhaustive investigation of pain, are clear in their statement that all chronic pain has myofascial trigger point activity as at least a part of its aetiology, and that in many instances trigger points are the major contributors to the pain.

A trigger point is a localized, palpable area of soft tissue that is painful on pressure and that refers symptoms, usually including pain, to a predictable target area some distance from itself. It is an area of local facilitation that has developed following a very similar aetiological pathway to that occurring in segmental (spinal) facilitated areas.

Facilitation paraspinally and in general muscle tissue can be the result of repetitive minor or single major traumatic influences or stress factors (as described in Ch. 1). The form of facilitation that is our main focus in this chapter is a localized area of hyperirritability – the trigger point.

Travell and Simons

Much research and clinical work has been done in recent years in this field by Janet Travell (Travell 1957, Travell & Simons 1983, 1992, Travell, Simons & Travell 1999), who is on record as stating that if a pain is severe enough to cause a patient to seek professional advice (in the absence of organic disease) referred pain is likely to be a factor, and therefore a trigger area is probably involved. She maintains that patterns of referred pain are constant in distribution in all people; only the intensity of referred symptoms or referred pain will vary.

Among the effects of an active trigger point, apart from pain, there may be numbness, tingling, weakness, lack of normal range of movement. The aetiological myofascial trigger point for a particular pain pattern is always located in a particular part of a particular muscle (Webber 1973). While eradication of the trigger, by whatever appropriate means, can remove all symptoms, treatment of the target or reference area is useless.

 Trigger points (Fig. 3.6)

Trigger points are localized areas of deep tenderness and increased resistance, and digital pressure on such a trigger will often produce twitching and fasciculation (see Fig. 3.6). Pressure maintained on such a point will produce referred pain in a predictable area. If there are a number of active trigger points, the reference areas may overlap.

What is distinctive about active trigger points (myofascial trigger points) is that, when active, they also refer sensations or symptoms to a distinct target area, and this target area is more or less reproducible in other individuals, when trigger points are located in similar positions. No other soft tissue dysfunction has this particular attribute.

Before an active trigger point exists there needs to be a period of evolution towards that unhappy state. This involves the development of soft tissue changes that are palpable and probably sensitive, or painful, but that, until sufficient localized stress has been involved, will not refer symptoms onwards. In other words, many localized muscular areas of sensitivity or pain, which do not refer pain or other symptoms, may be considered to be embryonic or evolutionary trigger points. A single trigger may refer pain to several reference sites and can give rise to embryonic, or satellite, triggers in those target areas. Travell (1981) describes, for example, how a trigger in the distal areas of the sternomastoid muscle can give rise to new triggers in the sternalis muscle, the pectoral muscle and/or serratus anterior.

Travell's description of a trigger point is:

> It lies in skeletal muscle, and is identified by localised deep tenderness, in a palpable firm band of muscle (muscle hardening); and at the point of maximum deep hyperalgesia, by a positive 'jump sign', a visible shortening of the part of the muscle which contains the band. To elicit the jump sign most effectively, one must place the relaxed muscle under moderate passive tension, and snap the band briskly with the palpating finger.

The trigger point must also refer symptoms or sensations, which are familiar to the patient, to a target area. Otherwise, rather than being active, it may be a latent trigger point, which could be activated by stress or strain on the tissues in which it lies (Box 3.2). The difference between most other areas of discrete palpable soft tissue dysfunction and an active trigger is this quality of referring symptoms. All other points may be prospective triggers, but are not active (Fig. 3.7).

Figure 3.6 Some common trigger points and their target areas.

Continued

Tibialis anticus

Long extensors

Gastrocnemius

Soleus

Peroneus longus

Abductor hallucis

Short extensors

Subscapularis

Deltoid

Middle finger extensor

Extensor carpi radialis

Supinators

Pectorals

Pectoralis major

Sternalis

Serratus anterior

Longissimus

Vastus medialus

Biceps femoris

Gluteus minimus

Vastus medialis

Figure 3.6—cont'd

Box 3.2 Active and latent trigger points defined (see Fig. 3.6)

- An active trigger point, when mechanically stimulated by compression, needling, stretch or other means, will refer to, or intensify, a target zone (referral pattern, usually of pain) which the person recognizes as being part of their current symptom picture.
- When a latent trigger point is stimulated, it refers a pattern that may be unfamiliar to the person, or that is an old pattern which they used to have but have not had for a while (previously active, reverted to latent).

All the same characteristics that denote an active trigger point may be present in the latent trigger point, with the exception of the person's recognition of their active pain pattern. The same signs as described for segmental facilitation, such as increased hydrosis, a sense of 'drag' on the skin,

loss of elasticity, etc., can be observed and palpated in these localized areas as well.

Travell & Simons (1983, 1992) use the term 'essential pain zone' to describe a referral pattern that is present in almost every person when a particular trigger point is active. Some trigger points may also produce a 'spill-over pain zone', beyond the essential zone or in place of it, where the referral pattern is usually less intense. These target zones should be examined, and ideally palpated, for changes in tissue 'density', temperature, hydrosis and other characteristics associated with satellite trigger point formation. Any appropriate manual treatment, movement or exercise programme that encourages normal circulatory function is likely to modulate these negative effects and reduce trigger point activity.

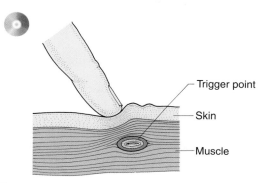

Figure 3.7 Trigger points are areas of local facilitation that can be housed in any soft tissue structure, most usually muscle and/or fascia. Palpation from the skin or at depth may be required to localize them.

 STAR or TART

In osteopathic medicine an acronym 'STAR' is used as a reminder of the characteristics of somatic dysfunction, which would include those relating to myofascial trigger points:

- Sensitivity (or 'Tenderness')
- Tissue texture change
- Asymmetry
- Range of motion reduced.

The acronym is modified in some texts to 'TART' (Tenderness – Asymmetry – Range of movement modified – Tissue texture change).

While the 'tenderness' and range of motion characteristics, as listed in the STAR acronym, hold true for trigger points, the following refinements have been detailed by Simons et al (1999):

- The soft tissues housing the trigger point will demonstrate a painful limit to stretch range of motion.
- A palpable taut band with exquisitely tender nodule should be located.
- Pressure on the tender spot elicits pain familiar to the patient and often a pain response ('jump sign').

Baldry (1993) noted that the commonest sites for trigger points are close to:

- muscular origins and insertions
- free borders of muscle
- muscle belly
- motor end-point
- body tissues other than muscle, including skin, fascia, ligament, joint capsule and periosteum, and also in scar tissue.

Simons et al (1999), in their latest research, place great emphasis on the distinct differences in treatment protocols for so-called 'attachment' and 'central' trigger points (see Box 3.3).

Box 3.3 Understanding and treating central and attachment trigger points (Chaitow & DeLany 2000, Simons et al 1999)

Simons, Travell and Simons' (1999) model of central trigger points

- Central trigger points form almost directly in the centre of the muscle's fibres, close to the motor endplate (neuromuscular junction).
- This formation is probably due to dysfunctional endplate activity.
- A metabolic crisis occurs and acetylcholine (ACh) is excessively released at the synapse, usually associated with overuse or strain, leading to release of calcium.
- The resulting ischaemia in the area creates an oxygen/nutrient deficit and a local energy crisis.
- Without available adenosine triphosphate (ATP), the calcium ions, which are keeping the gates open for ACh to keep flowing, cannot be removed.
- A chemically sustained contracture occurs. This is involuntary without motor potentials, and should be distinguished from a contraction, which is voluntary and involves motor potentials, and spasm, which is involuntary with motor potentials.
- As the endplate keeps producing this ACh flow, the actin/myosin filaments shorten and bunch in the immediate area of the motor endplate (centre of fibre).
- A contracture 'knot' forms the characteristic trigger point nodule.
- The remainder of the sarcomeres of that fibre are stretched, creating the equally characteristic taut band, which is usually palpable.
- When massage, stretch applications, injection or other modalities are applied, which disturbs the sarcomeres, alters the chemistry or possibly damages the endplate, the cycle is disrupted and the tissue relaxes, often in seconds – often permanently.

Simons, Travell and Simons' model of attachment trigger points

- Attachment trigger points form at junctures of myofascial and tendinous or periosteal tissues.
- Tension from taut bands on periosteal or connective tissues can lead to enthesopathy or enthesitis, as recurring concentrations of muscular stress may provoke inflammation, with a strong tendency towards subsequent fibrosis and calcific deposition.

Processes

- Central and attachment trigger points can both lead to referred and/or radiating pain; however, the local processes seem to be different and the two types of trigger point seem to respond to different therapeutic approaches.
- Until they have been examined thoroughly and tissue reactions noted, attachment trigger points should be addressed, with their tendency towards inflammation in mind.
- Central trigger points should be addressed with their contracted central sarcomeres and local ischaemia in mind.
- As the end of that taut band is likely to create enthesopathy, stretching the muscle before releasing its central trigger point might further inflame the attachments.
- Techniques should first be applied to relax the taut fibres before manual stretching (such as gliding strokes or myofascial release) is attempted.
- Stretches, particularly those involving active range of motion, should be applied gently until reaction is noted, to avoid further tissue insult.
- When passive stretching is applied, care should be taken to assess for tendinous or periosteal inflammation, in order to avoid placing more tension on already distressed connective tissue attachments.

Treatment choices for central trigger points

- Elongation of the tissue to its full length is, according to Simons et al (1999), critical to abolish the mechanism sustaining a trigger point.
- This may be achieved manually by application of gliding strokes from the centre of the fibres out to the attachment sites, stretching the tissue passively through its range of motion, or by having the person perform active range of motion, both during the treatment session and at home.
- Proprioceptive neuromuscular facilitation (PNF) techniques can be used to override the mechanisms causing the condition.
- Reciprocal inhibition (RI) and post-isometric relaxation (PIR) can accompany or precede range of motion movements and stretches to augment the benefits (see MET notes in Ch. 8).

Continued

> **Box 3.3   Understanding and treating central and attachment trigger points (Chaitow & DeLany 2000, Simons et al 1999)—cont'd**
>
> - Central trigger points seem to respond well to heat.
> - When compression techniques are used, local chemistry can change as a result of induced ischaemia, followed by flushing of the tissues when the compression is released (see Box 3.5).
> - The effects of thermal or other applications (skin irritants such as capsaicin, moxibustion, dry or wet needling, etc.) may induce the contracture to release.
> - Contrast hydrotherapy, employing alternating ice and heat, can be effective via its circulatory and/or neurological (reflex) influences.
>
> **Treatment choices for attachment trigger points**
> - Attachment trigger points seem to respond to ice applications rather than heat.
> - Gliding techniques should be applied from the centre of the fibres out towards the attachments, unless contraindicated (as in some extremity tissues).
> - By elongating the tissue toward the attachments, sarcomeres that are shortened at the centre of the fibre will be lengthened, and those that are overstretched near the attachment sites will have their tension released.

Trigger points: symptoms other than pain

While pain is the commonest symptom arising from the activity of trigger points, other symptoms may be noted, including lymphatic stasis and reduced mobility of joints.

Lymphatic stasis

Travell & Simons (1983, 1992) have identified triggers that impede lymphatic function.

The scalenes (in particular anticus) can entrap structures passing through the thoracic inlet. This is aggravated by the 1st rib (and clavicular) restriction, which can be caused by triggers in anterior and middle scalenes. Scalene trigger points have been shown reflexly to suppress lymphatic duct peristaltic contractions in the affected extremity, whereas triggers in the posterior axillary folds (subscapularis, teres major, latissimus dorsi) influence lymphatic drainage affecting the upper extremities and breasts. Similarly, triggers in the anterior axillary fold (pectoralis minor) can be implicated in lymphatic dysfunction affecting the breasts (Kuchera 1997).

Autonomic effects

(Travell & Simons 1983, 1992)

- Vasoconstriction (blanching)
- Coldness
- Sweating
- Pilomotor response
- Ptosis
- Hypersecretion.

Clinical symptoms other than pain

(Kuchera & McPartland 1997)

- Diarrhoea, dysmenorrhoea
- Diminished gastric motility
- Vasoconstriction and headache
- Dermatographia
- Proprioceptive disturbance, dizziness
- Excessive maxillary sinus secretion
- Localized sweating
- Cardiac arrhythmias (especially pectoralis major triggers)
- Goose flesh
- Ptosis, excessive lacrimation
- Conjunctival reddening
- Interstitial cystitis (Weiss 2001).

Linking symptoms to specific trigger points

(Simons 2002)

- Tension-type headache may derive from active triggers located in sternocleidomastoid, upper trapezius, posterior cervical musculature or temporalis.

- Frozen shoulder symptoms may be associated with trigger points in subscapularis, supraspinatus, pectoralis major and minor, and in the deltoid muscles.
- Epicondylitis may derive from trigger points present in the extensors of the fingers and hand, supinator and triceps brachii.
- Carpal tunnel syndrome may be associated with triggers in the scaleni and finger extensors.
- Atypical angina pectoris pain may be associated with active trigger points in left side pectoralis major or in the intercostals.
- Low back pain may involve trigger points in quadratus lumborum, iliopsoas, thoracolumbar paraspinals, rectus abdominis, piriformis, gluteus maximus and/or medius.

Reduced mobility

Joint restrictions have been noted as deriving from trigger point activity; for example, Kuchera (1997) has listed trigger points associated with shoulder restriction as shown in Table 3.1.

Production of trigger points

The causes of trigger point presence can relate to any combination of physical or psychic stress factors that result in alterations in normal tone in muscles, fascia and other soft tissues which, in turn, can effect changes in joint play, breathing, posture, etc. (Fig. 3.8). The progression from

Figure 3.8   Trigger points evolve in specific areas of stressed myofascial tissue. As these tissues compensate progressively towards an ever more dysfunctional fibrotic state, so the activity of associated trigger points increases.

hypertonicity to retained metabolic wastes and relative ischaemia, in muscles affected by, for example, poor posture, has been discussed previously (see Ch. 1). The feature of ischaemia and prolonged stress seems to be a major predisposing condition in the production of trigger points and their referred pain and dysfunction. Travell's research has shown that a series of embryonic trigger points develops in target/referred areas so that, in time, a chain reaction of triggers may be present.

Identifying trigger points

Kuchera & McPartland (1997) have described the major clinical characteristics of trigger points, based largely on the work of Travell and Simons. They report that, due to an apparent metabolic crisis involving impaired circulation and neural hyperreactivity (facilitation), a number of palpable signs are usually apparent:

- Altered cutaneous temperature (increased or decreased) (see Box 3.4)
- Altered cutaneous humidity (usually increased)
- Small nodular or spindle-shaped thickening representing trigger point locality

Table 3.1   Trigger points associated with shoulder restriction (Kuchera 1997)

Restricted motion	Muscle housing trigger point
Flexion	Triceps
Abduction	Subscapularis
	Infraspinatus
	Supraspinatus
	Teres major
	Levator scapulae
Internal rotation	Teres major
	Infraspinatus
External rotation	Subscapularis
	Pectoralis minor

Box 3.4 Thermography and trigger points (Baldry 1993)

Various forms of thermography have been used to identify trigger point activity, including infrared electrical or liquid crystal.

Swerdlow & Dieter (1992) found, after examining 365 patients with clinically demonstrable trigger points in the upper back, that 'although thermographic "hot-spots" are present in the majority, the sites are not necessarily where the trigger points are located.'

Is it possible that 'old' triggers lie in ischaemic tissue leading to 'cold spots' being noted?

Thermal examination of reference zones (target areas) usually shows that skin temperature is raised – but not always. Simons (1987) attributes this anomaly to different effects of triggers on the autonomic nervous system.

Barrall (1996) has shown that manual–thermal diagnosis is accurate with respect to 'heat' only 70% of the time. Apparently, when heat is noted during off-the-body scanning as when the hand moves over a truly warm area and then over a cooler area, the difference between the two areas provokes a sensation of 'heat', even though the area being scanned when this is noted may be appreciably cooler than surrounding tissues. This remains a valuable tool, however, as 'different' – whether hot or cold – suggests direct palpation of the area to be a useful next step.

- A 'jump' sign (or exclamation !) may accompany palpation because of extreme sensitivity
- A local twitch response may be elicited by stroking across the long axis of taut band housing trigger
- Local trophic changes or 'goose-flesh' may be evident overlying the trigger site.

Palpation might therefore involve (see Ch. 5 for a fuller presentation of assessment methods when using skin characteristics as a feature):

1. Off-body scan (manual thermal diagnosis), which may offer evidence of variations in local circulation; trigger point activity is more likely in areas of greatest 'difference' (see Box 3.4).
2. Movement of skin on fascia – resistance indicates the general locality of reflexogenic activity – a 'hyperalgesic skin zone' such as a trigger point (Lewit 1992).
3. Local loss of skin elasticity – refines definition of the location (Lewit 1992).
4. Light stroke, seeking 'drag' sensation (increased hydrosis), offers pinpoint accuracy of location (Lewit 1992).
5. Digital pressure (angled rather than perpendicular) into tissues seeks confirmation of active trigger (recognizable referred symptoms) or inactive, latent, trigger (local pain or unfamiliar referral pattern).
6. Use of NMT in its assessment mode (see Chs 5, 6, 11).

Obstacles to direct palpation of myofascial trigger points

Using skin characteristics (see Ch. 5) and thermal assessments (see Box 3.4) it is usually possible to identify the location of soft tissue somatic dysfunction. To establish whether the form that dysfunction takes involves a myofascial trigger point, palpatory pressure into the tissues is required (as in assessment mode NMT; see Chs 5 and 6 in particular). Apart from undeveloped, or unrefined, palpation skills, Simons (2002) suggests various reasons for failing to achieve direct palpation of myofascial trigger points, including:

- supervening layer(s) of fat
- intervening muscle(s), which may be hypertonic, indurated, fibrotic or simply too thick to allow palpation pressure to achieve contact with the trigger point
- intervening aponeurosis
- tense, thick, subcutaneous tissue
- spasm.

Trigger point features

The pathways that allow particular triggers to produce symptoms in target areas do not follow known neurological patterns, nor do they precisely mimic the pathways of traditional Chinese medicine meridians – although there is some overlap. Wall & Melzack (1989) have shown that approximately 80% of major trigger point sites are on established acupuncture points.

Travell & Simons (1983) have described the trigger point as follows:

In the core of the trigger lies a muscle spindle that is in trouble for some reason. Visualise a spindle like a strand of yarn in a knitted sweater … a metabolic crisis takes place which increases the temperature locally in the trigger point, shortens a minute part of the muscle (sarcomere) – like a snag in a sweater, and reduces the supply of oxygen and nutrients into the trigger point. During this disturbed episode an influx of calcium occurs and the muscle spindle does not have enough energy to pump the calcium outside the cell where it belongs. Thus a vicious cycle is maintained and the muscle spindle can't seem to loosen up and the affected muscle can't relax.

Simons (1994) has reviewed the work of others who have tested this concept and found that at the centre of the trigger points there is indeed a lack of oxygen compared with that in the muscles surrounding it (Simons 1994). Using sophisticated microdialysis equipment Shah & Gilliams (2008) have identified extreme ischaemia, hypoxia and acidity, as features of the local tissues in which trigger points are found. Distinct differences were noted between these conditions in active trigger points, latent trigger points and normal muscle.

Travell & Simons (1983, 1992) have confirmed that the following factors can all help to maintain and enhance trigger point activity:

- nutritional deficiency, especially vitamins C, B complex and iron
- hormonal imbalances (low thyroid hormone production, menopausal or premenstrual situations)
- infections (bacteria, viruses or yeast)
- allergies (wheat and dairy in particular)
- low oxygenation of tissues (aggravated by tension, stress, inactivity, poor respiration).

Trigger point deactivation

A number of methods exist for the deactivation of such trigger points, ranging from use of pharmacological agents such as novocaine or xylocaine, to coolant sprays and acupuncture techniques. It is noteworthy that direct digital pressure techniques can also effectively deactivate trigger points – if only temporarily in many instances. Clinical experience has shown that an absolute requirement for trigger point deactivation (apart from removal of the causes) involves the need to restore the muscle in which the trigger point lies to its normal resting length.

Trigger point deactivation may be achieved by (Chaitow & DeLany 2000, Kuchera 1997, Travell & Simons 1992):

- inhibitory compression as used in osteopathic soft tissue manipulation, neuromuscular therapy and massage (see Boxes 3.5 and 3.6)
- chilling techniques (spray, ice, possibly combined with stretching – 'spray & stretch')
- acupuncture, injection, etc. (Baldry 1993)
- positional release methods such as strain/counterstrain (Chaitow & Delany 2000, Jones 1981, Ibáñez-García 2009)
- muscle energy (stretch) techniques (Simons et al 1999)
- myofascial release methods (Barnes 1997)
- combination sequences such as integrated neuromuscular inhibition technique (INIT) (Chaitow 1994)
- correction of associated somatic dysfunction possibly involving high-velocity thrust (HVT) adjustments and/or osteopathic or chiropractic mobilization method (Liebenson 1996)
- education and correction of contributory and perpetuating factors (posture, diet, stress, breathing habits, etc.) (Bradley 1999)
- self-help strategies (stretching, etc.) (Simons et al 1999)
- microcurrent applications (McMakin 1998)
- ultrasound (Lowe & Honeyman-Lowe 1999).

Stretching

Clinical experience suggests that failure to restore the muscle containing the trigger point to its normal resting length means that treatment is likely to provide only short-term relief.

It is vital to remember that a trigger point is self-perpetuating, unless it is treated correctly and sufficiently. This means that, once symptoms have been relieved, the muscle containing the trigger should be stretched gently to its longest resting length. Failing this, symptoms will return, irrespective of the technique used (chilling, pressure, injection, acupuncture, etc.).

Box 3.5 Compression: method and effects (see Fig. 3.9)

Method 1

1. Apply firm digital compression to the trigger point sufficient to produce localized discomfort or pain, as well as symptoms in the target area.
2. Maintain this compression for 5 seconds.
3. Release for 2–3 seconds.
4. Reapply pressure (same level) and keep repeating '5 seconds on, 2–3 seconds off' until the patient reports a reduction in local or referred pain *or* an increase in pain (which is rare) *or* until 2 minutes have passed with no change in the pain level.
5. If using the INIT sequence (see Ch. 9), the next phase involves the positional release component.

Method 2

1. Apply firm digital pressure to the trigger point, sufficient to produce localized discomfort or pain, as well as symptoms in the target area.
2. Maintain the pressure for approximately 10 seconds.
3. Increase the degree of pressure slightly and maintain for a further 10 seconds.
4. Increase the degree of pressure once more and maintain for approximately 10 more seconds.
5. Slowly release pressure and, if utilizing the INIT sequence, the positional release component follows (see Ch. 9).

Manual contacts with trigger points

Tendons should be ignored when locating central trigger points. Only the actual length of the fiber is considered; for instance, the long tendon of either biceps brachii head is not included when assessing for central trigger points in this muscle; only the length of its belly is taken into account.

Central trigger points are usually palpable, with either flat palpation (against underlying structures), flat compression (between thumb and fingers like a clothes-peg) or pincer compression (between thumb and fingers like a C-clamp) (see upper trapezius treatment in Chapter 10).

A general thickening in the central portion of a muscle's belly will usually soften when a broad general pressure is applied by using a flat compression. Compressions may be applied wherever the tissue may be lifted without compressing neurovascular bundles.

A precise compression of individual fibres is possible by using the more specific pincer palpation or flat palpation, both of which capture specific bands of tissue.

Underlying structures, including neurovascular courses which might be impinged or compressed, and sharp surfaces such as foraminal gutters, determine whether pincer or flat palpation is more appropriate.

Compression techniques, between fingers and thumb, have the advantage of offering information from two or more of the examiner's digits simultaneously, whereas flat palpation against underlying tissues offers a more solid and stable background against which to assess the tissue.

Effects

The following effects are probable or possible during the application of sustained or intermittent digital compression of tissues:

- Ischaemia, which is reversed when pressure is released (Simons et al 1999).
- 'Neurological inhibition' results from sustained efferent barrage (Ward 1997). See Chapter 12 for details of the use of inhibitory pressure in a sequential manner when treating localized pain.
- A degree of mechanical stretching occurs as 'creep' of connective tissue commences (Cantu & Grodin 1992).
- Piezoelectric effects modify the 'gel' state of tissues to a more solute ('sol') state (Barnes 1997).
- Rapid mechanoreceptor impulses interfere with slower pain messages ('gate theory') (Wall & Melzack 1989).
- Pain-relieving endorphin and enkephalin release occurs (Baldry 2001), as does up-regulation of analgesic endocannabinoids (Klein 2005, McPartland & Simons 2007)
- Taut bands associated with trigger points release spontaneously (Simons et al 1999).
- Traditional Chinese medicine suggests modification of energy flow through tissues following pressure application (Zhao-pu 1991).

Digital pressure at 45° angle introduces ischaemic, inhibitory pressure.

Various models exist:

- ☑ Temporarily cuts off circulation, 'flushing' tissues when released
- ☑ Inhibition of neural activity
- ☑ Local mechanoreceptors stimulated, producing gating of pain messages
- ☑ Release of local endorphins and brain enkephalins
- ☑ Mechanical stretching of tissues
- ☑ Alters gel-like tissues to softer 'sol' state
- ☑ Taut bands associated with trigger points release
- ☑ Enhanced energy flow according to TCM

Trigger point

Figure 3.9   Schematic representation of myofascial trigger point.

Box 3.6   Algometrics: using appropriate pressure

When applying digital pressure to a tender point in order to ascertain its status ('Does it hurt?', 'Does it refer?', etc.), or when treating a trigger point, it is important to have some way of knowing that the pressure being applied is uniform.

It has been shown that, using a simple technology (bathroom scales), physical therapy students can be taught accurately to produce specific degrees of pressure on request. The students were tested applying posteroanterior pressure force to lumbar tissues. After training, using bathroom scales to evaluate pressure levels, the students showed significantly reduced error, both immediately after training and 1 month later (Keating et al 1993).

The term 'pressure threshold' is used to describe the least amount of pressure required to produce a report of pain and/or referred symptoms (Hong et al 1996). It is obviously useful to know how much pressure is required to produce pain and/or referred symptoms, and whether this degree of pressure is different before and after treatment, or at a subsequent clinical encounter. Without a measuring device such as an algometer there would be no means of standardized pressure application.

Use of an algometer is not really practical in everyday clinical work, but it becomes an important tool in research, as an objective measurement of a change in the degree of pressure required to produce symptoms. An algometer is also a useful tool for a practitioner to use in training themselves to apply a standardized degree of pressure when treating, and to 'know' how hard they are pressing.

An algometer is a hand-held, spring-loaded, rubber-tipped, pressure-measuring device, which offers a means of achieving standardized pressure application. Using an algometer, sufficient pressure to produce pain is applied to points, at a precise 90° angle to the skin. The measurement is taken when pain is reported.

Baldry (referring to research by Fischer) discusses algometer use (he calls it a 'pressure threshold meter') and suggests it should be employed to measure the degree of pressure required to produce symptoms 'before and after deactivation of a trigger point, for when this is successful, the pressure threshold over the trigger point increases by about 4 kg' (Baldry 1993, Fischer 1988).

Such stretching should be gradual and gentle, and the recommendation of Lewit (1992) and Travell & Simons (1992) is that muscle energy technique (MET), in which gentle isometric contractions followed by stretch are employed (see Ch. 8), is the method of choice to achieve that stretching. Lewit (1992) suggests that, in many instances, stretching is adequate in itself for deactivating trigger point activity.

Other views on trigger points

In order to gain further understanding of the significance of these widespread noxious entities, it is essential to be aware of the process of facilitation, as well as Selye's general and local adaptation syndromes (see Chs 1 and 9 on clinical applications of NMT). We need, also, to be aware of views of others who have tried to make sense of the myriad systems that have identified patterns of reflex activity in surface tissues (as discussed in Ch. 4).

Mennell

Mennell (1975) agrees that a muscle that can attain and maintain its normal resting length is a pain-free muscle. One that cannot (a muscle in spasm) is usually a source of pain, regardless of whether the source of the spasm is in that muscle or not. Whatever the means used to 'block' the trigger activity, and whatever the neuropathological routes involved, the critical factor in the restoration of pain-free normality is that, during any relief from the state of spasm or contraction, the affected muscle should have its normal resting length restored by stretching. Mennell defines trigger points as localized palpable spots of deep hypersensitivity from which noxious impulses bombard the central nervous system to give rise to referred pain. Mennell favours chilling the trigger area by vapocoolant or ice-massage – an approach supported by Travell and Simons, who now both advocate MET as well. Details of their recommended methods are given in Chapter 8.

Chaitow

Chaitow (1994) has proposed that a sequence of treatment to achieve trigger point deactivation – commencing with palpation/identification utilizing NMT, followed by ischaemic compression (also NMT), followed by adoption of a positional release posture (such as is used in osteopathic functional technique or strain/counterstrain; see Ch. 8) – should be followed by a stretching of the tissues housing the trigger point. The stretching in this sequence can follow a focused (to activate the fibres involved) isometric contraction, or be applied at the same time as the contraction – introducing an isolytic muscle energy approach into the methodology (see Ch. 8).

This sequence has been dubbed 'integrated neuromuscular inhibitor technique' (INIT) and is considered further in the chapters that deal with treatment.

Chaitow and Delany

Chaitow & Delany (2001) have hypothesized that there are times when the activity of a trigger point might be regarded as serving a useful physiological role, and that in such circumstances deactivation would be counterproductive. Treatment of trigger points may then best be left until after correction of the adaptational mechanisms that have caused their formation. An example involves the stabilization of the sacroiliac joint during the gait cycle. As the right leg swings forward, the right ilium rotates backwards in relation to the sacrum (Greenman 1996). Simultaneously, sacrotuberous and interosseous ligamentous tension increases to brace the sacroiliac joint in preparation for heel strike. Just before heel strike, the ipsilateral hamstrings are activated, thereby tightening the sacrotuberous ligament (into which they merge) to further stabilize the sacroiliac joint. In the case of an unstable or dysfunctional sacroiliac joint, a persistent bracing mechanism, involving a hypertonic biceps femoris, possibly including trigger point activity, might represent a potentially useful attempt to maintain stability in the joint. Deactivation of the trigger point, and/or release of the tight hamstring, could in such circumstances reduce stability, with undesirable results (van Wingerden et al 1997).

Bradley

New Zealand physiotherapist Dinah Bradley epitomizes those practitioners who use trigger points as monitors, rather than treating them. Bradley, an expert in breathing rehabilitation, palpates and identifies key trigger points in the intercostals and upper trapezius as a rule, at the outset of the patient's course of breathing rehabilitation. She asks them to ascribe a value out of 10 to the trigger point, while it is under digital pressure, before they commence their exercise and treatment programme (no direct treatment is given to the trigger points themselves), and periodically during the rehabilitation course, as well as at the time of discharge.

Bradley (1999) states:

I use trigger point testing as an objective measurement. Part of [the patient's] recovery is a reduction in musculoskeletal pain in these overused muscles. I use a numeric scale to quantify this. Patients themselves feel the reduction in tension and pain [over time], a useful subjective marker for them, and an excellent motivator.

This use of trigger points, in which they are not directly deactivated but are used as monitors of improved breathing function, highlights several key points (Fig. 3.10).

It is possible to draw various conclusions from this approach:

• As function and oxygenation improve, trigger points become less reactive and painful.

• Enhanced breathing function represents a reduction in overall stress, reinforcing the concepts associated with facilitation: as stress (of whatever kind) reduces, trigger points react less actively.

• Direct deactivation tactics are not the only way to reduce trigger point activity.

• Trigger points can be seen to be acting as 'alarm' signals, virtually quantifying the current levels of adaptive demand being imposed on the individual, or on the specific tissues.

The stress burden and trigger points

One of Selye's most important findings is commonly overlooked when the concurrent impact of multiple stressors on the system is being considered (Selye 1974).

Shealy (1984) summarizes as follows:

Selye has emphasized the fact that any systemic stress elicits an essentially generalized reaction, with release of adrenaline and glucocorticoids, in addition to any specific damage such stressor may cause. During the stage of resistance (adaptation), a given stressor may trigger less of an alarm; however, Selye insists that adaptation to one agent is acquired at the expense of resistance

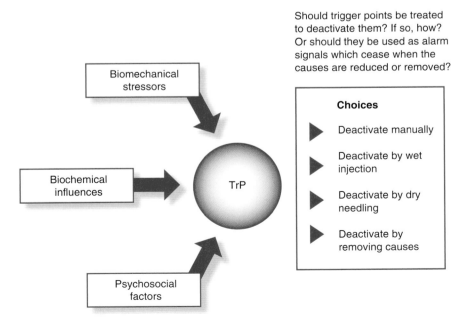

Figure 3.10   Schematic representation of trigger point deactivation choices.

to other agents. That is, as one accommodates to a given stressor, other stressors may require lower thresholds for eliciting the alarm reaction. Of considerable importance is Selye's observation that concomitant exposure to several stressors elicits an alarm reaction at stress levels that individually are sub-threshold. That is, one-third the dose of histamine, one-third the dose of cold, one-third the dose of formaldehyde, elicit an alarm reaction equal to a full dose of any one agent.

In short, therefore, as adaptation to life's stresses and stressors continues, pain thresholds drop, and a lesser stress load is required to produce responses (pain, etc.) from facilitated structures, whether paraspinal or myofascial.

Hyperventilation: an example of compound stress influences

There are few more complex functional stress influences than those that arise from altered breathing patterns, such as are manifest when upper chest breathing and/or hyperventilation is habitual. Chaitow et al (2002) have expressed this as follows:

Consider someone who is habitually breathing in an upper chest mode (for postural, habitual, emotional or other reasons), the stress of which will place adaptive demands on the accessory breathing muscles, with consequent hypertonicity, shortness, reciprocal inhibition, malcoordination, stiffness and pain, almost certainly involving trigger point activity, as well as joint dysfunction.

- The biomechanical changes which evolve from this functional chaos will modify the structure of the breathing apparatus to the extent that normal breathing function becomes difficult or impossible.
- In addition the individual will probably display evidence of anxiety as a direct result of respiratory alkalosis, deriving from CO2 imbalance ... caused by the breathing pattern. Or the breathing pattern may have been created because of a predisposing anxiety (Timmons 1994).
- This pattern of breathing, and the anxiety it encourages, feeds back into a cycle of

aggravated upper chest breathing, reinforcing the pattern.
- What may have started as an emotional state will have evolved into a chronic biochemical imbalance and a state of relative biomechanical rigidity.

It is easy to see how [therapeutic] interventions which focus on the anxiety would be helpful, as would focus on the biomechanical/structural imbalances: Interventions which reduce anxiety will help all associated symptoms. Such interventions might also involve biochemical modification (medication etc.), stress coping approaches or psychotherapy.

Interventions which improve breathing function, probably involving easing of soft tissue distress (including deactivation of trigger points) and/or joint restrictions, should also help to reduce the symptoms by allowing, with retraining, a more normal breathing pattern to be practiced.

The most appropriate approach will be the one which most closely deals with causes rather than effects, and which allows for long term changes that will reduce the likelihood of recurrence. Biochemistry, biomechanics and the mind are seen, in this example, to be inextricably bonded with each other.

The lesson to be learned from this all-too-common example is that treating pain and dysfunction in the neck, shoulders and thorax of such an upper chest breather, with trigger points as major features, might usefully involve manual methods, or relaxation/psychotherapy (if appropriate), or rebreathing retraining, or a combination of methods.

Pathophysiology of fibromyalgia/ fibrositis/myodysneuria

The changes that occur in tissue involved in the onset of myodysneuria/fibromyalgia, according to Gutstein (see earlier in this chapter), are thought to be initiated by localized sympathetic predominance, associated with changes in the hydrogen ion concentration and calcium and sodium balance in the tissue fluids (Petersen 1934). This is associated with vasoconstriction and hypoxia/ischaemia. Pain results, it is thought, from these alterations affecting the pain sensors and proprioceptors. Muscle spasm and hard nodular localized tetanic contractions of muscle bundles (Bayer 1950), together with vasomotor and musculomotor stimulation, intensify each other, creating a vicious cycle of self-perpetuating impulses. There are varied and complex patterns of referred symptoms that may result from such 'trigger' areas, as well as local pain and minor disturbances.

Such sensations as aching, soreness, tenderness, heaviness and tiredness may all be manifest, as may modification of muscular activity due to contraction resulting in tightness, stiffness, swelling, etc.

Recent research has resulted in strict guidelines for a diagnosis of fibromyalgia from the American College of Rheumatology (Wolfe et al 1990):
1. History of widespread pain.

Pain is considered widespread when all of the following are present: pain in the left side of the body, pain in the right side of the body, pain above the waist and pain below the waist. In addition there should be pain in the spine or the neck or front of the chest, or thoracic spine or low back.

2. Pain in 11 of 18 palpated tender point sites.
There should be pain on pressure (around 4 kg of pressure maximum) on not fewer than 11 of the following sites (Fig. 3.11):

- Either side of the base of the skull where the suboccipital muscles insert
- Either side of the side of the neck between the 5th and 7th cervical vertebrae – technically described as between the 'anterior aspects of inter-transverse spaces'
- Either side of the body on the midpoint of the muscle that runs from the neck to the shoulder (upper trapezius)
- Either side of the body on the origin of the supraspinatus muscle that runs along the upper border of the shoulder blade
- Either side, on the upper surface of the rib, where the 2nd rib meets the breast bone, in the pectoral muscle
- On the outer aspect of either elbow just below the prominence (epicondyle)
- In the large buttock muscles, either side, on the upper outer aspect in the fold in front of the muscle (gluteus medius)

Figure 3.11   Sites of the 18 fibromyalgia tender points as defined by the American College of Rheumatologists.

- Just behind the large prominence of either hip joint in the muscular insertion of piriformis muscle
- On either knee in the fatty pad just above the inner aspect of the joint.

A puzzle

Questions often asked include:

- Is fibromyalgia the same as myofascial pain syndrome (pain problems in which trigger points are clearly involved)?
- Do trigger points actually cause fibromyalgia?

The condition called myofascial pain syndrome (MPS) – a disorder in which pain of a persistent aching type is referred to a number of target areas by triggers lying some distance away – has long been recognized as a cause of severe and chronic pain. Since many experts insist that the 'tender' points that are palpated when diagnosing fibromyalgia need to refer pain elsewhere if they are to be taken seriously in the diagnosis (making them trigger points by definition), the question needs to be asked whether MPS is not the same thing as fibromyalgia syndrome (FMS)?

The answer is: not quite.

Scandinavian researchers showed in 1986 that around 65% of people with fibromyalgia had identifiable trigger points, and it is clear, therefore, that there is an overlap between FMS and MPS.

D. P. Baldry, a leading British physician/acupuncturist, has summarized the similarities and differences between these two conditions (Baldry 1993) as follows. The two conditions are *similar* or identical in that both fibromyalgia and MPS:

- are affected by cold weather
- may involve increased sympathetic nerve activity and may involve conditions such as Raynaud's phenomenon
- have tension headaches and paraesthesia as a major associated symptom
- are unaffected by anti-inflammatory pain-killing medication, whether of the cortisone type or standard formulations.

Fibromyalgia and MPS are *different* in that:

- MPS affects males and females equally; fibromyalgia mainly involves females.
- MPS is usually local to an area such as the neck and shoulders, or low back and legs,

although it can affect a number of parts of the body at the same time, whereas fibromyalgia is a generalized problem, often involving all four 'corners' of the body at the same time.
- Muscles containing areas that feel 'like a tight rubber band' are found in around 30% of people with MPS, but in more than 60% of people with FMS.
- People with FMS have poorer muscle endurance than people with MPS.
- MPS can sometimes be bad enough to cause disturbed sleep, whereas in fibromyalgia the sleep disturbance has a more causative role, and is a pronounced feature of the condition.
- MPS produces no morning stiffness whereas fibromyalgia does.
- Fatigue is not usually associated with MPS, while it is common in fibromyalgia.
- MPS can sometimes lead to depression (reactive) and anxiety, whereas, in a small proportion of fibromyalgia cases, depression/anxiety can be the trigger for the start of FMS.
- Conditions such as irritable bowel syndrome, dysmenorrhoea and a feeling of swollen joints are noted in fibromyalgia, but seldom in MPS.
- Low-dosage tricyclic antidepressant drugs are helpful in dealing with the sleep problems, and many of the symptoms of fibromyalgia, but not of MPS.
- Exercise programmes (cardiovascular fitness) can help some patients with fibromyalgia, according to experts, but this is not a useful approach in MPS.
- The outlook for people with MPS is excellent because the trigger points usually respond quickly to massage, manipulative or acupuncture techniques, whereas the outlook for those with fibromyalgia is less positive, with a lengthy treatment and recovery phase being the norm.

Schneider (1995) reports:

It is now clear that there are several important differences between fibromyalgia (FM) and myofascial pain syndrome (MFPS) ... local treatment applied to tender points [in FM] is ineffective, yet specific treatment of trigger points [in MFPS] is dramatically effective.

Simons (2002) has summarized the main differences between MPS and fibromyalgia (Table 3.2).

Table 3.2   Differences between MPS and fibromyalgia (Simons 2002)

Myofascial trigger points	Fibromyalgia
Muscular origin	Systemic or central nervous system origin
Female:male ratio 1:1	Female:male ratio 4–9:1
Local or regional pain	Widespread, general pain
Focal tenderness	Widespread tenderness of most of body
Muscle feels tense (taut bands)	Muscle feels soft and doughy
Restricted stretch range of motion	Commonly hypermobile
Examination for trigger points anywhere	Examination for prescribed tender points
Immediate response to trigger point injection	Delayed response to trigger point injection
May also have fibromyalgia	Nearly all also have myofascial trigger points
All myofascial trigger points are tender	Not all tender points are myofascial trigger points

Conclusion and hypothesis

We have seen how hyperreactive local (trigger point) and spinal areas can arise and be maintained and/or aggravated as a result of repetitive and continuous stress of one sort or another.

What we see in fibromyalgia is that areas of the brain behave in a facilitated manner, and that this hyperreactive brain activity could well be another version of this same phenomenon (facilitation). If so, we can learn much about fibromyalgia from our experience of handling localized facilitation processes such as trigger points.

Korr's studies, discussed previously, show that facilitated areas act as 'neurological lenses', focusing whatever stress impacts on the person as a whole through these sensitized tissues.

If that 'tissue' happens to be (a part of) the brain, we have a situation in which it becomes imperative for stress of all sorts (climatic, emotional, structural/postural, nutritional, toxic, infective, allergenic, etc.) to be minimized, and this includes tailoring therapeutic interventions to be as non-invasive as possible (deep massage causes increased muscle pain in fibromyalgia, whereas light massage does not).

Constitutional therapeutic approaches such as deep relaxation, non-stressful hydrotherapy, wellness massage and similar methods are more likely to be helpful than anything that makes adaptive demands on an already compromised individual.

Summary

Trigger points are certainly often part – in some cases the major part – of the pain suffered by people with fibromyalgia. When they are present (as they certainly are if pressure on the 'tender point' produces pain somewhere else in the body), we need to know more about them and how they can be treated successfully.

In the next chapter an overview is presented of other reflex systems, awareness of which should add to our comprehensive understanding of myofascial trigger points.

References

Baldry P: *Acupuncture trigger points and musculoskeletal pain*, Edinburgh, 1993, Churchill Livingstone.

Baldry P: *Myofascial pain and fibromyalgia syndromes*, Edinburgh, 2001, Churchill Livingstone.

Barnes M: The basic science of myofascial release, *Journal of Bodywork and Movement Therapies* 1(4):231–238, 1997.

Barrall JP: *Manual–thermal diagnosis*, Seattle, 1996, Eastland Press.

Bayer H: Pathophysiology of muscular rheumatism, *Zeitschrift für Raeumaforschung* 9:210, 1950.

Beal M: Palpatory testing of somatic dysfunction in patients with cardiovascular disease, *J Am Osteopath Assoc* 82(11):73–82, 1983.

Beal MC: Viscerosomatic reflexes: a review, *J Am Osteopath Assoc* 85(12):786–801, 1985.

Benatsen L: Central sensitization in tension-type headache – possible pathophysiological mechanisms, *Cephalalgia* 20(6):603–610, 2000.

Bradley D: Breathing retraining advice from three therapists, *Journal of Bodywork and Movement Therapies* 3(3):159–167, 1999.

Brugger A: Pseudoradikulare syndrome, *Acta Rheumatol* 19:1, 1962.

Cantu R, Grodin A: *Myofascial manipulation*, Gaithersburg, Maryland, 1992, Aspen Publications.

Chaitow L: Integrated neuro-muscular inhibition technique in treatment of pain and trigger points, *British Osteopathic Journal* XIII:17–21, 1994.

Chaitow L: *Fibromyalgia syndrome – a practitioner's guide to treatment*, Edinburgh, 2000, Churchill Livingstone.

Chaitow L, DeLany J: *Clinical applications of neuromuscular technique, Lower body*, vol. 2, Edinburgh, 2000, Churchill Livingstone.

Chaitow L, Bradley D, Gilbert C: *Multidisciplinary approaches to breathing pattern disorders*, Edinburgh, 2002, Churchill Livingstone.

Codere T, Katz J, Vaccarino A, et al: Contributions of central neuroplasticity to pathological pain: review of clinical and experimental evidence, *Pain* 52:259, 1993.

Cornelius A 1909 Die neurepunkt lehre. vol. 2. George Thins, Leipzig.

Denslow J, Korr I, et al: Quantitative studies of chronic facilitation, *Am J Physiol* 150:229–238, 1949.

Dittrich RJ: Somatic pain and autonomic concomitants, *Am J Surg*, 1954.

Dowling D: DiGiovanna E, editor: *An osteopathic approach to diagnosis and treatment*, Philadelphia, 1991, Lippincott.

Dowling D: Progressive neuromuscular inhibition technique (PINS), *J Am Osteopath Assoc* 100(5):285–298, 2000.

Dvorak J, Dvorak V: *Manual medicine diagnostics*, Stuttgart, 1984, Georg Thieme.

Fairbank J: Prolapsed intervertebral disc, *BMJ* 336(7657):1317–1318, 2008.

Feinstein B, Longton J, Jameson R, et al: Experiments on pain referred from deep somatic tissues, *J Bone Joint Surg* 36A:981, 1954.

Fischer A: Documentation of muscle pain and soft tissue pathology. In Kraus H, editor: *Diagnosis and treatment of muscle pain*, Chicago, 1988, Quintessence.

Greenman PE: *Principles of manual medicine*, ed 2, Baltimore, 1996, Williams & Wilkins.

Gutstein R: A review of myodysneuria (fibrositis), *Am Pract Dig Treat* 6(4):114–124, 1944.

Gutstein R: The role of abdominal fibrositis in functional indigestion, *Miss Valley Med J* 66:114–124, 1944.

Gutstein R: The role of craniocervical myodysneuria in functional ocular disorders, *Am Pract Dig Treat November*, 1956.

Hix E: Reflex viscerosomatic reference phenomena, *Osteopathic Annals* 4(12):496–503, 1976.

Hockaday M, Whitty CW: Patterns of referred pain in the normal subject, *Brain* 90:481–496, 1967.

Hong CZ, Chen YN, Twehouse D, et al: Pressure threshold for referred pain by compression on trigger point and adjacent area, *Journal of Musculoskeletal Pain* 4(3):61–79, 1996.

Ibáñez-García J, et al: Changes in masseter muscle trigger points following strain-counterstrain or neuro-muscular technique, *Journal of Bodywork and Movement Therapies* 13(1):2–10, 2009.

Ji RR, Kohno T, Moore KA, et al: Central sensitization and LTP: Do pain and memory share similar mechanisms? *Trends Neurosci* 26(12):696–705, 2003.

Jones L: *Strain and counterstrain*, Colorado Springs, 1981, Academy of Applied Osteopathy.

Keating J, Matuyas T, Bach T: The effect of training on physical therapists' ability to apply specified forces of palpation, *Phys Ther* 73(1):38–46, 1993.

Kellgren J: Observations on referred pain coming from muscle, *Clin Sci* 3:175–190, 1938.

Kellgren J: On the distribution of pain arising from deep somatic structures, *Clin Sci* 4:35–46, 1939.

Klein T: Cannabinoid-based drugs as anti-inflammatory therapeutics, *Nat Rev Immunol* 5(5):400–411, 2005.

Korr I: *Physiological basis of osteopathic medicine*, New York, 1970, Postgraduate Institute of Osteopathic Medicine and Surgery.

Korr I: Proprioceptors and somatic dysfunction, *J Am Osteopath Assoc* 74:638, 1975.

Korr I: Spinal cord as organiser of disease process, *Academy of Applied Osteopathy Yearbook*, 1976.

Korr I, editor: *Neurobiological mechanisms in manipulation*, New York, 1977, Plenum Press.

Korr I: Somatic dysfunction, *J Am Osteopath Assoc* 86(2):109–114, 1986.

Kuchera M: Travell & Simons myofascial trigger points. In Ward R, editor: *Foundations of Osteopathic Medicine*, Philadelphia, 1997, Williams & Wilkins.

Kuchera M, McPartland J: Myofascial trigger points. In Ward R, editor: *Foundations of Osteopathic Medicine*, Philadelphia, 1997, Williams & Wilkins.

Lavelle W, Lavelle E, Smith H: Interventional Techniques for Back Pain, *Clin Geriatr Med* 24(2):345–368, 2008.

Lewis T: Suggestions relating to the study of somatic pain, *Br Med J* 1:321–325, 1938.

Lewit K: *Manipulative therapy in rehabilitation of the locomotor system*, London, 1992, Butterworths.

Li J, Simone D, Larson A: Windup leads to characteristics of central sensitization, *Pain* 79:75–82, 1999.

Liebenson C: *Rehabilitation of the spine*, Baltimore, 1996, Williams & Wilkins.

Lowe JC, Honeyman-Lowe G: Ultrasound treatment of trigger points, *Medecine du Sud-est* 2:12–15, 1999 April–May–June.

McEachern JC, Shaw CA: The plasticity-pathology continuum: Defining a role for the LTP phenomenon, *J Neurosci Res* 58(1):42–61, 1999.

McMakin C: Microcurrent treatment of myofascial pain in head, neck and face, *Topics in Clinical Chiropractic* 5(1):29–35, 1998.

McPartland J, Simons D: Myofascial trigger points: translating molecular theory into manual therapy, *Journal Manual and Manipulative Therapies* 14:232–239, 2007.

Melzack R, Wall P: *Textbook of pain*, ed 2, London, 1989, Churchill Livingstone.

Mennell J: The therapeutic use of cold, *J Am Osteopath Assoc* 74:1146–1158, 1975.

Mense S, Simons D: *Muscle pain*, Philadelphia, 2001, Williams & Wilkins.

Patterson M: *Model mechanism for spinal segmental facilitation*, Academy of Applied Osteopathy Yearbook, 1976.

Petersen W: *The patient and the weather: autonomic disintegration*, Ann Arbor, 1934, Edward Bros.

Schneider M: Tender points – fibromyalgia vs. trigger points – myofascial pain syndrome, *J Manipulative Physiol Ther* 18(6):398–406, 1995.

Selye H: *Stress without distress*, Philadelphia, 1974, Lippincott.

Shah J, Gilliams E: Uncovering the biochemical milieu of myofascial trigger points using in vivo microdialysis: An application of muscle pain concepts to myofascial pain syndrome, *Journal of Bodywork and Movement Therapies* 12(4):371–384, 2008.

Shealy CN: Total life stress and symptomatology, *Journal of Holistic Medicine* 6(2):112–129, 1984.

Simons D: Myofascial pain due to trigger points, *International Rehabilitation Medicine Association* Monograph 1, 1987.

Simons D: Myofascial pain syndromes, *Journal of Musculoskeletal Pain* 2(2):113–121, 1994.

Simons D: Understanding effective treatments of myofascial trigger points, *Journal of Bodywork and Movement Therapies* 6(2):81–88, 2002.

Simons D, Travell J, Simons L: ed 2, *Myofascial pain and dysfunction: the trigger point manual*, vol. 1, Upper half of body. Baltimore, 1999, Williams & Wilkins.

Speransky A: *A basis for the theory of medicine*, New York, 1943, International Publishers.

Staud R: Biology and therapy of fibromyalgia: pain in fibromyalgia syndrome, *Arthritis Res Ther* 8:208, 2006.

Sutter M: Versuch einer Wesensbestimmung pseudoradikularer Syndrome, *Schweiz Rundsch Med Prax* 63:42, 1975.

Swerdlow B, Dieter N: Evaluation of thermography, *Pain* 48:205–213, 1992.

Timmons B: *Behavioral and psychological approaches to breathing disorders*, New York, 1994, Plenum Press.

Travell J: *Symposium on mechanism and management of pain syndromes*, 1957 Proceedings of the Rudolph Virchow Medical Society.

Travell J: Identification of myofascial trigger point syndromes, *Arch Phys Med* 62:100, 1981.

Travell J, Bigelow N: Role of somatic trigger areas in the patterns of hysteria, *Psychosom Med* 9(6):353–363, 1947.

Travell J, Simons D: *Myofascial pain and dysfunction: the trigger point manual*, vol. 1, Upper half of body. ed 1, Baltimore, 1983, Williams & Wilkins.

Travell J, Simons D: *Myofascial pain and dysfunction: the trigger point manual*, vol. 2, The lower extremities. Baltimore, 1992, Williams & Wilkins.

Travell J, Simons D, Travell L: *Myofascial pain and dysfunction: the trigger point manual*, vol. 1, ed 2, The upper extremities. Baltimore, 1999, Williams & Wilkins.

Van Wingerden J-P, Vleeming A, Kleinvensink G, Stoekart R: The role of the hamstrings in pelvic and spinal function. In Vleeming A, Mooney V, Dorman T, 1997.

Wall P, Melzack R: *Textbook of pain*, Edinburgh, 1989, Churchill Livingstone.

Ward R: *Foundations of osteopathic medicine*, Philadelphia, 1997, Williams & Wilkins.

Webber TD: Diagnosis and modification of headache and shoulder-arm-hand syndrome, *J Am Osteopath Assoc* 72:697–710, 1973.

Weiss J: Pelvic floor myofascial trigger points: manual therapy for interstitial cystitis and the urgency-frequency syndrome, *J Urol* 166(6):2226–2231, 2001.

Wolfe F, Smythe HA, Yunus MB, et al: The American College of Rheumatology 1990 Criteria for the Classification of Fibromyalgia, *Arthritis Rheum* 33:160–172, 1990.

Zhao-Pu W: *Acupressure therapy*, Edinburgh, 1991, Churchill Livingstone.

4

The variety of reflex points

CHAPTER CONTENTS

Reflex patterns and areas	**75**
Are all tender points trigger points?	76
Distinguishing features of myofascial trigger points	76
Mechanotransduction, fascial pathways, and endocannabinoid influences – some recent advances	77
Mechanotransduction	77
Fascial communication	77
Endocannabinoids	77
Summary	78
Acupuncture points	**78**
Acupuncture points and their morphology	78
Acupuncture and applied kinesiology	79
Ah Shi points	82
Alarm points, Associated points, Akabane points	82
Bennett's neurovascular reflex points	84
Chapman's reflexes	**86**
Connective tissue massage/manipulation	**89**
CTM: Method and mechanism	90
Jones' tender points	90
Periosteal pair points	93
Confusion?	**93**

Reflex patterns and areas

In this chapter some of the major systems that have identified and classified reflex areas on the body surface will be discussed, because many of the 'points' that these identify are bound to be accessed during the application of NMT in an assessment or a treatment mode.

Osteopathic physician Eileen DiGiovanna (1991) states: 'Today many physicians believe there is a relationship among trigger points, acupuncture points and Chapman's reflexes. Precisely what the relationship may be is unknown.' She quotes from a prestigious osteopathic pioneer, George Northup (1941), who stated as far back as 1941:

> One cannot escape the feelings that all of the seemingly diverse observations (regarding reflex patterns) are but views of the same iceberg the tip of which we are beginning to see, without understanding either its magnitude or its depth of importance.

Awareness of the reflex potential of the body surface widens the therapeutic potential of NMT, although deciding which of the many possible applications of reflex activity to utilize in diagnosis or treatment can be a daunting task. The discussion in this text of these reflex systems and classifications should not be taken as indicating recommendation for their use, merely recognition of the fact that they are widely used, and that NMT offers an additional means of access and employment of their potential.

Felix Mann (1983), one of the pioneers of acupuncture in the West, entered the controversy as to the existence, or otherwise, of acupuncture meridians (and indeed acupuncture points). Mann, in an effort to alter the emphasis that traditional acupuncture places on the specific charted positions of points, stated:

> McBurney's point, in appendicitis, has a defined position. In reality it may be 10cms higher, lower, to the left or right. It may be one centimetre in diameter, or occupy the whole of the abdomen, or not occur at all. Acupuncture points are often the same, and hence it is pointless to speak of acupuncture points in the classical traditional way. Carefully performed electrical resistance measurements do not show alterations in the skin resistance to electricity, corresponding with classical acupuncture points. There are so many acupuncture points mentioned in some modern books, that there is no skin left which is not an acupuncture point. In cardiac disease, pain and tenderness may occur in the arm however this does not occur more frequently along the course of the heart meridian, than anywhere else in the arm.

Hence, Mann concludes, meridians do not exist, or – more confusingly perhaps – the whole body is an acupuncture point!

Leaving aside the validity of Mann's comment, it is true to say that if all the multitude of points described in acupuncture, traditional and modern, together with those points described by Travell and co-workers, Chapman, Jones and Bennett (see later in this chapter), were to be placed together on one map of the body surface, we would soon come to the conclusion that the entire body surface is a 'potential acupuncture point'.

This realization is supported by Speransky's findings from the 1930s, as discussed in Chapter 3.

Are all tender points trigger points?

A number of respected researchers and clinicians are frequently in error when they describe localized soft tissue areas that palpate as sensitive, but that do not refer symptoms elsewhere, as trigger points.

Certainly a trigger point will always be palpable, and will always be sensitive to pressure, but then so will most other 'points', whether these be Chapman's reflexes, Gutstein's myodysneuria points, Jones's tender points, or acupuncture alarm points. *These, however, will not necessarily refer painful symptoms to distant sites in the obvious manner displayed by trigger points.*

This is not to say that any 'tender' or sensitive point cannot become a trigger point, since, clearly, before it is active, a trigger point has to evolve, and in its earlier stages will be painful, sensitive or tender, but may at the time of palpation not be sufficiently sensitized and hyperreactive to refer pain and other symptoms. If a point 'belonging' to any of the various classifications discussed below *does* refer symptoms in the manner of trigger points, then it can be so classified and treated.

Distinguishing features of myofascial trigger points

(modified from Simons 2002)

- Active myofascial trigger points produce regional pain complaints and not bodywide pain and tenderness.
- Not all tender points are myofascial trigger points, but all myofascial trigger points are tender.
- Referred tenderness, as well as referred pain, is characteristic of a myofascial trigger point.
- All myofascial trigger points are associated with a taut band.
- Not all taut bands are palpable (requires sufficient palpation skill and accessibility).
- All active myofascial trigger points cause a clinical pain (sensory disturbance) that is familiar to the patient.
- Only an active myofascial trigger point, when compressed, reproduces the clinical sensory symptoms that are familiar to the patient.
- However, a latent myofascial trigger point produces no clinical sensory (pain or numbness) complaint that is familiar to the patient.

Some of the major 'point' classifications involving reflex activity, and with a diagnostic potential, are considered in this chapter, in alphabetical order (not in order of apparent importance).

Mechanotransduction, fascial pathways, and endocannabinoid influences – some recent advances

Before looking at a selection of point classifications, involving reflex activity, the evidence of recent research relating to the process of mechanotransduction requires a brief introduction, as does introduction of endocannabinoid influences.

We have seen earlier in this chapter that there exist in many individuals discrete localized areas that generate pain, and/or other symptoms (often at a distance), as a result of local or central sensitization.

It is therefore important to be able to demonstrate evidence that these can:

1. be identified via palpation, and
2. be manipulated/treated manually via stretching or compression – for example – or by tool assisted means (e.g. acupuncture).

Assessment/palpation will be investigated in Chapter 5, while therapeutic approaches will be described in Chapters 6, 7, 8, 9, 10 and 11.

But what are the mechanisms associated with influencing symptoms and tissues at a distance?

As we have seen, neurological explanations have been at the forefront of attempts to explain reflex influences. However, there have been other recent developments in our understanding of how manual treatment can influence distant tissues, for example via the biochemical and other processes involved in what is termed mechanotransduction; and also via the release of endocannabinoids.

Mechanotransduction

Burkholder (2006) notes:

There are many ways by which deformation of a myofiber might be converted to a biochemical signal. When a deformation is imposed on a muscle, changes in cellular and molecular conformations link the mechanical forces with biochemical signals, and the close integration of mechanical signals with electrical, metabolic, and hormonal signaling may disguise the aspect of the response that is specific to the mechanical forces. The mechanically induced conformational change may directly activate downstream signaling and

may trigger messenger systems to activate signaling indirectly.

A veritable cascade of biochemical changes result from mechanical deformation of tissues, involving calcium, insulin and a variety of complex substances that signal to other tissues 'downstream'.

It seems probable that such signalling can be modulated, directed, to achieve positive changes, via appropriate manual methods of treatment (Levin 2000).

Fascial communication

Closely linked to these ideas is an increased awareness of fascial connections that link distant, as well as local, areas of the body (Myers 2008, Huijing & Baan 2001).

Langevin et al (2005) have proposed fascia/connective tissue as a communication system:

Connective tissue may function as a previously unrecognized whole body communication system. Since connective tissue is intimately associated with all other tissues (e.g. lung, intestine), connective tissue signaling may coherently influence (and be influenced by) the normal or pathological function of a wide variety of organ systems ... connective tissue functions as a body-wide mechanosensitive signaling network [involving] three categories of signals: electrical, cellular and tissue remodeling, each potentially responsive to mechanical forces over different time scales.

Khalsa et al (2005) report that 'Langevin's research describes a common feature of manual therapies – the application of mechanical forces to connective tissues. Immediate (viscoelastic and mechanotransduction) and delayed (remodeling) connective tissue effects of these forces may contribute to the mechanism of these therapies.'

Endocannabinoids

In the 1990s a new class of self-generated pain-relieving substances was identified in the body, the endocannabinoids. These substances mimic the pain-relieving and euphoria-generating effects of the use of cannabis, and help to explain its illegal use by many chronically pain-ridden individuals (Degenhardt 2007).

As McPartland & Simons (2007) explain:

The endocannabinoid (eCB) system, like the better-known endorphin system, diminishes nociception and pain, reduces inflammation in myofascial tissues, and plays a role in fascial reorganization. The overall role of the eCB system can be summarized as 'resilience to allostatic load,' a phrase synonymous with health. Practitioners wield several tools that upregulate eCB activity, including myofascial manipulation, diet and lifestyle [particularly exercise].

Summary

NMT (and other soft tissue approaches to treatment of somatic dysfunction) clearly 'deform' tissues (compression, shear, stretch, etc.), albeit briefly, and over and above the local effects on tissue, the signalling potential that follows remains an intriguing area for further research. At the same time endocannabinoid influences are likely candidates to explain at least some of the local and distant effects of manual treatment such as NMT.

Empirical clinical evidence certainly indicates that distant influences are achieved using NMT, and these current research areas appear to explain some of the mechanisms.

Acupuncture points

Soft tissue changes often produce organized discrete areas that act as generators of secondary problems. A repetitive question arises as to whether traditional acupuncture points are in fact the same as trigger points (Fig. 4.1).

The location of acupuncture points, with their fixed anatomical locations, are capable of corroboration by electrical detection, each point being evidenced by a small area of lowered electrical resistance.

When 'active', possibly due to reflex factors, these points become even more detectable, as the electrical resistance lowers further. The skin overlying them also alters and becomes hyperalgesic and not difficult to palpate as differing from surrounding skin. Active acupuncture points also become sensitive to pressure and this is of value to the therapist because the finding of sensitive areas during palpation or treatment is of diagnostic importance. Sensitive and painful areas that do not have detectable tissue changes as part of their make-up may well be 'active' acupuncture points, or *tsubo*, which means 'points on the human body' in Japanese (Serizawe 1976).

Not only are these points detectable and sensitive, but they are also amenable to treatment by direct pressure techniques. They therefore display, in almost all particulars, the same features as trigger points.

Acupuncture points and their morphology

Pain researchers Wall & Melzack (1989), and others (Travell & Simons 1992, Melzack et al 1977), maintain that there is little, if any, difference between acupuncture points and most trigger points.

Dorsher (2004), carefully compared the location of 255 trigger points, as identified by Travell and Simons, with 747 acupuncture points as identified by the Shanghai College of Traditional Medicine (Chen 1995):

Figure 4.1A, B   Location of some important acupuncture points on the head and neck. Research indicates that over 75% of defined acupuncture points are also sites of common trigger points.

Gall bladder   14
Gall bladder   1
Gall bladder   3
Gall bladder   20
Gall bladder   21

Common trigger point sites on the Bladder meridian

The findings were that 92% of TPs had anatomically corresponding acupuncture points, 83% of these points had similar regional pain indications, and 87% of myofascial TPs had referred pain patterns that are identical or nearly identical to the corresponding acupuncture points' meridian distributions.

The conclusion was: TPs are essentially a 'rediscovery' of the 2000-year-old acupuncture tradition (a subset of acupuncture points). As will be noted below, not all researchers or clinicians agree with these findings (Birch 2008).

The morphology of acupuncture points has been studied, notably by Bosey (1984).

Some of his major conclusions, in summary, are as follows:

- Points are situated in palpable depressions ('cupules').
- The skin (epiderm) over the point is a little thinner at the cupule level, under which lies a fibrous cone in which there is frequently found either a neurovascular formation, or simply a cutaneous neurovascular bundle.
- Free nerve endings are noted, and the presence, beneath the point, of Golgi endings and Pacini corpuscles is common.
- Connective tissues lie below at varying depths.
- Fascia and aponeurosis are noted and a passage of vessels and nerves, through the fascia, is very often found under the acupuncture point.

The practice of manipulating the needle in acupuncture imposes a degree of traction on the underlying (muscular) tissue, which imposes stimulation on underlying receptor organs. Fat is also a common factor in the morphology of points, and this, and the connective tissue, is thought to be a key factor in the achievement of the 'acupuncture sensation' that accompanies successful treatment. The conclusion reached is that a number of tissues are simultaneously affected needling – a phenomenon confirmed by Langevin (2006), supporting the mechanotransduction mechanisms discussed earlier.

Some points, when dissected, showed that neurovascular structures lie immediately below the point, which could account for the particular effects noted by such points being treated. This is of interest to those using Bennett's neurovascular points. The implications for those practitioners not employing needles, and who rely on pressure techniques in order to provide stimulus or sedation to such areas, is that, if accurately applied, the effects of pressure should be identical (to needle acupuncture), especially in relation to pain control.

Acupuncture and applied kinesiology

An attempt to correlate the various reflex systems and methods has been made by the American chiropractor George Goodheart. His system of applied kinesiology involves testing muscle groups for weaknesses and then, depending upon the results of such tests, using various massage and pressure techniques applied to specific locations (points) in order to normalize function. These points correspond to Chapman's reflexes, acupuncture points and other less well known reflex systems. Many of Goodheart's techniques, theories and methods support and utilize methods that are in line with NMT.

Acupressure and pain thresholds

It has been shown that pain thresholds can be dramatically raised by pressure techniques applied to specific points. Researchers at the Peking Medical College conducted complex experiments which demonstrated that finger pressure acupuncture produced a rise of 133% in pain threshold of rabbits (using radiant heat as the painful stimulus). When cerebrospinal fluid was perfused from one rabbit to another after such experiments, the recipient rabbit was found to have achieved a rise in pain threshold of up to 80%. This suggested the presence of hormone-like substances produced by the brain in response to the original acupressure stimulus. These substances are now known to be enkephalins and endorphins, and these play a role in NMT pain control. The point used in these tests was equivalent to the acupuncture point known as Bladder 60, posterior to the ankle (externally) and just anterior to the Achilles tendon.

Acupuncture points and trigger points: not all agree that they are the same phenomenon

As outlined earlier, because they spatially occupy the same positions in at least 75% of cases (Wall & Melzack 1989, Dorsher 2004, Dorsher & Fleckenstein 2008) there are strong indications that trigger points are in fact no more than active acupuncture points. Wall & Melzack (1989) have concluded that: 'trigger points and acupuncture points when used for pain control, though discovered independently and labelled differently, represent the same phenomenon'.

Baldry (1993) does not agree, however, claiming differences in their structural make-up. He states:

> It would seem likely that they are of two different types, and their close spatial correlation is because there are A-delta afferent-innervated [fast transmitting receptors with a high threshold and sensitive to sharply pointed stimuli or heat produced stimulation] acupuncture points in the skin and subcutaneous tissues immediately above the intramuscularly placed, predominantly C afferent-innervated [slow transmitting, low threshold, widely distributed and sensitive to chemicals – such as those released by damaged cells – mechanical or thermal stimulus] trigger points.

Clearly, stimulation of an area that has, beneath the contacting instrument or digit, both an acupuncture and a trigger point will influence both types of neural transmission and both 'points'. Which route of reflex stimulation is producing a therapeutic effect, or whether other mechanisms altogether are at work – endorphin or endocannabinoid release, as examples – is therefore open to debate. This debate can be further widened if we include the vast array of other reflex influences identified by other systems and workers, as discussed later in this chapter.

Whereas traditional oriental concepts focus on 'energy' imbalances in reaction to acupuncture points, there exist also a number of Western interpretations.

Melzack et al (1977) have assumed that acupuncture points represent areas of abnormal physiological activity, producing a continuous low-level input into the central nervous system

(CNS). They suggested that this might eventually lead to a combining with noxious stimuli deriving from other structures, innervated by the same segments, to produce an increased awareness of pain and distress. They found it reasonable to assume that trigger points and acupuncture points represented the same phenomenon, having found that the location of trigger points on Western maps, and acupuncture points used commonly in painful conditions, showed a remarkable 75% correlation in position.

It is interesting that the link between the source of pain or tender points, and the referred area of pain noted in trigger points, in many instances seems to travel along the routes of traditional acupuncture meridians, but certainly not always. Spontaneous pain in such a point, according to acupuncture tradition, indicates the need for urgent attention. It is not the intention of this book to provide instruction in acupuncture methodology, nor necessarily to endorse the views expressed by traditional acupuncture in relation to meridians and their purported connection with organs and systems. However, it would be shortsighted to ignore the accumulated wisdom that has led many thousands of skilled practitioners to ascribe particular roles to these points, for example Alarm, Associated and Akabane points as described in this chapter.

As far as a manual therapy is concerned, there seems to be value in having awareness of the reported roles of particular acupuncture points, and of incorporating this into diagnostic and therapeutic settings.

As we palpate and search through the soft tissues, in basic neuromuscular technique, we are bound to come across areas of sensitivity that relate to these points. They are also often found to overlap with neurolymphatic and neurovascular points, as described elsewhere in this text.

For example, reflex number 19 in Chapman's reflexes, which relates to the urethra, is identical to the neurovascular point of the bladder, and the acupuncture alarm point of the Bladder meridian. Careful comparison shows many such overlaps.

General guidance as to how to treat acupuncture points, which are sensitive, must relate to whether a stimulating or sedating effect is desired. The body often seems to utilize therapeutic stimulation to its best advantage.

Selye has shown us (see Ch. 1) that homeostatic mechanisms are at work, so that any stimulus, if appropriate and not excessive, can result in a beneficial response. In accord with the methods used in treating neurolymphatic and neurovascular points (described elsewhere in this chapter) it is suggested that, to some extent, the 'feel' of the tissues be allowed to guide the practitioner. A change (in the sense of a release of tension, or a softening, or a sensing of a gentle pulsation in the tissues) is often an indication of an adequate degree of therapy. In order to sedate what is an overactive point, up to 5 minutes of sustained or intermittent pressure, or rotary contact, may be required.

For stimulation, the timing could involve between 20 seconds and 2 minutes. By this time, some degree of change should be palpable. As must be clear, if pressure is sustained beyond a certain point quite the opposite effect will be achieved. This is a common natural phenomenon which occurs in response to all factors in life that are initially stimulating. If prolonged, they become enervating or exhausting, and in terms of therapy this is undesirable unless anaesthesia is required.

A short cold (water) application, for example, will stimulate, whereas a long one will sedate, and too much can kill. The words of Speransky and Selye should be recalled and the minimum effort used, consistent with achieving a response.

We have noted previously that many of the different reflex systems have points that seem to be interchangeable, and that many of these are traditional acupuncture points. In terms of local pain, the view of Chifuyu Takeshige (Takeshige 1985), Professor of Physiology at Showa University, is that: 'The acupuncture point of treatment of muscle pain is the pain-producing muscle itself.'

Respected acupuncture clinicians, such as George Ulett, suggest that 'acupuncture points are nothing more than time honoured muscle motor points'. Professor C. Chan Gunn, however, finds this too simple an explanation, and states: 'Calling acupuncture points "motor points" or "myofascial trigger points" is too simple. They are Golgi tendon organs.' These, and other researchers, are quoted by Stephen Botek, Assistant Professor of Clinical Psychiatry, New York Medical College (Ernst 1983).

Botek (1985) believes that 'myofascial needling' is the term of choice to define the type of acupuncture that dispenses with traditional explanations as to the effects of acupuncture. The points utilized in one study were Large Intestine 4 (Hoku) in the web between thumb and the first finger, and Stomach 36 (Tsu san li) below the knee. The study recorded skin temperature of the face, hands and feet. It was found that, compared with a resting period, both manual and electrical stimulation of both points induced a general warming effect. This was immediate in the face (Lewith & Kenyon 1984) and appeared after 10–15 minutes in hands and feet. The temperature increase was notably more marked after manual acupressure than after electrical stimulation. Manual stimulation of these points was shown to be more effective than other forms of stimulation.

Lewith & Kenyon (1984) point to a variety of suggestions having been made as to the mechanisms via which acupuncture, or acupressure, achieves pain-relieving results. These include neurological explanations such as the 'gate control theory'. This, and variations on this theme, look at the various structures of the CNS and the brain in order to define the precise mechanisms involved in acupuncture's pain-relieving action.

This, in itself, is seen to be an incomplete explanation, and humoral (endorphin, endocannabinoid release, etc.) and psychological factors, are also shown to be involved in modifying the patient's perception of pain.

A combination of reflex and direct neurological elements, as well as the involvement of a variety of secretions, such as enkephalins and endorphins, is thought to be the modus operandi of acupressure, and probably of all of the various systems of reflex activity discussed in this section (neurolymphatics, etc.).

Many of the points of referred pain and tenderness used in Western medical diagnosis are also acupuncture points, for example:

- Head's zones could be shown to include most acupuncture points, especially the Alarm and Associated points (given below).

- The points noted as being 'tender' in appendicitis, such as McBurney's, Clado's, Cope's, Kummel's, Lavitas's, are on the Stomach, Spleen and Kidney meridians of traditional acupuncture, and these are used by acupuncturists in treating appendicitis.
- Patients with a gastric ulcer produce tenderness at a site known as Boas' point, and this is sited precisely on Bladder point 21, which is the Associated point of the Stomach meridian.
- Brewer's point, in Western medicine, is noted in kidney infection, and this is Bladder point 20, the Associated point for the Spleen (in traditional acupuncture this has a controlling role over water, the element of the kidneys).

The degree of overlap between these well-known points can also be noted when comparing other classification systems of points.

Ah Shi points

Acupuncture methodology also includes the treatment of points that are not listed on the meridian maps, and that are known as Ah Shi points. These include all painful points that arise spontaneously, usually in relation to particular joint problems or disease. For the duration of their sensitivity they are regarded as being suitable for needle or pressure treatment. These points may therefore be thought of as identical to the 'tender' points described by Lawrence Jones in his strain/counterstrain method, discussed later in this chapter.

Alarm points, Associated points, Akabane points

There are, in traditional acupuncture, a number of key points that are most likely to become painful in relation to particular visceral dysfunction. These have been classified as Alarm points. They are presented below, and the following general information may make their employment easier:

- The Alarm points are found only on the ventral surface of the body, each point being associated with one of the 12 meridians and its functions. Six of the points are on the

midline, the others are bilateral. Tenderness elicited by palpation of an Alarm point may indicate dysfunction of the organ related to the point. In traditional acupuncture, if sensitivity is noted on light pressure, there is an associated energy deficiency. If heavy pressure is required, the condition relates to an energy excess.
- Associated points lie on the back of the body, and these are all on the Bladder meridian, which runs parallel to the spine, bilaterally. Each Associated point is related to one of the meridians and its function. The same assumed relationship with energy deficit or excess exists, as in Alarm points (sensitivity on light pressure = deficiency, and on heavy pressure = excess). There are also a few extra Associated points, as illustrated (see Fig. 4.3). Spontaneous pain at any of these listed points indicates a disorder in that meridian, and in its associated organ or function.
- Akabane points are found on the fingers and toes, being the terminal points of the meridians. Sensitivity of any of these is said to relate to dysfunction and imbalance of energy in that meridian. Electronic measurement of these points (Melzack et al 1977) is performed in a number of modern electroacupuncture systems such as electroacupuncture according to Voll (EAV). Manual testing is common, and was obviously the method used before electrical methods arrived on the scene. These points are all bilateral.

Location of Alarm points

Alarm points (Table 4.1, Fig. 4.2) are on the anterior surface of the body. Spontaneous pain at any point is considered to indicate a disorder of the affiliated meridian. If tenderness is elicited on light pressure, a deficiency of energy in the meridian is assumed, whereas tenderness elicited on heavy pressure indicates an excess of energy in the meridian.

These are reflex points for meridian function, and awareness of the roles apparently played by the various meridians in body energy economics is necessary to evaluate the significance of reactions that produce tenderness in Alarm points.

Table 4.1 Alarm points

			Acupuncture point
Point 1	Lung		LU1
Point 2	Liver		LV14
Point 3	Gall bladder	Bilateral	GB24
Point 4	Kidney		GB25
Point 5	Spleen		LV13
Point 6	Large intestine		ST25
Point 7	Heart constrictor		VC17
Point 8	Heart		VC14
Point 9	Stomach		VC12
Point 10	Triple heater		VC5
Point 11	Small intestine		VC4
Point 12	Bladder		VC3

Location of Associated points

Associated points are on the dorsum of the body (Fig. 4.3). Spontaneous pain is thought to indicate a disorder in the meridian associated with it. Tenderness elicited on light pressure indicates a deficiency in energy in that meridian, and tenderness elicited on heavy pressure indicates an excess of energy in the associated meridian. These points are all on the Bladder meridian and their associations are given in Table 4.2. The points are slightly lateral to the median line bilaterally and are also reflex points for the meridians with which they are associated.

Location of Akabane points

Akabane points (Table 4.3, Fig. 4.4) represent the terminal points of the meridians. Sensitivity of these is thought to relate to imbalance in the

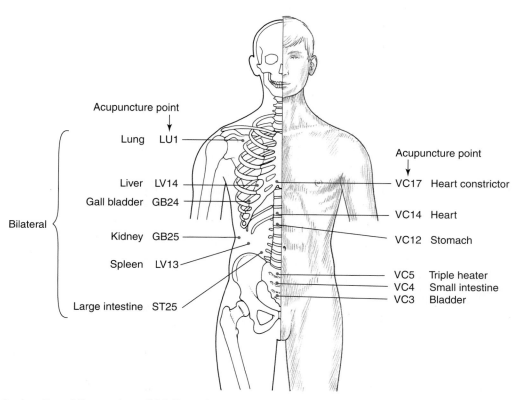

Figure 4.2 Location of Alarm points, which lie on the anterior surface of the body. If spontaneous pain develops in any alarm point, the associated meridian is thought to be involved. If light pressure produces tenderness, an 'energy deficiency' is considered to exist; if heavy pressure produces tenderness, an 'energy excess' is assumed. An understanding of the organs and functions associated with particular meridians is necessary in order to utilize these points therapeutically or diagnostically.

Figure 4.3   Location of Associated points, which lie on the dorsal surface of the body slightly lateral to the median line bilaterally. If spontaneous pain develops in any associated point, the allied meridian is thought to be involved. If light pressure produces tenderness, an 'energy deficiency' is considered to exist; if heavy pressure produces tenderness, an 'energy excess' is assumed. An understanding of the organs and functions associated with particular meridians is necessary in order to utilize these points therapeutically or diagnostically.

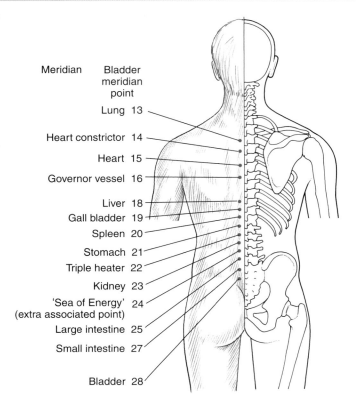

Meridian   Bladder
                meridian
                point

Lung 13
Heart constrictor 14
Heart 15
Governor vessel 16
Liver 18
Gall bladder 19
Spleen 20
Stomach 21
Triple heater 22
Kidney 23
'Sea of Energy' 24
(extra associated point)
Large intestine 25
Small intestine 27
Bladder 28

Table 4.2   Associated points

Meridian		Bladder meridian point
Point 1	Lung	B13
Point 2	Heart constrictor	B14
Point 3	Heart	B15
Point 4	Governor vessel	B16
Point 5	Liver	B18
Point 6	Gall bladder	B19
Point 7	Spleen	B20
Point 8	Stomach	B21
Point 9	Triple heater	B22
Point 10	Kidney	B23
Point 11	'Sea of Energy'	B24 (extra associated point)
Point 12	Large intestine	B25
Point 13	Small intestine	B27
Point 14	Bladder	B28

Table 4.3   Akabane points

Points on feet	Points on hands
1. Spleen	7. Large intestine
2. Liver	8. Heart constrictor
3. Stomach	9. Triple heater
4. Gall bladder	10. Heart
5. Kidney	11. Small intestine
6. Bladder	12. Lung

energy of the meridian. Comparative sensitivity shows relative imbalance in organ (energy) systems. Manual or electronic testing is possible.

Bennett's neurovascular reflex points

(Martin 1977)

A wide degree of clinical experience resulted in an American chiropractor, Terrence Bennett, reaching the conclusion that there was a group

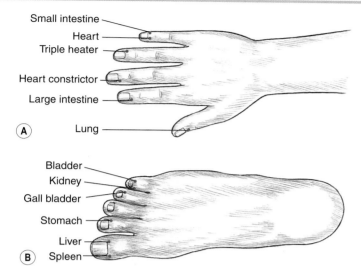

Small intestine
Heart
Triple heater
Heart constrictor
Large intestine
(A) Lung

Bladder
Kidney
Gall bladder
Stomach
Liver
(B) Spleen

Figure 4.4A,B Location of Akabane points, which represent the terminal points of the 12 meridians. Sensitivity of the points is thought to relate to imbalance in related organs (energy) systems. Both manual and electronic testing of these points is possible.

of previously unknown reflexes available for diagnostic and therapeutic use, which he termed neurovascular reflexes. He described his work in a series of lecture notes, which were compiled and published by Ralph Martin, after Bennett's death, as *Dynamics of Correction of Abnormal Function* (Martin 1977). The major points are listed in Chapter 5, which deals with diagnostic procedures.

Bennett describes the tissues that are palpated as altered in texture, being contracted or indurated, in much the same way as Chapman's reflexes (described below). His method of treatment calls for a slight degree of pressure, which he describes as 'only minimal, enough to render the tissues semi-anaemic, which is adequate stimulus'.

Experience indicates that the light pressure should be accompanied by slight stretching of the skin. In accordance with the views of Karel Lewit (1992), gentle stretching of the skin induces reflex activity when hyperalgesic (sensitized) skin zones are used therapeutically (see Ch. 5). When hyperalgesia occurs, skin becomes less elastic, with greater adherence to the underlying fascia and with lowered resistance to electricity.

In Bennett's system the skin is stretched with the minimum of force, so as to take up the slack, by the fingertips being drawn lightly apart. In most cases, if the area involves any degree of soft

tissue dysfunction, a lack of anticipated elasticity will be noted in the skin as this distraction takes place. By maintaining the slight stretch on the tissues (in effect a 'mini' myofascial release), a yielding occurs, and it is after this that a pulsation sensation should normally be felt. John Thie (1973) describes this pulsation sensation thus:

A few seconds after contact is made, a slight pulse can be felt, at a steady rate of 70 to 74 beats per minute. This pulse is not related to the heartbeat, but is believed to be the primitive pulsation of the microscopic capillary bed, in the skin.

Bennett insisted that the contact be maintained until a response was noted in the form of the tissue altering, relaxing and, most importantly, until the operator became aware of the presence of pulsation. This could arrive within a few seconds or take some minutes to emerge, depending on the patient and his or her condition. Bennett termed the pulsation felt as the 'arteriole pulse' because, he stated:

It is the beginning of the system, at the junction of the artery and the arteriole, that controls the metabolism. The sensation of pulsation is essential . . . It has to be there, or else we are not accomplishing anything.

Together with this, the change in tissue feel is important:

The tissues under your fingers begin to relax as you work for a few moments; you sense the degree of tension releasing. When it releases that is all you can do.

Some points are purely diagnostic, others are used for treatment, and some are both.

For example, the coronary reflex in the 2nd thoracic interspace on the left, which is a palpable area of tissue change and which is sensitive to the patient, is only diagnostic (not illustrated). Awareness of Bennett's reflex areas may be found to be a useful addition to the range of available therapeutic and diagnostic knowledge. In using NMT in its diagnostic mode, the tissues being evaluated will yield a multitude of sensitive points. Some of these may correlate with Bennett's findings, and they may then be used as part of an overall assessment of the nature of the dysfunction affecting the patient. They may, of course, also be used, as Bennett intended, as a system in their own right, for assessing and treating visceral and functional physiological changes and pathology. A number of Bennett's points have been incorporated into the methods of applied kinesiology, notably the points on the cranium, which are used for treating emotional disturbances.

Among the cautions issued by Bennett are:

- Do not overtreat the points on the cranium (2–3 minutes is a maximum).
- In hyperthyroid patients, do not treat the thyroid and pituitary reflexes at the same visit (one should be treated, and alternated with the other at a subsequent visit).
- If the heart is enlarged then the 3rd rib, at the mid-clavicular line, should not be treated.
- Aortic sinus reflex should be treated before any of the brain reflexes are contacted.
- If the ovary is being treated, the thyroid should receive prior attention.

A list of Bennett's reflex points can be found in Chapter 5, which considers diagnostic applications of NMT.

Chapman's reflexes

(Kuchera 1997, Mannino 1979, Owens 1980, Patriquin 1997, Walther 1988)

In the 1930s, Chapman and Owens described a 'neurolymphatic' reflex pattern, now widely used in osteopathic and chiropractic methodology. Chaitow (1965) discussed these reflexes as follows:

The reflexes of Chapman that I intend to discuss are not the whole picture – being only a part of the visible portion of the iceberg – but of immense value nonetheless. Drs Chapman and Owens first reported on Chapman's original findings in the late 1930s. A revised edition of their work has been published by the Academy of Applied Osteopathy. The surface changes of a Chapman's reflex are palpable. They may best be described as contractions located in specific anatomical areas and always associated with the same viscera. In describing each organ reflex Chapman normally indicated tissue reflex areas, occurring anteriorly and posteriorly. These reflexes found in the deep fascia are described as 'gangliform' contractions. These contractions vary in size from a pellet to a large bean and are located anteriorly in the intercostal spaces near the sternum. Similar tissue changes are found in those reflexes occurring on the pelvis. The tissue changes found in reflexes located on the lower extremities are described as 'stringy masses' or 'amorphous shotty plaques'. Those reflexes occurring posteriorly along the spine, midway between the spinal processes and the tips of the transverse processes are of a more oedematous nature.

Characteristics

Patriquin (1997) describes the characteristics of Chapman's reflexes as:

- small
- smooth
- firm
- discretely palpable
- approximately 2–3 mm in diameter.

Sometimes they are described as feeling like small pearls of tapioca, lying, partially fixed, on the deep aponeurosis or fascia.

Clinical value of the reflexes

Because the location of these palpable tissue changes is relatively constant in relation to specific viscera, it is possible to establish the location of pathology without knowing its nature. The value of these reflexes is threefold:

1. As diagnostic aids – Patriquin (1997) points out that some of the reflexes, such as that for appendix (tip of 12th rib on the right; see point 38 on Fig. 5.8B) are invaluable in helping with differential diagnosis when faced with right lower abdominal pain: 'Today, Chapman's reflexes are more likely to be used as an integral part of osteopathic physical examination than as a specific therapeutic intervention.'
2. They can be utilized to influence the motion of fluids, mostly lymph.
3. Visceral function can be influenced through the nervous system. '[The] reflexes can be clinically manipulated to specifically reduce adverse sympathetic influence on a particular organ or visceral system ... patients with frequent bowel movements from the effects of IBS report they have normal or near normal function for days to months after soft tissue treatment over the iliotibial bands and/or the lumbosacral paraspinal tissues and associated Chapman's reflexes' (Patriquin 1997). (See point 24, anterior and posterior, in Figs 5.8A and 5.8C.)

Mechanism of the reflexes

Regarding the mechanism whereby these reflexes act, it would appear that, in so far as the intercostal reflexes are concerned, stimulation of the receptor organs that lie between the anterior and posterior layers of anterior intercostal fascia acts through the intercostal nerve, which enervates the external and internal intercostal muscles and thus, through the sympathetic fibres, affects the intercostal arteries, veins, lymph nodes, etc. Stimulation thus causes afferent and efferent vessels draining these tissues to increase or decrease, permitting lymph flow to be increased or decreased, thus affecting the drainage of the entire lymph system in the area. Through the sympathetic fibres associated with these tissues, the lymph nodes of the vital organs are also affected.

Explaining results of neuromuscular technique

These reflexes seem to offer explanations for the sometimes startling results obtained through neuromuscular technique. Stanley Lief placed great emphasis on normalizing the tissues of the intercostal spaces and the paravertebral areas – sites of many major neurolymphatic reflexes. He also stressed the importance of not overtreating, a consideration that cannot be repeated too often.

Research evidence supports Chapman's reflex usefulness

- Caso (2004) reported a case study involving chronic constipation and low back pain. Use of Chapman's NL reflexes was seen to be useful diagnostically as well as therapeutically. 'The rather remarkable outcome from the application of this relatively simple, yet valuable, diagnostic and therapeutic procedure represents a thought-provoking impetus for future study and clinical application.'
- Lines et al (1990) treated 30 asymptomatic individuals, on four separate occasions, employing stimulation of the neurolymphatic reflexes theorized to relate to the diaphragm. Spirometric assessment of respiratory function before and after each treatment was performed. Measurements of forced vital capacity (FVC) and forced expiratory volume in 1 second (FEV1) over the whole sample showed no significant improvement following the treatment regimen. However eight of the 30 subjects had lower than predicted initial FVC and FEV1 values. *When the results for the group of eight subjects were analysed separately, it was found that a significant improvement was attained from the first pretreatment FVC to last posttreatment.*
- In a trial conducted to assess the effects of forms of manipulation on blood pressure, one of the methods used was stimulation of a Chapman's reflex (Mannino 1979). A specific effect attributable to this treatment was noted. The point chosen for treatment was the one related to adrenal function. The trial involved treatment of this point, or a sham point, in which pressure was applied to either the real or a false point, for a total of 2 minutes, in a

make-or-break circular motion. The point is located in the intertransverse space, on both sides of the 11th and 12th thoracic vertebrae, midway between the spinous processes and the tips of the transverse processes (see point 37 on Fig. 5.8F). The sham treatment involved the area between the 8th and 9th thoracic vertebrae, which relates to small intestine problems, and would have no effect on the sort of condition being assessed in these trials. The results showed no immediate effect on blood pressure, but did indicate fascinating alteration in aldosterone levels and subsequent blood pressure drop. Abnormalities in aldosterone levels have been shown in populations with essential hypertension. Following treatment of the reflexes there was a demonstrable and consistent fall in aldosterone levels within 36 hours of stimulation of the Chapman reflex for the adrenals, but no change at all in the levels when the sham points were stimulated. A drop of 15 mmHg systolic and 8 mmHg diastolic was noted some 36 hours after treatment of the adrenal points. The delay in response suggested that the treatment had a tendency to interrupt, or damp down, a feedback to the adrenal medulla by the sympathetic nervous system (Patriquin 1997).

Nimmo's dismissal of the Chapman reflexes

An element of disinformation has emerged regarding Chapman's neurolymphatic reflexes.

Vannerson & Nimmo (1971) writing in *The Receptor* – the journal of the organization that used (in the 1960s) to teach Nimmo's receptor-tonus technique (see Ch. 2) – stated:

Research has not borne out the presumption [by Chapman] of a neurolymphatic reflex. Muscle fibres, which alone have the specific function of constricting vessels, do not exist in the walls of lymph vessels, except for a few fibres in the thoracic duct, and a few large trunks. These are sparsely located, and have little effect in lymph fluid propulsion.

These two authors then deride Chapman's assertion that the reflexes could exist at specific sites, an idea that they call 'fantastic'.

Vanneron & Nimmo's first point is in contradiction to *Gray's Anatomy* (Gray 1973), which tells us that lymph moves in a number of ways. Filtration occurs, generated by filtration of fluid from the capillaries. There is also a degree of movement engendered by contraction of surrounding muscles, which compress lymph vessels, the movement of which is determined by the presence of valves. This muscular contraction is dependent upon normal activity, and muscular contraction–relaxation sequences. Lymph is further capable of being moved, in such regions, according to Gray, by massage movements. Pulsating arterial vessels, in close proximity, also assist lymph movement, as does respiratory movement. Also in contradiction of Vanneron & Nimmo, Gray states: 'The smooth muscle in the walls of the lymphatic trunks is most marked just proximal to the valves; stimulation of sympathetic nerves accompanying the trunks, results in contraction of the vessels; the intrinsic muscle of the vessels thus probably aids the flow of the lymph.'

In 1979, rhythmic pulse waves were recorded from the lymphatic vessels of five healthy, upright, motionless males at a rate of 8–10 per minute, asynchronous with respiration or leg movement (Oszeweski & Engeset 1979). Degenhardt & Kuchera (1996) describe the process as follows: 'The regulation of the intrinsic contractility of the lymphatic system is based on transmural distension of the vessel walls and neural and humoral mediators.'

They comment:

The physiology of the lymphatic system is quite complex. Research has only begun to demonstrate the many factors that influence lymphatic flow. The extrinsic compression of the myofascia on the lymphatics has been the focus of many manipulative techniques ... Studies now consistently demonstrate contractility in the lymphatic vessels. This intrinsic pumping has been shown to be under autonomic control, modulated locally by soft tissue chemicals and systemically produced hormones. Currently it appears that intrinsic contractions have more influence on lymph flow than extrinsic forces.

This evidence, therefore, suggests that the term 'neurolymphatic reflex', as described by

Chapman, may indeed be an accurate description of the phenomenon.

Vanneron & Nimmo's second observation (relating to the specificity of the reflex sites) may be more valid, especially if anatomical individuality is taken into account. Points of the body surface are never likely to be precisely identifiable by description of anatomical position. However, a general identification as to site is possible. McBurney's point, for example, if present in appendicitis, is usually located within a few degrees of its commonly described location. There are exceptions, of course, and in the inscrutable manner of the Orient, the Chinese have taken this well into account, in describing the locations of acupuncture points. The invention of the 'human inch', which takes account of the individual anatomical proportions of each person, allows for such individualization. In terms of the charts and maps to be found in this text, the same factor should be borne in mind. The positions are approximate, because variations exist from person to person.

Dysfunction in soft tissues is, however, palpable, and not dependent upon maps. Thus, the general guidelines provided by charts are useful, but cannot take the place of palpatory skills.

A complete illustrated list of Chapman's reflexes is found in Chapter 5, which deals with diagnosis and treatment using NMT.

Palpating for, and treating, the neurolymphatic points

Kuchera (1997) suggests: 'If Chapman's [neurolymphatic] myofascial tender points are to be tested, palpate them early in the examination because motion of the myofascial tissues in their area decreases their sensitivity. In this case their diagnostic clue, tenderness with palpation, may not be evident.'

If, during NMT assessment mode application to the anterior thorax and abdominal region (see Ch. 7) unusual tenderness is noted in the region of the umbilicus, this may relate to bladder, kidney or adrenal dysfunction (see points 15, 16 and 37 on Figs 5.8A & 5.8B); similarly, tenderness in the area if an anterior point is noted in the left fifth or sixth intercostal interspace (see points 13 and 14 on Fig. 5.8A), the patient may usefully

be asked about, for example, stomach or digestive symptoms.

Treatment of the lymphatic aspects of these dysfunctional organs or functions (should their existence be corroborated by other clinical evidence) might usefully include gentle applications of rotary pressure to the posterior points, in the sequence described in Chapter 5.

Arbuckle (1977) writes of Chapman's reflexes:

The diagnostic value of these reflexes is amazing. For instance, a female having severe pain in the right lower quadrant of the abdomen, presents several possibilities, but the offending organ may well be located by means of the reflexes, the positive one showing whether the disturbance is due to appendix, cecum, tube or ovary. With a degree of understanding of the interrelation of the endocrine glands, and of the importance of the lymphatics and the autonomic distribution, the therapeutic value of these considerations can be shown clinically. There is a definite sequence, which must be followed, in the management of these reflexes, to produce desired results, and, if not so applied, just as surely as the misapplication of any other therapy, further confusion of the body mechanism will result.

Connective tissue massage/manipulation

Another system that uses reflex effects diagnostically as well as therapeutically is connective tissue massage (CTM). CTM involves 'rolling' (or stretching using shear forces, or lifting) the tissues in order to achieve reflex and local effects.

Citak-Karakaya (2006) evaluated the use of CTM on 20 female patients with fibromyalgia (FMS). The results showed that:

Statistical analyses revealed that pain intensity, impact of FMS on functional activities, and complaints of non-restorative sleep improved after the treatment program.

Additional studies using CTM have demonstrated benefit in cases of:

• Migraine (Akbayrak et al 2001)
• Tension-type headache (Akbayrak et al 2002, Demiturk et al 2001)

- Fibromyalgia (Citak et al 2001)
- Raynaud's disease (Demiturk et al 2000)
- Autonomic imbalance (Reed 1988)
- Anxiety (McKechnie A et al 1983).

CTM: Method and mechanism

According to Ebner (1962), the palpable reflex tissue changes that are identified in diagnosis and treatment involving CTM, can take any of the following forms:

- drawn-in bands of tissue
- flattened areas of tissue
- elevated areas, giving the impression of localized swelling
- muscle atrophy or hypertrophy
- osseous deformity of the spinal column.

The common 'zones' of influence involving such changes are illustrated and discussed further in Chapter 5 (see Fig. 5.3). The digital strokes used in CTM pull and stretch the tissues, and it is suggested that the method's effectiveness is based on a viscerocutaneous reflex.

Bischof & Elmiger (1960) explain:

The specific mechanical stimulation of the pull on connective tissue seems to be the adequate stimulus to elicit the nervous reflex. Connective tissue massage/manipulation acts first on the sympathetic terminal reticulum in the skin. The smallest branches of the autonomic nervous system contact the impulses activated by the pulling strokes to the sympathetic trunk and the spinal cord. The impulses travel from the skin either through a somatosensory spinal nerve via a posterior root ganglion to the grey matter or over the vascular plexus to the same segmental sympathetic ganglion or to the ganglion of the neighbouring segment, through the ramus communicans albus to the posterior root and grey matter of the spinal cord. They terminate either directly or by means of the internuncial neurons at the efferent autonomic root cells.

In the efferent pathway the impulses travel from the autonomic lateral horn, or the intermediolateral column, over the anterior root, ramus communicans albus, to the segmental sympathetic ganglion or to the ganglion of the

neighbouring segment and finally to the diseased organ. The origin of the connective tissue reflex zones and the influence of the CTM depend on the relationship between the function of the internal organs, vessels, and nerves as well as the tissues of the locomotor apparatus, which descend from the same metamere.

Some of the reactions to CTM are normal autonomic responses such as pleasant fatigue, bowel movements and diuresis. Oedema is markedly reduced and hormonal distribution is seen to achieve a degree of balance. Aspects of CTM are similar to those of NMT, and the 'skin rolling' methods used in some body areas are virtually identical in application. The effects are therefore interesting from a comparative point of view.

Jones' tender points (Fig. 4.5)

(Jones 1980)

In his evolution of the 'strain and counterstrain' (SCS) functional manipulative approach to the normalization of hypertonicity, Lawrence Jones described a series of 'points' that he had identified. These sensitive areas were, Jones discovered, related to specific strains and stresses in the musculoskeletal system, and were used by the therapist as monitors while the areas were being guided into a position of ease, during which process there was both a reduction in sensitivity in the palpated tender point as well as a relaxation (increased ease) of the stressed tissues associated with it. The tender points as described by Jones and the methods of treating them fall within the umbrella term 'positional release techniques' (Chaitow 2001, D'Ambrogio & Roth 1997, Deig 2001). The methodology of SCS is summarized in Chapter 8, and is incorporated into the integrated (INIT) sequence for trigger point deactivation, as described in Chapter 9.

In many ways these 'tender' points, while sensitive to palpation, are not usually areas in which the patient was previously aware of pain. They are therefore similar to Ah Shi – spontaneously tender – points in traditional Chinese medicine (Chaitow 1991).

Significantly perhaps, as the area being treated is positioned in 'ease' so that tenderness vanishes

Connective tissue massage/manipulation 91

Squamosal
Nasal
Masseter-temporo-mandibular

Supra-orbital nerve
Infra-orbital nerve

Anterior 1st thoracic
Anterior acromio-clavicular
Latissimus dorsi

Anterior 7th cervical
Anterior 8th cervical
Depressed upper ribs

Anterior 7th thoracic
Anterior 8th thoracic
Anterior 9th thoracic
Anterior 10th thoracic
Anterior 11th thoracic
Anterior 2nd lumbar
Anterior 5th lumbar
Low ilium, flare out

Medial and lateral coronoid
Radial head
Anterior 12th thoracic
Anterior 1st lumbar
Iliacus
Anterior lateral trochanter
Low ilium
Thumb and fingers

Medial and lateral meniscus

Media and lateral patella

Media and lateral extension strain
of meniscus
Tibialis anticus, medial ankle

Media and lateral hamstrings

Flexion strain of ankle

Ⓐ

Figure 4.5A   Jones' points on the anterior body surface, commonly relating to flexion strains.

Figure 4.5   Location of Jones' tender points, which are bilateral in response to specific strain (acute or chronic) but are shown on only one side of the body in these illustrations. The point locations are approximate and will vary within the indicated area, depending upon the specific mechanics and tissues associated with the particular trauma or strain.

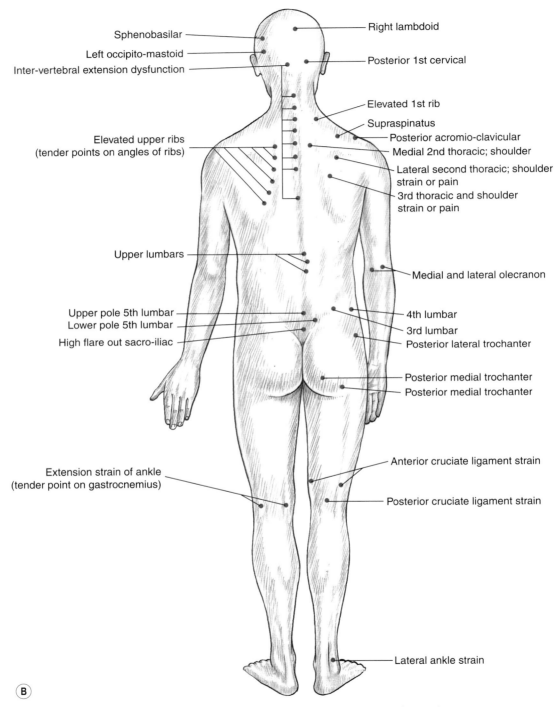

Sphenobasilar

Left occipito-mastoid

Inter-vertebral extension dysfunction

Right lambdoid

Posterior 1st cervical

Elevated 1st rib

Supraspinatus

Posterior acromio-clavicular

Medial 2nd thoracic; shoulder

Lateral second thoracic; shoulder strain or pain

3rd thoracic and shoulder strain or pain

Elevated upper ribs
(tender points on angles of ribs)

Upper lumbars

Medial and lateral olecranon

Upper pole 5th lumbar

Lower pole 5th lumbar

High flare out sacro-iliac

4th lumbar

3rd lumbar

Posterior lateral trochanter

Posterior medial trochanter

Posterior medial trochanter

Extension strain of ankle
(tender point on gastrocnemius)

Anterior cruciate ligament strain

Posterior cruciate ligament strain

Lateral ankle strain

B

Figure 4.5B   Jones' points on the posterior body surface, commonly relating to extension strains.

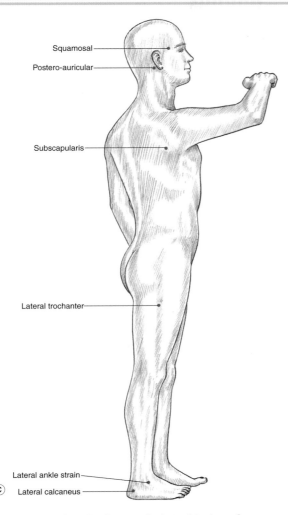

Squamosal

Postero-auricular

Subscapularis

Lateral trochanter

Lateral ankle strain

(c) Lateral calcaneus

Figure 4.5C Jones' points on the lateral body surface, commonly relating to strains involving side-bending or rotation.

Periosteal pain points

(Adapted from Lewit 1992)

These painful areas (Table 4.4) usually relate to acute or chronic contraction of associated muscles and tendons.

Felix Mann, pioneer acupuncture researcher and author, describes periosteal acupuncture as being more effective than ordinary acupuncture in a number of conditions (Mann 1963). He lists the sites given in Table 4.5 amongst the common sites usefully employed in this approach. Clinical experience indicates that NMT ischaemic compression techniques and muscle energy methods are as likely as traditional needling to produce benefit when treating these points.

Confusion?

The soft tissues are of major importance to the body's economy, structural integrity and well-being. They are also a major source of pain and dysfunction and, as must now be obvious, of reflex disturbances.

The various theories, methods and descriptive terminologies relating to the many point systems and classifications of 'points' are significant inasmuch as NMT offers the opportunity to access and use their potential. If we accept that there are many ways of looking at and interpreting the same phenomenon, then it will be an easy step to acknowledging that an acupuncture point and a trigger point and a Chapman's reflex point, for example, can all be the self-same point, but with different aspects of its reflex potential being considered in each classification.

NMT can (with other modalities) be used as an effective measure to detect and eliminate noxious trigger points and areas that generate or help to maintain dysfunction, or that influence reflexive activity. Such dysfunction can take the form of muscular weakness, muscular contraction, pain, vasodilatation, vasoconstriction, tissue degeneration, gastrointestinal disturbances, sympathetic nervous system abreactions, respiratory and a myriad other disorders including

from the tender point, a degree of ischaemic compression/inhibitory pressure/acupressure would be taking place. It is worth considering that the benefits noted, in terms of pain relief and reduction in contraction or spasm, could relate in some part to the resulting inhibitory/endorphin release action as well as to the subsequent improvement in circulation and possible neural influences, through the tissues and neurological modulation produced by the placing of the tissues into a situation of 'ease'.

Table 4.4   Periosteal pain points (adapted from Lewit 1992)

Site	Muscular/joint implication
Pain on head of metatarsals	Dropped arch, flat foot
Spur on calcaneum (pain on pressure)	Tight plantar aponeurosis
Pain on tubercle of tibia	Tight long adductor/possible hip dysfunction
Pain on head of fibula	Biceps femoris tightness
Posterior superior iliac spine tenderness	Various possible implications, involving low back, gluteal and sacroiliac region
Lateral aspects of symphysis pubis	Adductors tight. Hip or sacroiliac dysfunction
Pain on coccyx	Gluteus maximus tightness, possibly piriformis or levator ani involvement
Crest of ilium – pain	Tight quadratus lumborum/gluteus medius and/or lumbodorsal dysfunction
Pain on greater trochanter	Tight abductors/hip dysfunction
Pain on lumbar spinous processes (especially L5)	Tight paraspinal muscles
Pain mid-dorsal spinous processes	Lower cervical dysfunction
Pain spinous process of C2	Levator scapulae tight: C1–2, 2–3, dysfunction
Pain on xyphoid process	Rectus abdominus tight. 6–8 rib dysfunction
Pain on ribs, on mammary or axillary line	Pectoralis tightness. Visceral dysfunction referred to here
Pain at sternocostal junction upper ribs	Scalenus tightness
Pain on clavicle, medial aspect	Tight sternocleidomastoid
Pain transverse process of atlas	Tight sternocleidomastoid and/or recti capitis lateral. Atlanto-occipital dysfunction
Pain on occiput	Upper cervical or atlas dysfunction
Pain on styloid process of radius	Elbow dysfunction
Pain on epicondyles	Local muscular or elbow dysfunction
Pain at deltoid attachment	Scapulohumeral dysfunction
Mandibular condyles painful	Temporomandibular joint dysfunction. Tight masticators

emotional and 'psychological' disorders such as anxiety.

Noxious (pain producing) points that are the end result of various forms of stress imposed on the tissues housing them may reside in either hypertonic or hypotonic muscle, or in ligamentous or fascial tissues, or in apparently normal tissues. When active, such points will always be sensitive to correctly applied pressure and can often be neutralized by manual pressure or a combination of chilling and manual pressure and stretching.

In the treatment sections there will be discussion of methods for locating and treating such points; however, what effects each therapist attempts to achieve by manipulating reflexively active points depends on the individual's professional training and beliefs.

Table 4.5   Periosteal acupuncture points and associations

Site	Associated with
1. Appropriate transverse cervical process	Headache, migraine, interscapular pain and cervical spondylosis
2. Area of sacroiliac joint	Low back pain, sciatica without neurological deficit, testicular pain
3. Coracoid process	Painful shoulder joint
4. Medial condyle tibia	Knee pain, without advanced pathology
5. Neck of femur	Hip pain, without major changes evident on radiography
6. Lateral aspect of posterior spine of lower lumbar vertebrae	If sacroiliac joint (2 above) does not yield benefit, these areas may be used

References

Akbayrak T, Citak I, Demirturk F, et al: Manual therapy and pain changes in patients with migraine—an open pilot study, *Adv Physiother* 3:49–54, 2001.

Akbayrak T, Akarcal VI, Karabudak R, et al: The results of connective tissue manipulation in the treatment of tension type headache, *Pain Clin* 13:343–347, 2002.

Arbuckle B: 1977, The selected writings of Beryl Arbuckle, *National Osteopathic Institute and Cerebral Palsy Foundation.*

Baldry P: *Acupuncture, trigger points and musculoskeletal pain,* Edinburgh, 1993, Churchill Livingstone.

Birch S: On the impossibility of trigger point-acupoint equivalence: a commentary on Peter Dorsher's analysis, *J Altern Complement Med* 14(4):353–359, 2008.

Bischof I, Elmiger G: Connective tissue massage. In Licht E, editor: *Massage, manipulation and traction,* New Haven, Connecticut, 1960.

Bosey J: *Acupunct Electrother Res* 9(2):79–106, 1984.

Botek S: *Acupunct Electrother Res* 10(3):241, 1985.

Burkholder T: Mechanotransduction in skeletal muscle, *Front. Biosci* 12:174–191, 2006.

Caso M: Evaluation of Chapman's neurolymphatic reflexes via applied kinesiology: a case report of low back pain and congenital intestinal abnormality, *J Manipulative Physiol Ther* 27(1):66–72, 2004.

Chaitow L: An introduction to Chapman's reflexes, *British Journal of Naturopathy* (Spring) 1965.

Chaitow L: *Acupuncture treatment of pain,* Vermont, 1991, Healing Arts Press.

Chaitow: *Positional release techniques,* ed 2, Edinburgh, 2001, Churchill Livingstone.

Chen E: *Cross-sectional anatomy of acupoints,* Edinburgh, 1995, Churchill Livingstone.

Citak I, Akbayrak T, Akarcali I, Demirturk F: Connective tissue manipulation in treatment of fibromyalgia syndrome: a pilot study, *Turk J Physiother Rehabil* 12:110–114, 2001.

Citak-Karakaya I, et al: Short and long-term results of connective tissue manipulation and combined ultrasound therapy in patients with fibromyalgia, *J Manipulative Physiol Ther* 29:524–528, 2006.

D'Ambrogio K, Roth G: *Positional release therapy,* St Louis, Missouri, 1997, Mosby.

Degenhardt B, Kuchera M: Update on osteopathic medical concepts and the lymphatic system, *J Am Osteopath Assoc* 96(2):97–100, 1996.

Degenhardt B, et al: Role of osteopathic manipulative treatment in altering pain biomarkers: a pilot study, *Journal American Osteopathic Association* 107:387–394, 2007.

Deig D: *Positional release technique,* Boston, 2001, Butterworth-Heinemann.

DiGiovanna E: *An osteopathic approach to diagnosis and treatment,* Philadelphia, 1991, Lippincott.

Demirturk F, Akbayrak T, Citak, et al: Acute effects of connective tissue manipulation on skin temperature and blood flow rate in a patient with Raynaud's disease, *Turkish J Physiother Rehabil* 11:159–160, 2000.

Demirturk F, Akarcali I, Akbayrak T, et al: Results of two different manual therapy techniques in chronic tension type headache, *Pain Clin* 14:121–128, 2001.

Dorsher P: (Poster 196) Myofascial pain: rediscovery of a 2000-year-old tradition? *Arch Phys Med Rehabil* 85(9):e42, 2004.

Dorsher P, Fleckenstein J: 2008, Trigger Points and Classical Acupuncture Points, *Deutsche Zeitschrift fuer Akupunktur* 51(4):6–11.

Ebner M: *Connective tissue massage,* Edinburgh, 1962, Churchill Livingstone.

Ernst M: *Acupunct Electrother Res* 8(3/4):343, 1983.

Gray H: *Gray's anatomy,* ed 35, London, 1973, Longman.

Huijing P, Baan G: Myofascial force transmission causes interaction between adjacent muscles and connective tissue: effects of blunt dissection and compartmental fasciotomy on length force characteristics of rat extensor digitorum longus muscle, *Arch Physiol Biochem* 109:97–109, 2001.

Jones L: Strain and counterstrain, Boulder, Colorado, 1980, Academy of Applied Osteopathy.

Khalsa P, et al: The 2005 Conference on the Biology of Manual Therapies, *J Manipulative Physiol Ther* 29:341–346, 2005.

Kuchera W: Lumbar and abdominal region. In Ward R, editor: *Foundations for osteopathic medicine,* Baltimore, 1997, Williams & Wilkins.

Langevin HM, Bouffard NA, Badger GJ, et al: Dynamic fibroblast cytoskeletal response to subcutaneous tissue stretch ex vivo and in vivo, *Am J Physiol Cell Physiol* 288(3):C747–C756, 2005.

Langevin H: Connective tissue: A body-wide signaling network, *Med Hypotheses* 66(6):1074–1077, 2006.

Levin SM: Put the shoulder to the wheel: a new biomechanical model for the shoulder girdle. In Ribreau C, editor: *MechanoTransduction,* Paris, 2000, Societe Biomechanique, pp 131–136.

Lewit K: *Manipulative therapy in rehabilitation of the locomotor system,* London, 1992, Butterworths.

Lewith G, Kenyon J: *Soc Sci Med* 19(12):1367–1376, 1984.

Lines D, McMillan A, Spehr G: Effects of soft tissue technique and Chapman's neurolymphatic reflex stimulation on respiratory function, *J Aust Chiropr Assoc* 20:17–22, 1990.

McKechnie A, et al: Anxiety states: A preliminary report on the value of connective tissue massage, *J Psychosom Res* 27(2):125–129, 1983.

McPartland JM, Simons DG: Myofascial trigger points: translating molecular theory into manual therapy, *Journal Manual and Manipulative Therapies* 2007(14):232–239, 2007.

Mann F: *The treatment of disease by acupuncture,* London, 1963, William Heinemann Medical.

Mann F: 1983, International Conference of Acupuncture and Chronic Pain, September 1983.

Mannino J: The application of neurological reflexes to the treatment of hypertension, *J Am Osteopath Assoc* 79(4):225–230, 1979.

Martin R, editor: *Dynamics of correction of abnormal function*, Sierra Madre, 1977, Ralph Martin.

Melzack R, Stillwell D, Fox E: Trigger points and acupuncture points of pain, *Pain* 3:3–23, 1977.

Myers T: *Anatomy Trains*, ed 2, Edinburgh, 2008, Churchill Livingstone.

Northup G: The role of the reflexes in manipulative therapy, *J Am Osteopath Assoc* 40:521–524, 1941.

Oszeweski W, Engeset A: Intrinsic contractility of leg lymphatics in man, *Lymphology* 21:81–84, 1979.

Owens C: *An endocrine interpretation of Chapman's reflexes.* Newark, Ohio, 1980, American Academy of Osteopathy.

Patriquin D: Chapman's reflexes. In: Ward R, editor: *Foundations for osteopathic medicine*, Baltimore, 1997, Williams & Wilkins.

Reed B, Held J: Effects of sequential connective tissue massage on autonomic nervous system of middle aged and elderly adults, *Phys Ther* 68:1231–1234, 1988.

Serizawe K: *Tsubo: vital points for oriental therapy*, San Francisco, 1976, Japan Publications.

Simons D: Understanding effective treatments of myofascial trigger points, *Journal of Bodywork and Movement Therapies* 6(2):81–88, 2002.

Takeshige C: *Acupunct Electrother Res* 10(3):195–203, 1985.

Thie J: *Touch for health*, California, 1973, DeVorss.

Travell J, Simons D: *Myofascial pain and dysfunction*, vol 2, Baltimore, 1992, Williams & Wilkins.

Vannerson J, Nimmo R: Specificity and the law of facilitation in the nervous system, *The Receptor* 2(1):1971.

Wall P, Melzack R: *Textbook of pain*, Edinburgh, 1989, Churchill Livingstone.

Walther D: *Applied kinesiology*, Pueblo, 1988, SDC Systems.

5

Diagnostic methods

CHAPTER CONTENTS

Neuromuscular technique – assessment   **97**
and diagnosis
         Palpation   **98**
    Palpatory diagnosis   99
Mackenzie's abdominal reflex areas   104
Skin: reflex effects and hyperalgesic   **104**
skin zones
    Lifting skin folds (assessment)   105
Stretching superficial tissue (assessment)   106
Skin distraction (diagnostic and therapeutic)   109
Chapman's reflexes in diagnosis   **110**
and treatment
    Chapman's neurolymphatic reflexes   110
Bennett's neurovascular reflexes   **117**
          Conclusions   **117**
    Finding 'points' using NMT   121

In previous chapters we have dipped into the vast amount of information that exists in relation to the neuromuscular component of the human body.

A great many diagnostic aids exist for discovering just what is happening when aspects of this network of tissues malfunction. The great beauty of neuromuscular technique, as devised by Lief, is the way in which diagnostic and therapeutic processes are combined. The thumb, as it glides close to the spinal attachments of the paraspinal musculature, is assessing the tissue tone, density, temperature, etc., and at the same moment is capable of treating any tissues that display evidence of dysfunction (see discussion of STAR characteristics – sensitivity, tissue texture alteration, asymmetry, reduced range of motion – in Ch. 3). The response of the searching thumb or finger to whatever information the tissues impart can be immediate. The use of greater or lesser degrees of pressure, varying in direction and duration, allows the practitioner to judge and treat at the same time, and with great accuracy (Figs 5.1 & 5.2).

If treatment of musculoskeletal dysfunction is to be focused and meaningful, a diagnostic or assessment plan is required. Whilst local muscular changes will become more apparent as treatment progresses, an overall diagnostic picture is required to enable a coherent plan to emerge and for prognosis and progress to be judged.

Neuromuscular technique – assessment and diagnosis

If therapeutic intervention is to be structured and organized – and something other than hit and

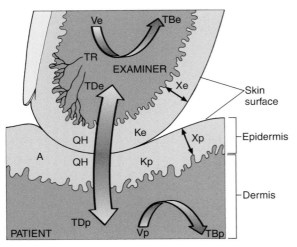

Figure 5.1   This diagram depicts some of the physical and physiological factors that affect the thermoreceptor (TR) discharge rate and consequently the temperature sensed in an examiner's skin in contact with a patient's skin. The temperature and rate of change of the examiner's thermoreceptors are functions of the net effects of the time that the tissues are in contact, their contact area (A), the temperatures (TBe and TBp) and volume flow rates (Ve and Vp) of blood perfusing the examiner's and patient's skin, epidermal thickness (Xe and Xp) and thermal conductivity (Ke and Kp) of both, dermal temperature (TDe and TDp) of both, as well as of the net heat exchange rate (QH) between the two tissues. QH is strongly affected by the heat transfer properties of material trapped between the two skin surfaces, for example air, water, oil, grease, hand lotion, dirt, tissue debris and fabric (Adams, Steinmetz, Heisey, Holmes & Greenman 1982).

Figure 5.2   Light 'skin on skin' palpation can give indications of deeper dysfunction due to modification of sympathetic and circulatory activity.

miss – there is a basic need for evaluation and assessment of the way in which the mechanical component of the body is adapting to its current situation, of the extent of changes from the norm, and of the ways in which patterns of pain, malcoordination and restriction are interacting. These changes might involve reflexively active structures such as myofascial trigger points, locally traumatized areas, fibrotic alterations, shortened and/or weakened muscles, joint restrictions and/or general or systemic factors (such as exist in arthritic conditions).

NMT provides a diagnostic/assessment tool and also offers, when it switches from assessment to actively therapeutic mode, a means whereby precisely focused and modulated degrees of force

can be directed towards influencing restricted tissues. Myofascial release techniques, as well as ischaemic compression (osteopathic inhibitory technique), can be applied to precise targets via the contacting thumb or finger in NMT. Perhaps NMT's greatest usefulness in assessment relates to the opportunity it offers for the identification of local soft tissue dysfunction in a gentle noninvasive manner. In the USA, as well as in the UK, the focus of many therapists utilizing NMT in recent years has been towards the identification and treatment of myofascial trigger points (and the often widespread musculoskeletal dysfunction that produces or is associated with them).

Palpation

There is no valid substitute for skilful palpatory diagnosis in ascertaining the relatively minute structural changes – primary or reflex – that often have far-reaching effects on the body's economy.

It is generally agreed that the pads of the fingers are the most sensitive portion of the hand available for use in diagnosis. Indeed, the combination of the thumb and first two fingers is the finest mechanism, and can be adapted to conform with the variable areas under palpatory consideration.

Palpatory diagnosis

(Baldry 1993, Beal 1983, DiGiovanna 1991, Travell & Simons 1983, 1992)

Skin assessment before adding lubricant

One of the most successful methods of palpatory diagnosis is to run the pads of a finger or several fingers extremely lightly over the (unlubricated) area being assessed, feeling for changes in the skin texture that may indicate alterations in the tissues below. After localizing any changes in this way, deeper periaxial structures can be evaluated by means of the application of greater pressure. There are a number of specific changes to be sought in light palpatory examination in both acute and chronic dysfunction.

Skin changes (Lewit 1992). Over an area of acute or chronic dysfunction, skin will feel tense, and will be relatively difficult to move or glide over the underlying structures. The skin above reflexively active structures will therefore be more adherent to the underlying fascia, something that will be evident in any attempt to glide or roll it, compared with skin covering normal areas. By applying a series of bilateral 'pushes' of skin on fascia, assessment is possible for asymmetry of movement.

The skin overlying reflexively active areas such as trigger points (or active acupuncture points) tends to produce a sensation of 'drag' as it is lightly stroked, because of increased hydrosis. There is also an apparent – very slight – sensation of undulation, a rising and falling, palpable on a light stroke, described illustratively as 'hills and valleys'.

Over areas of reflexogenically induced dysfunction, the skin will also lose its fully elastic quality, so that on light stretching (taking an area of skin to its easy resistance barrier on stretching) it will test as less elastic than neighbouring skin.

Methods for assessing these skin changes are described in more detail later in this chapter.

Assessment after adding lubricant

Dysfunctional patterns revealed by means of assessment of skin changes should become apparent in the application of neuromuscular palpation/assessment strokes, as described in detail in Chapters 6 & 7.

Induration. A slight increase in diagnostic pressure will show whether or not the superficial musculature has an increased indurated feeling ('dense', 'firm', less elastic). When chronic dysfunction exists, the superficial musculature will demonstrate a tension and immobility, indicating fibrotic changes within and below these structures. These changes are discussed further in the text dealing with the application of basic spinal and abdominal NMT (Chapters 6 & 7).

Temperature changes. In acute dysfunction, a localized increase in temperature may be evident. In chronic lesion conditions there may, because of relative ischaemia, be a reduced temperature of the tissues. This usually indicates that fibrotic changes have occurred.

Tenderness. Tenderness requires investigation. Is the tissue inflamed? Is the local area reflexively active? What is the nature and cause of the tenderness?

Oedema. An impression of swelling, fullness and congestion can often be obtained in the overlying tissues in acute dysfunction. In chronic dysfunction this is usually absent, having been replaced by fibrotic changes.

Localized contractures. Local - sometimes very small – areas, may display evidence of trigger point activity with the presence of taut bands, or minute contracture 'knots', that are exquisitely painful on pressure, and which may refer pain to distant areas.

Key questions

The questions that need to be asked when palpation elicits the sort of changes briefly outlined above, include:

- What tissues am I feeling?
- What significance does what I can feel have in relation to the patient's condition or symptoms?

- How does this relate to any other areas of dysfunction I have noted elsewhere?
- Is what I can feel acute or chronic?
- Is this a local problem, or part of a larger pattern of dysfunction?
- What do these palpable changes mean?

Deeper palpation: Peter Lief's perspective

In deeper NMT palpation, the pressure of the palpating fingers or thumb needs to increase sufficiently to make contact with structures such as the periaxial (paravertebral) musculature, without provoking a defensive response. The changes that might be noted could include immobility/rigidity, tenderness, oedema, deep muscle tension, fibrotic and interosseous changes. Apart from the fibrotic changes, that are characteristic of chronic dysfunction, all these changes can be found in either acute or chronic problems.

As Peter Lief (1963), son of the innovator of NMT, explains:

Palpation is the main method of detection. Gross lesions are easily palpable, but sometimes they are so minute that their detection presents considerable difficulty, especially to the beginner. It sometimes takes many months of practice to develop the necessary sense of touch, which must be firm, yet at the same time sufficiently light, in order to discern the minute tissue changes that constitute the palpable neuromuscular lesion.

The presence of a lesion is always revealed by an area of hypersensitivity to pressure, an area which may be better described as being 'a painful spot'. After these have been detected and noted, specific attention is given to them in the subsequent treatments.

Note: the word 'lesion' as used by Lief and Youngs (see below) refers to what is now described as 'somatic dysfunction'.

Youngs' NMT description: tissue changes and objectives

Youngs (1964) has described what it is that the palpating fingers are seeking and finding and, as in NMT diagnosis and treatment often take place together, what they are achieving:

The changes which are palpable in muscles and soft tissues associated with reflex effects have been listed by Stanley Lief. They are essentially 'congestion'. This ambiguous word can be interpreted as a past hypertrophic fibrosis. Reflex cordant contraction of the muscle reduces the blood flow through the muscular tissue and in such relatively anoxic regions of low pH and low hormonal concentration, fibroblasts proliferate and increased fibrous tissue is formed. This results in an increase in the thickness of the existing connective tissue partitions – the epimysia and perimysia, and also this condition probably infiltrates deeper between the muscle fibres to affect the normal endomysia. Thickening of the fascia and subdermal connective tissue will also occur if these structures are similarly affected by a reduced blood flow. Fat may be deposited, particularly in endomorphic types, but fibrosis is most pronounced in those with a strong mesomorphic component – a useful pointer for both prognosis and prophylaxis.

Fibrosis seems to occur automatically in areas of reduced blood flow, e.g., in a sprained ankle – where swelling is marked and prolonged, in the lower extremities where oedema of any origin has been constant over a period, in the gluteals where prolonged sitting is a postural factor, and in the neck and upper dorsal region where psychosomatic tension is frequent to a marked degree – depending upon the constitutional background. Where tension is the aetiological factor, fibrosis seems teleological.

Many devices have been developed to ease the strain on muscles which tend to be permanently contracted, e.g., locking of the knee joint, or the exact balance of the head on the shoulders, where only gentle contraction is needed to maintain postural integrity. If postural integrity is lost through some cause or another, then the strain on the muscle may be eased by structural alteration and the increase of fibrous tissue in the muscles acts to maintain normal position of the head. Fibrous tissue can then take the strain instead of the muscle fibres. It is this long-term homeostatic reflex which apparently operates in all cases of undue muscle contraction, whether due to strain or tension.

From this one can amplify Stanley Lief's beneficial effects of neuromuscular treatment as follows:

1. *To restore muscular balance and tone.*
2. *To restore normal trophicity in muscular and connective tissues by altering the histological picture from a patho-histological to a physiologic–histological pattern with normal vascular and hormonal response.*
3. *To affect reflexively the related organs and viscera and to tonify them naturally.*
4. *To improve drainage of blood and lymph through the areas subject to gravitational or postural stasis, e.g., abdominal vessels not necessarily connected with viscera.*
5. *To reduce fatty deposits.*

Thus the hyperaemia, resulting from [NMT] treatment automatically operates to reverse the original patho-histological picture and consequently normality will be approached.

Trigger points

In clinical terms it is safe to say that a chronic state of dysfunction exists if soft tissues have been consistently stressed for more than a few weeks, for after such a short period fibrotic adaptations begin to be palpable.

There is clinical evidence that trigger points have a consistent distribution, and their localization can be predicted by studying the patterns of referred dysfunction and pain to which they give rise. Similarly patterns of referred pain are predictable if the trigger point can be located (Travell 1957, Travell & Simons 1992).

A patient with unexplained pain, the examination of which reveals no local cause, may well have trigger points feeding pain messages into the target area. Thus the point at which the patient feels pain, and the point at which the pain originates, are often not the same, and knowledge of the reference patterns as illustrated in Chapter 3 (see Fig. 3.6) is therefore important.

Whether treatment of trigger points consists of anaesthetic injections, acupuncture, cryotherapy, or pressure and stretch techniques (NMT), or combinations such as INIT (see Ch. 9), the diagnostic aspect remains the same. Deep palpation and pressure on the located point must reproduce the symptoms in the target area in order to 'prove' the connection.

Zones of dysfunction: connective tissue changes

As well as trigger points there exist a number of palpable and often visible (Box 5.1) zones of soft tissue alteration, possibly involving viscerosomatic activity, in which diseased or stressed organs negatively influence soft tissues paraspinally and elsewhere (Bischof & Elmiger 1960). Viscerosomatic reflexes and the processes of facilitation (sensitization) were discussed in Chapter 3. Some of these zones overlap and incorporate 'trigger' points, so a general awareness and knowledge of their existence is useful if an understanding of what can be achieved in NMT is to be more complete (Fig. 5.3).

As organs mainly receive their autonomic supply homolaterally, changes of a reflex nature will normally be found on the same side of the body surface:

- On the right side will be found the connective tissue reflex zones from the liver, gall bladder, duodenum, appendix, ascending colon, ilium, etc.
- On the left side will be found the reflex zones from the heart, stomach, pancreas, spleen, jejunum, transverse colon, descending colon, rectum, etc.
- Central zones occur as a result of dysfunction in the bladder, uterus and head.
- Changes on the homolateral side of the body occur due to dysfunction of the lungs, suprarenal glands, ovaries, kidneys, blood vessels and nerves on that side.

According to Teiriche-Leube & Ebner (quoted in Teiriche-Laube 1960), these changes in the connective tissue and muscles can take the following forms:

- drawn-in bands of tissues
- flattened areas of tissue
- elevated areas, giving the impression of localized swelling
- muscle atrophy or hypertrophy
- osseous deformity of the spinal column.

Box 5.1 Assessing the dominant eye

In making a visual diagnosis it is important for the practitioner/therapist to be sure of the information he or she is acquiring. American osteopathic physician Edward Stiles (1984) made a valuable contribution to this area by pointing out that it is often for reasons of position, in observing structure, that a student or practitioner fails to see what is obvious:

> By being so positioned as to bring into play the non-dominant eye this becomes far more likely. The orientation of the subject in the field of view is determined by the position of the dominant eye, and thus it is essential to initially ascertain which eye this is.

Hold your hands straight in front of you with the palms facing each other. Bring them together to make an aperture (gap) of about 1–2 inches across. Looking through this aperture, focus on an object across the room from you. Close first one eye and then the other. When the non-dominant eye is closed the image you see through the aperture will not change. When you close the dominant eye the image shifts out of the field of vision.

The dominant eye is not always on the same side as the dominant hand. If dominant hands and eyes are on different sides, this can lead to problems of accurately assessing palpatory findings, and the advice given is to palpate with eyes closed, where possible, in such cases.

When assessing visually, make sure that the dominant eye is lined up with the area or object being viewed. In an example where assessment of the chest is being made, Stiles suggested that, because most accurate visual information would be gained when the dominant eye was over the midline, the observation of the supine patient should be from the head of the table, and that this should be approached from the side that brings the dominant eye closest to the patient.

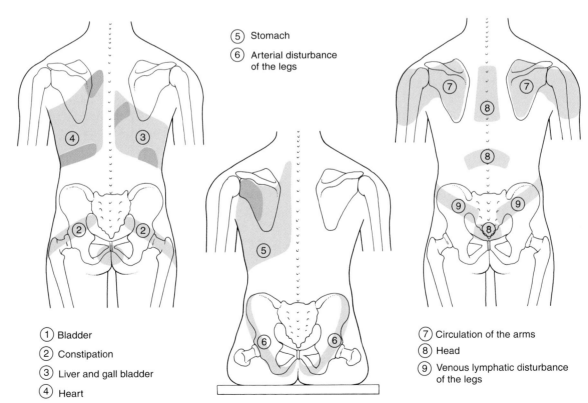

(5) Stomach
(6) Arterial disturbance of the legs

(1) Bladder
(2) Constipation
(3) Liver and gall bladder
(4) Heart

(7) Circulation of the arms
(8) Head
(9) Venous lymphatic disturbance of the legs

Figure 5.3 Connective tissue reflex zones (after Ebner).

For Teiriche-Leube & Ebner's description of some of these zones, see Box 5.2.

Using NMT in its assessment mode, as described in Chapters 6 & 7, or in specialized skin diagnosis (see below), these and other areas of soft tissue dysfunction can be readily located, identified and treated, even if no obvious symptoms of the associated conditions or diseases are present. It is clear that soft tissue changes often precede the appearance of symptoms of underlying pathology, and in this alone the diagnostic value of these zones is evident.

Practitioners using German connective tissue massage/manipulation (CTM) claim that it is often possible to beneficially influence symptoms of organ dysfunction, and to improve the function of these organs (liver, stomach, etc.), by treatment of the congested fibrotic reflex zone. This is not, however, to be considered an end in itself because it is clear that underlying causative factors and pathology (nutrition, infection, etc.) should also be dealt with. However, the value of this neuromuscular modality should not be underestimated.

Box 5.2   Altered connective tissue zones resulting from disturbed organs and functions

1. **Bladder**
   Small 'drawn in' area above anal cleft. Iliotibial tract may be drawn in. Swelling lateral aspect of ankles.
   Symptoms – Bladder dysfunction. Cold feet and legs (below the knee). Rheumatic diagnosis.

2. **Constipation**
   'Drawn in' band 2–3 inches (5–8cm) wide, running from middle third of the sacrum downwards and laterally.
   Symptoms – Tendency to, or actual, constipation.

3. **Liver and gall bladder**
   Large 'drawn in' zone over right thoracic region and a band along lateral costal border on the right side. Small 'drawn in' area between lower vertebral border of scapula to spine at the 5th and 6th dorsal level. 7th cervical area appears swollen or congested.
   Symptoms – Liver and gall bladder dysfunction and anyone who has suffered from hepatitis.

4. **Heart**
   Tension over left thoracic region including lower costal margin. If hepatic circulation is involved, right costal margin will also be affected. The area between the left scapula and 2nd and 3rd dorsal vertebrae will be indurated. Posterior aspect of axilla appears thickened.
   Symptoms – Coronary and valvular diseases of the heart.

5. **Stomach**
   (a) Overlapping the heart zones (above).

Symptoms – Stomach dysfunction.
   (b) Localized tension area below lateral aspect of the left scapular spine.
   Symptoms – Gastric ulcer and gastritis.

6. **Arterial disease of legs**
   A V-shaped configuration of the buttocks is noticed when sitting, rather than the normal rounded shape.
   Symptoms – Circulatory disturbance accompanied by angiospasm.

7. **Arms**
   'Drawn in' areas over scapula extending over posterior deltoid.
   Symptoms – Circulatory arm and hand problems. Neuritis paraesthesia.

8. **Head**
   (a) Thoracic area between scapulae.
   Symptoms – Insomnia and all types of headache.
   (b) Lower third of sacrum just above bladder zone.
   Symptoms – Headaches related to digestive dysfunction.
   (c) Just below origin of trapezius.
   Symptoms – Headaches due to tension.

9. **Venous lymphatic disturbance of the legs**
   A tight band from middle third of sacrum, parallel to iliac crest laterally and anteriorly over gluteus medius.
   Symptoms – Cramp. Swollen legs in summer, varicose veins and paraesthesia.

Mackenzie's abdominal reflex areas

Youngs (1964) points out that Sir James Mackenzie established a clear relationship between the abdominal wall and the internal abdominal organs (Mackenzie 1909). Mackenzie showed that organs that cannot react directly to painful stimuli (i.e. the majority) react by producing spasm and paraesthesia in the reflexively related muscle wall (the myotome), often augmented by hyperaesthesia of the overlying skin (dermatome) (see Figures 5.4A, B, C).

The reflexes involved occur via the autonomic nervous system and may be viscerosomatic or – as has been shown by many researchers, including Lief – the origin may be somatic and the reflex, therefore, somaticovisceral.

Mackenzie's abdominal reflex areas are as illustrated in Fig. 5.4C and, although there is sometimes a degree of individualization, it is reasonable to state that the presence in abdominal muscles and connective tissues of contracted or sensitive areas indicates (in the absence of recent trauma or strain) some underlying dysfunction that is causing or resulting from the soft tissue lesion. (See also discussion in Chapter 7 of Pain variables in somatic abdominal tissues.)

Skin: reflex effects and hyperalgesic skin zones

The work of Mackenzie early in the 20th century, as well as research into connective tissue zones

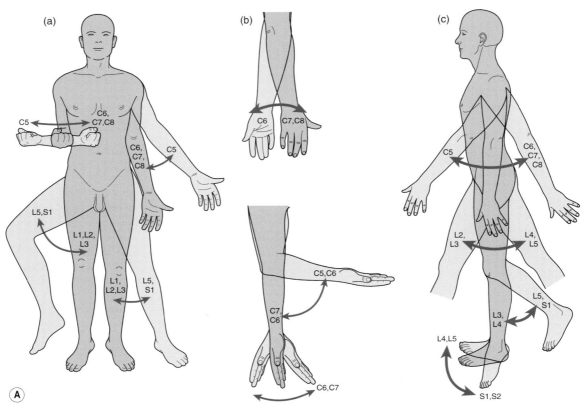

Figure 5.4A   Reflex myotomes: These examples show which spinal nerves innervate the skeletal muscles that produce the movements indicated by the arrows. **A,** Rotation and abduction/adduction of the arm and hip. **B,** Flexion/extension of the hand and wrist; pronation/supination of the hand. **C,** Flexion/extension/hyperextension of the arm, hip, and knee; dorsiflexion and plantar flexion of the foot. *C,* Cervical spinal nerves; *L,* lumbar spinal nerves; *S,* sacral spinal nerves; *T,* thoracic spinal nerves. (From Thibodeau GA, Patton KT: *Anatomy and Physiology,* ed 5, St Louis, 2003, Mosby.)

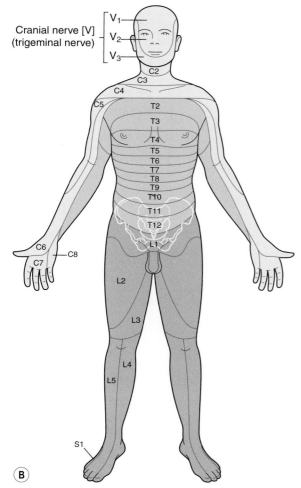

Cranial nerve [V]
(trigeminal nerve)

Figure 5.4B Anterior view of Dermatomes. Relating to the relationship between the spinal nerve & skin.

evolving out of Bindegewebsmassage in Germany, demonstrates that the surface of the body offers evidence of internal dysfunction (see Fig. 5.4C), and that it is possible to influence the interior by application of reflexively powerful stimuli from the surface.

Koizumi (1978) found that stimulation of the skin of the abdomen produced profound inhibition of intestinal movement. Stimulation of the skin produces an increase in sympathetic activity associated with the intestine, thereby inhibiting peristalsis. Koizumi noted that this was a strong effect, and that the intestine often became completely quiescent.

Stimulation of other skin areas, notably the neck, chest, forelimbs and hindlimbs, inhibited sympathetic activity, and therefore actually augmented intestinal motility. Vagal involvement in these changes was thought to be minimal, for when the vagi were sectioned the same responses were still noted. Reflexes disappeared, however, when the sympathetic nerve supply to the intestine (the splanchnic nerves) was sectioned. If we consider the involvement of these mechanisms in affecting internal function, via stimulus applied to the skin, we may better appreciate the findings of Chapman (Owen 1980), Bennett (Arbuckle 1977) and others, in their work on the multitude of reflex areas, that they have so painstakingly charted, and which are discussed later in this chapter.

The sometimes dramatic effects obtained by the use of CTM (see previous chapter) can also be seen to relate to the patterns of therapeutic and diagnostic opportunities that this knowledge offers. For example, various techniques are available to us in diagnosing from, and treating, the cutaneous structures for reflex effect. These include skin rolling, as well as the delicate 'skin distraction' or stretching method, advocated by Lewit (1992, 1999). Lewit discusses hyperalgesic skin zones that are likely to be present in the skin overlying most areas of reflex activity. He points out a major advantage afforded by an awareness of hyperalgesic skin zones (HSZs): unlike the eliciting and mapping of areas, points or zones, which rely upon the subjective reporting of the patient, these areas are palpable to the operator.

A popular method of identifying relative tension in skin is to 'roll' it.

A fold of skin is formed, and this is rolled between the fingers (see Fig. 8.17). This method may produce some discomfort, or even transient pain (a sharp 'cutting' sensation is often reported), but is useful in that the increased tension, and visibly thicker skin fold thus produced (compared with surrounding tissues) can then be diagnostic of a HSZ.

 Lifting skin folds (assessment)

The assessment methods used in CTM are designed to obtain a picture of the mobility of the various layers of the connective tissue, as well

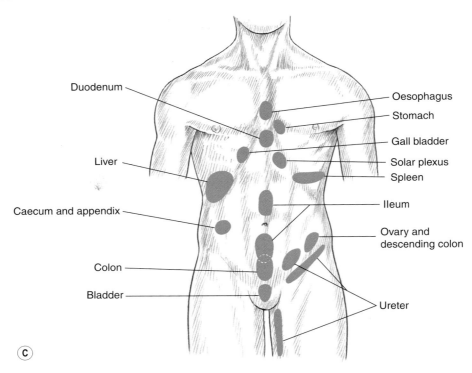

Figure 5.4C Reflex abdominal areas (after Mackenzie).

as an idea of their consistency. One such method involves the lifting of skin folds, with the patient sitting. The skin is gripped between thumb and fingers, with care being taken not to pinch the fold (Fig. 5.5). The fold comprises sufficient tissue to allow it to be lifted away from the fascial layer. This is usually performed by starting at the lower costal margin and going up as far as the region of the shoulders. In some areas, especially overlying the mid-dorsal region, if there is any dysfunction involving the liver, gall bladder, stomach or heart, restriction of tissue elasticity will be noted. By lifting two folds simultaneously, right and left, it is possible to compare the relative freedom of these tissues.

 ### Stretching superficial tissue (assessment)

A second method may be used, in which relatively smaller areas are assessed, with the patient prone or seated.

- With fingers lightly flexed, and using only enough pressure to produce adherence

between the fingertips and the skin, a series of short pushing motions are made simultaneously with both hands, which stretches the tissues to their elastic barrier (Fig. 5.6).
- Usually the pattern of testing goes from inferior to superior, sometimes in an obliquely diagonal direction towards the spine.
- If the patient is seated and the operator works from behind, tissues from the buttocks to the shoulders may be tested, always comparing the sides for symmetry of range of movement to the elastic barrier.

Two quite different evaluations can be performed simultaneously:

1. Becoming aware of asymmetry and noting areas of interest for more refined assessment, wherever skin does not slide as easily on the underlying tissue on one side, compared with the other
2. Additionally and alternatively, the possible organ or system reflexes may be noted, if that is of interest to the therapist (see Box 5.1).

Areas investigated, direction of stretch of tissues, and possible implications of reduced elasticity include:

1. The buttocks – stretching tissue from the ischial region towards the lateral borders of the sacrum (arterial and constipation zone).
2. From the posterior aspect of the trochanters, towards the iliac crests (venous lymphatic and arterial disturbances of legs).
3. From the trochanters, towards sacroiliac joints (venous lymphatic zone).
4. Over the sacrum, working from the apex towards the upper sacral segments (bladder and headache zones).
5. Over the lumbar region, on either side of the spine, working upwards (kidney zone).

(A)

Figure 5.5A   Skin folds can be lifted from the underlying fascial layer to test for restrictions, which may indicate local or reflexive dysfunction.

(B)

Figure 5.5B   Lifting skin fold on abdomen as part of CTM assessment

(A)

Figure 5.6A   Testing and comparing skin and fascial mobility as bilateral areas are 'pushed' to their elastic barriers.

Figure 5.6B   These lines indicate directions of application of CTM using tension, shear, bending and torsion forces, in assessment and treatment. Restricted mobility of superficial tissue-on-fascia will be evident when dysfunction exists, giving similar feedback to that noted in use of the 'pushing' methods illustrated in Figure 5.6A, and skin rolling approaches described above and illustrated in Figure 8.17.

6. Bilaterally up the spine, from lower costal region to the mid-thoracic level (liver and gall bladder zone (right side), and heart, stomach (left) and pulmonary (bilateral)).
7. Between the scapulae (headache zone).
8. Over the scapulae, from inferior angle, towards spine of scapula (arm zone).

Normal variations will exist independent of reflex activity, and in individuals carrying increased adipose tissue a generally greater

degree of tension or adherence will be noted, compared with a thinner individual.

An older person's skin will feel looser, in comparison with that of a younger individual. The skin over the lumbar region is naturally less mobile than that in other regions.

Note that it is adherence ('*tightness of tissues to each other*') that is being assessed, and this may or may not be accompanied by sensitivity. In connective tissue massage assessment of this sort is made regularly, as it is seen to be both diagnostic and prognostic, showing the rate of progress or lack of it, and providing a possible insight into visceral and functional status.

Skin distraction (diagnostic and therapeutic)

Lewit (1992) describes a method that he finds reliable, painless and therapeutically very useful. Any area of skin may be assessed in this way, large or small, with fingertip or hand contact.

In a small area, the fingertips (both index fingers) or index and middle fingertips of both hands, are placed close together, resting on the tissues to be tested. By separating the fingers, the skin is pulled apart and stretched to its easy elastic barrier (Fig. 5.7).

A minimum of force is used, in order simply to take out the slack in the skin. The 'easy' end-position is noted, as is the degree of 'springing' available in the tissues. This is compared in several directions, over the area being assessed, and

Figure 5.7 Hyperalgesic skin zones that lie above reflexive dysfunction (e.g. trigger points) are identified by means of the sequential stretching to their elastic barrier of local areas of skin. A series of such stretches indicates precisely those areas where elasticity is reduced in comparison to surrounding tissues. These are then tested for sensitivity and potential to cause referred pain by the application of ischaemic compression (inhibition).

comparison is also made with the presumably healthy tissue on the contralateral side.

If a hyperalgesic skin zone (HSZ) is present, then a greater degree of resistance will be noted after the slack has been taken up. Where there is such resistance, if the end-position of stretch is held for between 10 and 20 seconds, the resistance will be felt to ease, and the normal physiological degree of springing will then be noted. This is a measurable phenomenon and, by marking the first stretch position with a skin pencil and marking the stretch position available after 'release of the tissue', a significant increase is usually noted.

The techniques may be used for even small areas (e.g. between the toes). These may be stretched by fingertip (light) pressure and separation. Larger areas, such as regions of the back, may be contacted by the ulnar border of the hands in order to introduce separation stretch. The hands are crossed and placed on the tissue to be tested or treated. Separation of the hands introduces stretch to take up the slack. (See Figs 8.20A and 8.20B.)

Having introduced this initial degree of stretch, resistance (end-feel) is then noted. If the tissues are resistant to stretch, and springiness is absent, the maintenance of the stretch (painless) achieves a release of the tissues over a period of less than half a minute as a rule.

All trigger points, tender points, connective tissue zones, Mackenzie's abdominal areas, etc. are characterized by the presence of such a HSZ in the overlying tissues. This very useful tool allows easy identification of reflex activity and is itself an ideal form of treatment of these reflexes in sensitive individuals, and further provides accurate evidence of the subsequent situation. Techniques for treating skin and superficial tissue are further discussed in Chapter 8.

Scar tissue often leads to the presence of HSZs around the scar, and these frequently become focal points of reflex activity. Specific release methods, as described in Chapter 8, may be used to alter the status of tissues affected by scar tissue (Lewit & Olšanská 2004). Acupuncture can also be a useful method of treating very sensitive aspects of the scars themselves (Baldrey 1993).

Chapman's reflexes in diagnosis and treatment

The reflexes described by Chapman are now commonly termed 'neurolymphatic' reflexes. These can be used in diagnosis and treatment, and as a guide to the effectiveness of treatment. See additional discussion of these reflexes in Chapter 4.

In 1965 I described the technique for using these as follows (Chaitow 1965):

> Treatment applied through these reflexes, as advocated by Chapman and Owens, consists of a firm but gentle rotary pressure imparted by the index or middle finger. The finger should not be allowed to slip. As these areas are acutely sensitive great care should be taken not to overtreat as the reflex will become fatigued and no benefit will be derived.

My current view coincides with the above method except that I now use a variable thumb pressure that fits in with the general neuromuscular technique. Knowledge of the exact location of the reflexes is of primary importance.

Methodology

- By gentle palpation, the practitioner/ therapist should first ascertain the presence of involved reflexes. (See Table 5.1 and Figs 5.8A–F.)
- The anterior reflexes should be tested first.
- If found to be present, the anterior reflex should be treated first, then the posterior counterpart of the involved anterior reflexes should be treated.
- The anterior reflex has, therefore, a dual role: namely, for assessment, and then to initiate the reflex treatment.
- The anterior reflex is later of value to ascertain the effectiveness of treatment (after both anterior and posterior reflexes have been treated).
- If, on re-palpating the reflexes, there is no change in the feel or tenderness, the treatment should be repeated.
- If there is again no change, this indicates either that the pathology is too great for rapid change, or that pathology is irreversible.

- It may also indicate that some musculoskeletal factor is maintaining the reflex.
- Primary treatment should then be directed at this factor rather than the reflex.
- The degree of treatment should be ascertained by palpation.

Chapman and Owens described dosage of treatment in terms of seconds, but in practice I feel that anyone experienced in neuromuscular treatment would have the degree of sensory awareness required to 'feel' when sufficient treatment had been given.

I would stress that I have found the reflexes of Chapman useful in differential diagnosis, and in the treatment of various conditions from spastic constipation to migraine – but always as a part of a broader approach to the patient as a whole. That they can influence lymphatic drainage dramatically, I have no doubt. I am less sure of the effect on visceral conditions, but have found that the reflexes themselves provide an excellent guide to progress. If they are no longer present, then invariably the condition is progressing well. These personal observations are confirmed by Patriquin (1997).

Chapman's neurolymphatic reflexes
(Fig. 5.8A–F)

The research evidence for, and the possible mechanisms relating to, Chapman's neurolymphatic reflexes, were presented in Chapter 4.

In this chapter the method used in their application, as well as their positions, are discussed.

Chapman (Owen 1980) suggested a vibratory treatment in stimulating the neurolymphatic reflexes, lasting 10–15 seconds. He used fingertip pressure to impart the required energy, although thumb pressure of varying intensity is just as effective. This can be applied as a gradually intensifying pressure building up over 5–8 seconds, easing for 2 or 3 seconds and then repeated. Altogether this should not take more than half a minute.

These points can be overtreated and the optimum time would seem to be from 15 to 30 seconds with the pressure (or squeeze) of a variable nature. If the patient is able to report a referred pain resulting from the pressure, then

Table 5.1   Location of Chapman's neurolymphatic reflexes

No.	Symptoms/area	Anterior	Fig.	Posterior	Fig.
1.	Conjunctivitis and retinitis	Upper humerus	5.8A	Occipital area	5.8C
2.	Nasal problems	Anterior aspect of first rib close to sternum	5.8A	Posterior the angle of the jaw on the tip of the transverse process of the 1st cervical vertebra	5.8C
3.	Arms (circulation)	Muscular attachments pectoralis minor to 3rd, 4th & 5th ribs	5.8A	Superior angle of scapula and superior third of the medial margin of the scapula	5.8C
4.	Tonsillitis	Between 1st and 2nd ribs, close to sternum	5.8A	Midway between spinous process and tip of transverse process of 1st cervical vertebra	5.8E
5.	Thyroid	Second intercostal space close to sternum	5.8A	Midway between spinous process and tip of transverse process of 2nd thoracic vertebra	5.8C
6.	Bronchitis	Second intercostal space close to sternum	5.8A	Midway between spinous process and tip of transverse process of 2nd thoracic vertebra	5.8E
7.	Oesophagus	As no. 6	5.8A	As no. 6	5.8E
8.	Myocarditis	As no. 6	5.8A	Between the 2nd and 3rd thoracic transverse processes. Midway between the spinous process and the tip of the transverse process	5.8D
9.	Upper lung	3rd intercostal space close to sternum	5.8A	As no. 8	5.8D
10.	Neuritis of upper limb	As no. 9	5.8A	Between the 3rd and 4th transverse processes, midway between the spinous process and the tip of the transverse process	5.8D
11.	Lower lung	4th intercostal space, close to sternum	5.8A	Between 4th and 5th transverse processes. Midway between the spinous process and the tip of the transverse process	5.8D
12.	Small intestines	8th, 9th & 10th intercostal spaces, close to cartilage	5.8A	8th, 9th & 10th thoracic intertransverse spaces	5.8C
13.	Gastric hypercongestion	6th intercostal space to the left of the sternum	5.8A	6th thoracic intertransverse space, left side	5.8C
14.	Gastric hyperacidity	5th intercostal space to the left of the sternum	5.8A	5th thoracic intertransverse space, left side	5.8F
15.	Cystitis	Around the umbilicus and on the pubic symphysis, close to the midline	5.8A	Upper edge of the transverse processes of the 2nd lumbar vertebra	5.8F
16.	Kidneys	Slightly superior and lateral to the umbilicus	5.8A	In the intertransverse space between the 12th thoracic and the 1st lumbar vertebra	5.8F
17.	Atonic constipation	Between the anterior superior spine of the ilium and the trochanter	5.8A	11th costal–vertebral junction	5.8C
18.	Abdominal tension	Superior border of the pubic bone	5.8A	Tip of the transverse process of the 2nd lumbar vertebra	5.8D
19.	Urethra	Inner edge of pubic ramus near superior aspect of symphysis	5.8A	Superior aspect of transverse process of 2nd lumbar vertebra	5.8F

Continued

Table 5.1   Location of Chapman's neurolymphatic reflexes—Cont'd

No.	Symptoms/area	Anterior	Fig.	Posterior	Fig.
20.	Depuytren's contracture, and arm and shoulder pain	None		Anterior aspect of lateral margin of scapulae, inferior to the head of humerus	5.8F
21.	Cerebral congestion (related to paralysis or paresis)	(On the posterior aspect of the body). Lateral from the spines of the 3rd, 4th & 5th cervical vertebrae	5.8A	Between the transverse processes of the 1st and 2nd cervical vertebrae	5.8E
22.	Clitoral irritation and vaginismus	Upper medial aspect of the thigh	5.8A	Lateral to the junction of the sacrum and coccyx	5.8D
23.	Prostate	Lateral aspect of the thigh from the trochanter to just above the knee. Also lateral to symphysis pubis as in uterine conditions (see no. 43)	5.8A	Between the posterior superior spine of the ilium and the spinous process of the 5th lumbar vertebra	5.8D
24.	Spastic constipation or colitis	Within an area of an inch or two wide extending from the trochanter to within an inch of the patella	5.8A	From the transverse processes of the 2nd, 3rd & 4th lumbar vertebrae to the crest of the ilium	5.8C
25.	Leucorrhoea	Lower medial aspect of thigh, slightly posteriorly (on the posterior aspect of the body)	5.8A & 5.8C	Between the posterior/superior spine of the ilium and the spinous process of the 5th lumbar vertebra	5.8D
26.	Sciatic neuritis	Anterior and posterior to the tibiofibular junction	5.8A	1. On the sacroiliac synchondrosis 2. Between the ischial tuberosity and the acetabulum 3. Lateral and posterior aspects of the thigh	5.8C
27.	Torpid liver (nausea, fullness, malaise)	5th intercostal space, from the mid-mammillary line to the sternum	5.8B	5th thoracic intertransverse space on the right side	5.8C
28.	Cerebellar congestion (memory and concentration lapses)	Tip of coracoid process of scapula	5.8B	Just inferior to the base of the skull on the 1st cervical vertebra	5.8E
29.	Otitis media	Upper edge of clavicle where it crosses the 1st rib	5.8B	Superior aspect of 1st cervical transverse process (tip)	5.8C
30.	Pharyngitis	Anterior aspect of the 1st rib close to the sternum	5.8B	Midway between the spinous process and the tip of the transverse process of the 2nd cervical vertebra	5.8E
31.	Laryngitis	Upper surface of the 2nd rib, 2–3 inches (5–8 cm) from the sternum	5.8B	Midway between the spinous process and the tip of the 2nd cervical vertebra	5.8E
32.	Sinusitis	Lateral to the sternum on the superior edge of the 2nd rib in the first intercostal space	5.8B	As no. 31	5.8E
33.	Pyloric stenosis	On the sternum	5.8B	10th costovertebral junction on the right side	5.8F
34.	Neuraesthenia (chronic fatigue)	All the muscular attachments of pectoralis major on the humerus, clavicle, sternum, ribs (especially 4th rib)	5.8B	Below the superior medial edge of the scapula on the face of the 4th rib	5.8D

Table 5.1 Location of Chapman's neurolymphatic reflexes—Cont'd

No.	Symptoms/area	Anterior	Fig.	Posterior	Fig.
35.	Wry neck (torticollis)	Medial aspect of upper edge of the humerus	5.8B	Transverse processes of the 3rd, 4th, 6th & 7th cervical vertebrae	5.8E
36.	Splenitis	7th intercostal space close to the cartilaginous junction, on the left	5.8B	7th intertransverse space on the left	5.8C
37.	Adrenals (allergies, exhaustion)	Superior and lateral to umbilicus	5.8B	In the intertransverse space between the 11th and 12th thoracic vertebrae	5.8F
38.	Mesoappendix	Superior aspect of the 12th rib, close to the tip, on right	5.8B	Lateral aspect of the 11th intercostal space on the right	5.8C
39.	Pancreas	7th intercostal space on the right, close to the cartilage	5.8B	7th thoracic intertransverse space on the right	5.8F
40.	Liver and gall bladder congestion	6th intercostal space, from the mid-mammillary line to the sternum (right side)	5.8A	6th thoracic intertransverse space, right side	5.8F
41.	Salpingitis or vesiculitis	Midway between the acetabulum and the sciatic notch (this is on the posterior aspect of the body)	5.8F	Between the posterior, superior spine of the ilium and the spinous process of the 5th lumbar vertebra	5.8D
42.	Ovaries	Round ligaments from the superior border of the pubic bone, inferiorly	5.8B	Between the 9th and 10th intertransverse space and the 10th and 11th intertransverse space	5.8D
43.	Uterus	Anterior aspect of the junction of the ramus of the pubis and the ischium	5.8B	Between the posterior superior spine of the ilium and the 5th lumbar spinous process	5.8D
44.	Uterine fibroma	Lateral to the symphysis, extending diagonally inferiorly	5.8B	Between the tip of the transverse process of the 5th lumbar vertebra and the crest of the ilium	5.8C
45.	Rectum	Just inferior to the lesser trochanter	5.8B	On the sacrum close to the ilium at the lower end of the iliosacral synchondrosis	5.8F
46.	Broad ligament (uterine involvement usual)	Lateral aspect of the thigh from the trochanter to just above the knee	5.8B	Between the posterior, superior spine of the ilium and the 5th lumbar spinous process	5.8D
47.	Groin glands (circulation and drainage of legs and pelvic organs)	Lower quarter of the sartorius muscle and its attachment to the tibia	5.8B	On the sacrum close to the ilium at the lower end of the iliosacral synchondrosis	5.8F
48.	Haemorrhoids	Just superior to the ischial tuberosity. (These areas are on the posterior surface of the body)	5.8D	On the sacrum close to the ilium, at the lower end of the iliosacral synchondrosis	5.8D
49.	Tongue	Anterior aspect of 2nd rib at the cartilaginous junction with the sternum	5.8A	Midway between the spinous process and the tip of the transverse process of the 2nd cervical vertebra	5.8E

pressure/treatment can be continued for up to 1 minute, with fluctuations in the degree of pressure, until the patient indicates a diminution in the referred pain or until the time has elapsed.

It is important to realize that the objective 'feel' of these contractions is unlikely to change during such treatment. Any changes resulting from the treatment will occur later, when homeostatic forces have come into operation.

Figure 5.8A, B   Chapman's neurolymphatic reflexes. Symptom/area numbers are described in Table 5.1.

The variation in pressure during the treatment is more desirable than a constantly held degree of pressure, which may irritate and exacerbate the condition. In the foreword to Owen's book *An Endocrine Interpretation of Chapman's Reflexes* (1980), in which Owen describes his and Chapman's research, noted osteopathic researcher Fred Mitchell recommends that pressure should be applied by the pad of the middle finger. This should be maintained as a light direct pressure,

Figure 5.8C, D, E Chapman's neurolymphatic reflexes. Symptom/area numbers are described in Table 5.1.

(F)

Figure 5.8F   Chapman's neurolymphatic reflexes. Symptom/area numbers are described in Table 5.1.

Reflexes that are not painful should not be treated: only an active (and therefore sensitive) reflex point requires attention.

The reflexes may be treated as part of a general neuromuscular treatment, or on their own in accordance with the recommendations of Chapman, Owen and Mitchell, which suggest the treating of the reflexes by light digital pressure of the anterior reflex followed by the corresponding posterior reflex.

- The anterior point should then be re-examined and, if there has been a palpable change, or sensitivity has diminished, then no more action is required.
- If no such change is found, the treatment to the anterior and then the posterior points is again carried out and, if still no change is noted, it is assumed that pathology is too great for a rapid change or is irreversible, or that there is a musculoskeletal factor maintaining the dysfunction.

If this approach is adopted, the grouping of reflexes into systems, is a useful method. If one of a group is found to be active then all others in the group should be examined and, if active, treated; for example:

- The endocrine group comprises: prostate, gonads, broad ligaments, uterus, thyroid and adrenals.
- The gastrointestinal group comprises the colon, thyroid, pancreas, duodenum, small intestine and liver.
- The infections group comprises liver, spleen and the adrenals.

The advice, therefore, is to use reflexes intelligently, treating only what is palpable and sensitive. Some of the anterior reflexes (the ones that should, in theory, be treated first) lie on the posterior aspect of the body.

These include those for:

- haemorrhoids (no. 48)
- cerebellar congestion (no. 21)
- leucorrhoea (no. 25)
- salpingitis (no. 41).

in an effort to decongest the fluid content of the palpable reflex point. Mitchell believed that the determining factor for the amount of treatment is whether a decrease in oedema takes place, or whether a dissolution of the gangliform contraction occurs, together with reduction in the sensitivity of the point over a period of between 20 and 120 seconds.

The stimulation threshold is being raised in these points, by such stimulation, and inhibition of noxious impulses is being achieved. There is nothing to be gained from achieving local pressure anaesthesia (numbing) by exaggerated effort.

It is suggested that reference be made to Owen (1980) for more detailed study. Table 5.1 gives the reflex by name, number and description of location, together with an indication of the figure on which it is indicated (it was not possible to incorporate all the drawings on to one picture without creating a confusing series of overlaps). It is also suggested that practitioners learn to search appropriate areas for the type of sensitive tissue changes that represent the superficial manifestation of these reflexes, and to use Fig. 5.8A–F and Table 5.1 to become familiar with the patterns and groups of these important aids to healing.

The illustrations will aid in locating these useful diagnostic and therapeutic areas.

Bennett's neurovascular reflexes

(Note these will be sensitive to light pressure if active.) (See Figs 5.9A–C & Box 5.3.)

The way in which Bennett's neurovascular (NV) reflex points are used depends largely on the therapeutic objective: as diagnostic indicators; to influence specific muscle function; or to ease symptoms, particularly those deriving from emotional causes.

As with Chapman's neurolymphatic points, neurovascular points might be seen as useful additional sources of information regarding the organ, structure or function to which they appear to be linked. If the region of the point palpates as sensitive, further confirmation should be sought of the dysfunction indicated by the reflex.

Applied kinesiology methodology tends to use these neurovascular points as a means of modifying specific muscles with which they are purported to be reflexly linked.

Walther (1988) explains:

A specific muscle responds to only one [neurovascular] reflex, but most reflexes influence more than one muscle. Bennett's reflexes are primarily on the anterior surface of the trunk and on the head. The reflexes on the head are those used in applied kinesiology, with few exceptions.

The way in which these reflexes are treated is as follows:

1. The point is located and a contact is made with the pad or tip of one finger.
2. The skin overlying the point is 'tugged' lightly and the finger contact is maintained until a pulsation is noted.
3. If the pulsation does not appear, the direction in which the skin 'tug' is made is varied until a pulsation is noted.
4. After the pulsation is noted, the finger contact is maintained for a further 15–20 seconds.

Walther (1988) describes how neurovascular points can be used to treat symptoms related to emotional causes:

Many of the emotional problems dealt with by this technique are those found in general examination to determine the reason for a recurring [problem]. It is not necessary ... to know the precise emotional factor ... Ask the person to think about the problem with the eyes closed, and watch for rapid eye movement (REM) which [may be] associated with the emotional experience ... The NV reflex is located bilaterally on the frontal bone eminence [see point 28 (frontal-emotional) on Fig. 5.9C and description in Box 5.3] and is treated with a light tugging contact [see above] ... until a maximum pulsation is felt. It may be necessary to hold the contact points for several minutes.

Conclusions

Speransky (1943) stated that 'the nervous system contains a record of the past history of the organism'. For the practitioner, the signs present in the musculoskeletal system constitute a map of past and present dysfunctions. It presents him or her with the opportunity to treat, alleviate and prevent further dysfunction.

Apart from palpation for tissue changes and reflex trigger areas, diagnosis should involve an evaluation of the gross stress patterns and postural factors. Each patient is an individual challenge, and indeed this challenge is renewed at each visit. Thus, whilst the mechanics of

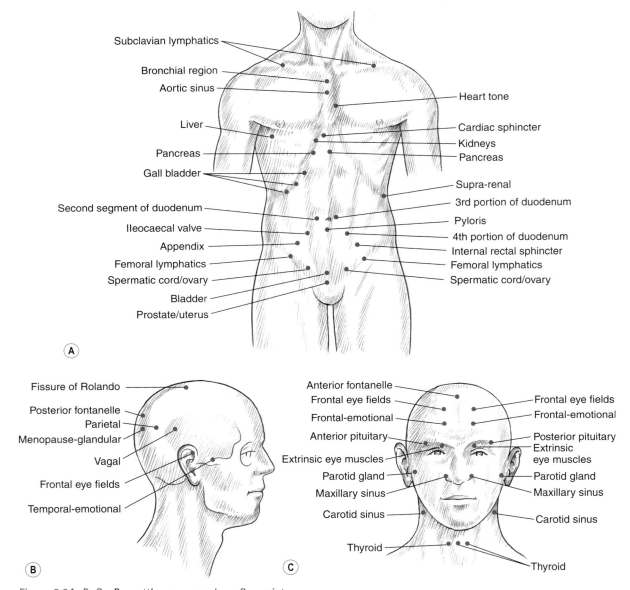

Figure 5.9A, B, C   Bennett's neurovascular reflex points.

treatment are similar, the emphasis will probably be different at each visit. It is important that the patient understands this, and the nature of the problem as well as the goals being aimed for. A cooperative patient will accept the time and effort required to achieve that goal.

- Observation of the dynamic posture, or body in motion, gives an idea of balance,

posture, gravitational stress, gross structural anomalies, etc.
- Observation of certain body areas in individual movement will then help the understanding of their stress patterns, restrictions, and so on.

We need to learn to appreciate the arrangement of the various body structures and their

Box 5.3   Bennett's neurovascular reflexes

Reflex name	Site
1. **Parotid gland**	Raised area on masseter when jaw clenched *Diagnostic and treatment point.* Associated conditions: prostate problems, mumps, premenstrual problem, mastitis, lymphatic stasis.
2. **Cardiac sphincter**	Tip of xyphoid process *Diagnostic and treatment point.* If sensitive may relate to incompetent sphincter, heartburn.
3. **Liver**	Midclavicular line; right 5th intercostal *Diagnostic and treatment point.*
4. **Gall bladder**	Below costal cartilages right 9th, 10th, 11th ribs *Diagnostic and treatment point.* All points mentioned are treatment points; only 11th rib point is diagnostic. Pain may be noted as far lateral as mid-axillary line.
5. **Pancreas**	Medial to 6th and 7th rib heads. 1 inch below xyphoid process *Diagnostic point.* 5th and 6th costal cartilages right and left.
6. **Pyloris**	Lower border of umbilicus *Diagnostic and treatment point.*
7. **2nd segment of duodenum**	1 inch and 45° above umbilicus on right *Diagnostic and treatment point.* *Note*: Order of treatment in this region should follow sequence of pyloris–duodenum–pancreas–liver–gall bladder.
8. **3rd portion of duodenum**	1 inch and 45° above umbilicus on left *Diagnostic and treatment point.*
9. **4th portion of duodenum**	1 inch and 45° lateral and below umbilicus (left) *Diagnostic and treatment point.*
10. **Kidneys**	Tip of 8th rib. Bilateral *Diagnostic and treatment point.*
11. **Ileocaecal valve**	On right side midway between anterior–superior iliac spine and umbilicus *Diagnostic and treatment point.*
12. **Internal rectal sphincter**	On left midway between anterior/superior iliac spine and umbilicus *Diagnostic and treatment point.*
13. **Appendix**	Directly over the organ *Diagnostic and treatment point.*
14. **Bladder**	Just above pubic arch on midline *Diagnostic and treatment point.*
15. **Prostate/uterus**	Symphysis pubis *Diagnostic and treatment point.*
16. **Spermatic cord/ovary**	Approx. 1–1½ inches either side of bladder reflex (*Note*: thyroid to be treated when ovaries receiving attention) *Diagnostic and treatment point.*
17. **Supra-renal**	One finger-width below tip 12th rib. Diagnostic point is tip of 12th rib. *Diagnostic and treatment point.*
18. **Anterior pituitary**	Right, lateral aspect of eyebrow *Diagnostic and treatment point.*
19. **Posterior pituitary**	Left, lateral aspect of eyebrow *Diagnostic and treatment point.*

Continued

Box 5.3   Bennett's neurovascular reflexes—cont'd

20. **Thyroid**	Over the organ *Diagnostic and treatment point.*
21. **Carotid sinus**	On carotid artery, below angle of jaw *Diagnostic and treatment point.*
22. **Aortic sinus**	Manubriosternal junction on ridge, or just inferior *Diagnostic and treatment point.*
23. **Heart tone**	Sternal end of 3rd rib. Contact on cartilage (left) *Diagnostic and treatment point.*
24. **Subclavian lymphatics**	Just inferior to and slightly medial to midpoint of clavicle *Diagnostic and treatment point.*
25. **Femoral lymphatics**	On Poupart's ligament. Midway between symphysis pubis and anterior superior iliac spine *Diagnostic and treatment point.*
26. **Maxillary sinus**	Lateral to nares; bilaterally *Diagnostic and treatment point.*
27. **Bronchial region**	Midway between manubrium sternum and episternal notch *Diagnostic and treatment point.*
28. **Frontal-emotional**	Frontal eminences of forehead *Diagnostic and treatment point.*
29. **Vagal**	2 inches superior and 2 inches posterior to external auditory meatus *Diagnostic and treatment point.*
30. **Parietal**	2 inches superior and 3 inches posterior to external auditory meatus *Diagnostic and treatment point.*
31. **Temporal-emotional**	Midway between outer aspect of eye and external auditory meatus. Just superior to zygomatic bone *Diagnostic and treatment point.*
32. **Anterior fontanelle**	Over anatomical area *Diagnostic and treatment point.*
33. **Mid-sylvian**	1 inch superior to anterior aspect of external auditory meatus *Diagnostic and treatment point.*
34. **Fissure of Rolando**	Approx. 1½ inches posterior to anterior fontanelle *Diagnostic and treatment point.*
35. **Frontal eye fields**	1½ inches superior to frontal eminences *Diagnostic and treatment point.*
36. **Extrinsic eye muscles**	Superior to eyelids with closed eyes *Diagnostic and treatment point.*
37. **Posterior fontanelle**	Over anatomical area *Diagnostic and treatment point.*
38. **Menopause-glandular**	½ inch inferior and lateral to posterior fontanelle *Diagnostic and treatment point.*

All the points on the cranium are useful for treating emotional and stress conditions. Those marked 'emotional' are the strongest. Light pressure only is suggested. Reference to these reflexes will be found in the chapter on treatment techniques (Ch. 6).

interrelationships so that myofascial tensions can then be visualized. When these gross and local postural patterns, in active and passive modes, have been observed, an overall impression can be added to the palpatory impressions, both superficial and deep, which the hands evaluate with the patient standing, supine or prone.

- By lightly passing the hands over the various structures, alterations in tissue density and configuration can be felt.
- The deeper palpation to localize the dysfunction can then be performed or left to the neuromuscular treatment, where diagnosis coincides with treatment.

A history will have been taken before observation, palpation and mobility tests, and such history should be comprehensive, taking note of traumatic incidents, habits, occupational positions and postures, emotional state and history, congenital deformity and surgery, as well as general medical history and specific details of the presenting problems.

Mobility tests form part of the diagnostic procedures in soft tissue assessment and, because all manual therapists are concerned with joint mobility, these tests will also be part of any overall assessment. Active motion, movement of one part of the body in relation to another, powered by conscious muscular effort as well as passive motion in which an outside force acts on the body to induce movement, are both of diagnostic importance. Eventually it is possible to distinguish between healthy tissue, and tissue in which there is dysfunction. This can be learned only by experience.

Observation, static and active; palpation, superficial and deep; a comprehensive and detailed history; mobility tests as required; localization of trigger areas; re-evaluation during the course of treatment; and an intelligent cooperative understanding of the patient's problems, are the diagnostic tools with which to undertake the task in hand.

Finding 'points' using NMT

Knowledge of Chapman's neurolymphatic areas, Bennett's reflexes, Mackenzie's reflex areas, connective tissue zones, and trigger points, might appear a massive task for the memory – and so it is.

However, the application of the general knowledge of their existence enables treatment to be effective even without precise knowledge of all the individual reflexes involved. The aim of this chapter has been to try to classify some of the more obvious diagnostic indicators, so that the practitioner's awareness of the range of diagnostic and therapeutic possibilities can be broadened.

References

Arbuckle B: *Selected writings*, National Osteopathic Institute, 1977.

Baldry P: *Acupuncture, trigger points and musculoskeletal pain*, London, 1993, Churchill Livingstone.

Beal M: Palpatory testing for somatic dysfunction in patients with cardiovascular disease, *J Am Osteopath Assoc* 82:822–831, 1983.

Bischof I, Elmiger G: Connective tissue massage. In Licht E, editor: *Massage, manipulation and traction*, Connecticut, 1960, New Haven.

Chaitow L: An introduction to Chapman's reflexes, *British Naturopathic Journal* 6(4):111–113, 1965.

DiGiovanna E, editor: *An osteopathic approach to diagnosis and treatment*, Philadelphia, 1991, Lippincott.

Koizumi K: Autonomic system reactions, caused by excitation of somatic afferents: study of cutaneo-intestinal reflex. In Korr I, editor: *The neurobiological mechanisms in manipulative therapy*, New York, 1978, Plenum Press.

Lewit K: *Manipulative therapy in rehabilitation of the locomotor system*, ed 2, London, 1992, Butterworths.

Lewit K: *Manipulative therapy in rehabilitation of the locomotor system*, ed 3, London, 1999, Butterworths.

Lewit K, Olšanská S: Clinical importance of active scars: abnormal scars as a result of myofascial pain, *J Manipulative Physiol Ther* 27:399–402, 2004.

Lief P: *British Naturopathic Journal* 5(10):304–324, 1963.

Mackenzie J: 1909, *Symptoms and their interpretations*, London.

Owen C: *An endocrine interpretation of Chapman's reflexes.* Newark, Ohio, 1980, American Academy of Osteopathy.

Patriquin D: Chapman's reflexes. In Ward R, editor: *Foundations for osteopathic medicine*, Baltimore, 1997, Williams & Wilkins.

Speransky A: *A basis for the theory of medicine*, New York, 1943, International Publishers.

Stiles E: *Patient Care*, 15 May:16–87; 15 August: 117–164, 1984.

Teiriche-Leube H: *Grundriss der Bindesgewebsmassage*, Stuttgart, 1960, Fisher.

Travell J: Symposium on mechanisms and management of pain syndromes. In *Proceedings of the Rudolph Virchow Medical Society*.

Travell J, Simons D: *Myofascial pain and dysfunction*, vol 1, Baltimore, 1983, Williams & Wilkins.

Travell J, Simons D: *Myofascial pain and dysfunction*, vol 2, Baltimore, 1992, Williams & Wilkins.

Walther D: *Applied kinesiology*, Pueblo, Colorado, 1988, SDC Systems.

Youngs B: NMT of lower thorax and low back, *British Naturopathic Journal* 5(11):176–190, 340–358, 1964.

6

Basic spinal NMT

CHAPTER CONTENTS

Defining NMT	**123**
Unique aspects of NMT	**124**
Most used NMT approaches – and 'variable pressure'	**125**
Thumb considerations	**125**
NMT thumb technique	125
NMT finger technique	127
Use of lubricant	128
Lief's basic spinal treatment	**129**
Practitioner's posture	129
The mechanics of NMT – achieving economy of effort	130
Variable pressure – the key to painless pressure	131
Posterior reflex centres	132
Origins and insertions	133
Duration of treatment	133
Adopting a new position	133
Trapezius and sternomastoid muscles	134
Left-side trunk treatment	135
Right-side treatment	135
Left hip position	137
Lateral thigh and gluteal structures	139
Completion of treatment	139

Defining NMT

NMT, as the term is used in this book, is summarized in Box 6.1.

In this text the 'European' version of NMT, as developed by Stanley Lief, based partly on traditional Ayurvedic massage, is one of two areas of NMT focus.

The other NMT version described is the American NMT model, that resulted from the original work of Nimmo, Simons and Travell – with further development by St John and Walker, among others (see Chapters 10 and 13).

A confusing element relating to the term NMT emerges, because of its use by Dvorak et al (1988), when they describe what are, in effect, variations on the theme of the use of isometric contractions in order to encourage a reduction in hypertonicity. These methods, all of which form part of what is known as muscle energy technique (MET) in osteopathic medicine and proprioceptive neuromuscular facilitation (PNF) in physiotherapy, are described briefly in Chapter 8, and form the focus of a further title in the series of which this book is part (Chaitow 2001, 2006).

Dvorak et al (1988) have listed various MET methods (as NMT) as follows:

1. Methods that involve self-mobilization by patient action, to encourage movement past a resistance barrier, are described as 'NMT 1'.
2. Isometric contraction and subsequent passive stretching of agonist muscles, involving postisometric relaxation, are called 'NMT 2'.
3. Isometric contraction of antagonists, followed by stretching, involving reciprocal inhibition, are described as 'NMT 3'.

- Neuromuscular technique, as the term is used in this book, refers to the manual application of specialized pressure and strokes, usually delivered by a finger or thumb contact, which have a diagnostic (assessment mode) or therapeutic (treatment mode) objective.
- Therapeutically, NMT aims to produce modifications in dysfunctional tissue, encouraging a restoration of normality, with a primary focus of deactivating focal points of reflexogenic activity such as myofascial trigger points.
- An alternative focus of NMT application is towards normalizing imbalances in hypertonic and/or fibrotic tissues, either as an end in itself or as a precursor to joint mobilization/rehabilitation.
- NMT utilizes physiological responses involving neurological mechanoreceptors, Golgi tendon organs, muscle spindles and other proprioceptors, in order to achieve the desired responses.
- Insofar as they integrate with NMT, other means of influencing such neural reporting stations, including positional release (strain/counterstrain) and muscle energy methods (such as reciprocal inhibition and post-isometric relaxation induction) are seen to form a natural set of allied approaches.
- Traditional massage methods that encourage a reduction in retention of metabolic wastes and enhanced circulation to dysfunctional tissues are included in this category of allied approaches.

Use of the terms NMT 1, 2 and 3 in these ways, by Dvorak et al (1988), in order to describe these methods, succeeds in adding to, rather than reducing, semantic confusion, and it is hoped that this aberrant set of descriptors will not persist.

Unique aspects of NMT

What is unique to NMT, as discussed in this book, is its concentration on the soft tissues, not just to give reflex benefit to the body, not just to prepare for other therapeutic methods such as exercise or manipulation, not just to relax and normalize tense fibrotic muscular tissue, and not just to enhance lymphatic and general circulation and drainage, but to do all these things and, at the same time, to be able to offer the practitioner diagnostic information via the palpating and treating instrument, which is usually the thumb.

NMT can usefully be integrated in treatment that is aimed at postural reintegration, tension release, pain relief, improvement of joint mobility, reflex stimulation/modulation or sedation. There are many variations of the basic technique, as developed by Stanley Lief, the choice of which will depend upon particular presenting factors, or personal preference. Similarities between some aspects of NMT and other manual systems (see Ch. 8) should be anticipated, as techniques have been borrowed and adapted from other systems where appropriate. For example, in Chapter 11 Dennis Dowling demonstrates the clinical value of using progressive inhibition of neuromuscular structures (PINS), a unique way of utilizing NMT effects, in pain control. Use of PINS in pain control offers an example of the evolution of new applications of the basics, which NMT provides (Dowling 2000).

And just as there are current evolutionary paths involving NMT principles, so there have been parallel evolutions of methods that derive from similar backgrounds. In Chapter 12 Howard Evans describes Thai yoga massage methods that are truly a blend of the model of manual care that evolved in Thailand, based on the same root approaches deriving from Ayurvedic massage which let to Lief's NMT. Evans' approach is further influenced by having studied Lief's methods giving him a useful Western and Eastern set of approaches which he has fused and described (Evans 2009).

NMT can be applied generally, or locally, and in a variety of positions (with the patient seated, supine, prone, side-lying, etc.). The order in which body areas are dealt with is not regarded as critical in general treatment, but seems to be of some consequence in postural reintegration (Rolf 1977).

In Chapter 13, Cohen describes both the historical work of Raymond Nimmo, and the continuing evolution of his methods, which form a major part of American Version NMT, as described by DeLany in Chapter 10.

Most used NMT approaches – and 'variable pressure'

The basic spinal NMT treatment and the basic abdominal (and related areas) NMT treatment (see Ch. 7) are the most commonly used, and will be described in detail in this and the next chapter. The methods described are in essence those of Stanley Lief ND DC and Boris Chaitow ND DC, both of whom achieved a degree of skill in the application of NMT that is unsurpassed. The inclusion of data on reflex areas and effects, together with basic NMT methods, provides the practitioner with a useful therapeutic tool, the limitations of which will be determined largely by the degree of intelligence and understanding with which it is employed.

As Boris Chaitow has written (personal communication, 1983):

The important thing to remember is that this unique manipulative formula is applicable to any part of the body for any physical and physiological dysfunction and for both articular and soft tissue lesions.

To apply NMT successfully it is necessary to develop the art of palpation and sensitivity of fingers by constantly feeling the appropriate areas and assessing any abnormality in tissue structure for tensions, contractions, adhesions, spasms.

It is important to acquire with practice an appreciation of the 'feel' of normal tissue so that one is better able to recognise abnormal tissue. Once some level of diagnostic sensitivity with fingers has been achieved, subsequent application of the technique will be much easier to develop. The whole secret is to be able to recognise the 'abnormalities' in the feel of tissue structures. Having become accustomed to understanding the texture and character of 'normal' tissue, the pressure applied by the thumb (in general), especially in the spinal structures, should always be firm, but never hurtful or bruising. To this end the pressure should be applied with a 'variable' pressure, i.e. with an appreciation of the texture and character of the tissue structures and
according to the feel that sensitive fingers should have developed. The level of the pressure applied should not be consistent because the character and texture of tissue is always variable. These variations can be detected by one's educated 'feel'. The pressure should, therefore, be so applied that the thumb is moved along its path of direction in a way which corresponds to the feel of the tissues.

This variable factor in finger pressure constitutes probably the most important quality any practitioner of NMT can learn, enabling him to maintain more effective control of pressure, develop a greater sense of diagnostic feel, and be far less likely to bruise the tissue.

Variation of applied digital pressure during the application of NMT is probably the most important single feature that deserves emphasis and re-emphasis to anyone learning or using these methods. This feature of NMT is discussed again later in this chapter.

Thumb considerations

 NMT thumb technique (Fig. 6.1)

Thumb technique as employed in NMT, in either assessment or treatment modes, enables a wide variety of therapeutic effects to be produced.

The tip of the thumb can deliver varying degrees of pressure, via any of four facets; the very tip may be employed or the medial or lateral aspect of the tip can be used to make contact with angled surfaces.

For more general (less localized and less specific) contact, of a diagnostic or therapeutic nature, the broad surface of the distal phalange of the thumb is often used. It is usual for a light non-oily lubricant to be used to facilitate easy, non-dragging, passage of the palpating digit.

- For balance and control, the hand should be spread, the tips of fingers providing a fulcrum or 'bridge' in which the palm is arched in order to allow free passage of the thumb towards one of the fingertips as the thumb moves in a direction that takes it away from the practitioner's body.

(A)

(B)

Figure 6.1   NMT thumb technique.

- During a single stroke, which covers between 2 and 3 inches (5–8 cm), the fingertips act as a point of balance, while the chief force is imparted to the thumb tip via controlled application through the long axis of the extended arm of body weight.
- The thumb, therefore, never leads the hand but always trails behind the stable fingers, the tips of which rest just beyond the end of the stroke.
- Unlike many bodywork/massage strokes, the hand and arm remain still as the thumb, applying variable pressure (see below), moves through its pathway of tissue.
- The extreme versatility of the thumb enables it to modify the direction of imparted force in accordance with the indications of the tissue being tested or treated.
- As the thumb glides across and through those tissues it becomes an extension of the practitioner's brain. In fact, for the clearest assessment of what is being palpated, the

practitioner should have the eyes closed, in order that every minute change in the tissue can be felt and reacted to.
- The thumb and hand seldom impart their own muscular force, except in dealing with small localized contractures or fibrotic 'nodules'.
- In order that pressure/force be transmitted directly to its target, the weight being imparted should travel in as straight a line as possible, which is why the arm should not be flexed at the elbow or the wrist by more than a few degrees. The positioning of the practitioner's body in relation to the area being treated is also of the utmost importance in order to facilitate economy of effort and comfort.
- The optimal height vis-à-vis the couch, and the most effective angle of approach to the body areas being addressed, must be considered and the descriptions and illustrations will help to make this clearer.
- The degree of pressure imparted will depend on the nature of the tissue being treated, with a great variety of changes in pressure being possible during strokes across and through the tissues. When being treated, the patient should not feel strong pain, but a general degree of discomfort is usually acceptable as the seldom stationary thumb varies its penetration of dysfunctional tissues.
- A stroke or glide of 2–3 inches (5–8 cm) will usually take 4–5 seconds – seldom more unless a particularly obstructive indurated area is being dealt with. If reflex pressure techniques are being employed, a much longer stay on a point will be needed, but in normal diagnostic and therapeutic use the thumb continues to move as it probes, decongests and generally treats the tissues.
- It is not possible to state the exact pressures necessary in NMT application because of the very nature of the objective, which in assessment mode attempts to meet and match the tissue resistance precisely, to vary the pressure constantly in response to what is being felt.
- In subsequent or synchronous (with assessment) treatment of whatever is uncovered during evaluation, a greater degree

of pressure is used and this too will vary, depending upon the objective – whether this is to inhibit, to produce localized stretching, to decongest and so on. Obviously, on areas with relatively thin muscular covering, the applied pressure would be lighter than in tense or thick, well covered areas such as the buttocks.

- Attention should also be paid to the relative sensitivity of different areas and different patients. The thumb should not just mechanically stroke across or through tissue but should become an intelligent extension of the practitioner's diagnostic sensitivities so that the contact feels to the patient as though it is sequentially assessing every important nook and cranny of the soft tissues. Pain should be transient and no bruising should result if the above advice is followed.
- The treating arm and thumb should be relatively straight because a 'hooked' thumb, in which all the work is done by the distal phalange, will become extremely tired and will not achieve the degree of penetration possible via a fairly rigid thumb.

Hypermobile thumbs

Some practitioners have hypermobile joints and it is difficult for them to maintain sustained pressure without the thumb giving way and bending back on itself. This is a problem that can be overcome only by attempting to build up the muscular strength of the hand or by using a variation of the above technique; for example, a knuckle or even the elbow may be used to achieve deep pressure in very tense musculature. Alternatively, the finger stroke as described below can take over from a hypermobile thumb.

Alternatively an instrument such as the 'T'-bar (see Ch. 10, Fig. 10.1B,C) may be used to ease mechanical stress on the thumb joints.

 ### NMT finger technique (Fig. 6.2)

In certain localities, the width of the thumb prevents the degree of tissue penetration needed for successful assessment and/or treatment. In such regions the middle or index finger can usually be suitably employed. The most usual area for use of finger, rather than thumb, contact is in the intercostal

Figure 6.2　NMT finger technique.

musculature, and in attempting to penetrate beneath the scapula borders in tense fibrotic conditions.

- The middle or index finger should be slightly flexed and, depending on the direction of the stroke (most usually toward the practitioner) and density of the tissues, supported by one of its adjacent members.
- As the treating finger strokes with a firm contact, and usually a minimum of lubricant, a tensile strain is created between its tip and the tissue underlying it.
- This is stretched and lifted by the passage of the finger which, like the thumb, should continue moving unless or until dense, indurated tissue prevents its easy passage. When treating, these strokes can be repeated once or twice, as tissue changes dictate.
- The angle of pressure to the skin surface is between 40° and 50°.
- The fingertip should never lead the stroke but should always follow the wrist, the palmar surface of which should lead, as the hand is drawn towards the practitioner. It is possible to impart a great degree of 'pull' on underlying tissues, and the patient's reactions must be taken into account in deciding on the degree of force to be used. Transient pain, or mild discomfort, is to be expected, but no more than that. All sensitive areas are

indicative of some degree of dysfunction, local or reflex, and are thus important, and their presence should be recorded. The patient should be told what to expect, so that a cooperative, unworried attitude evolves.

- As mentioned above, unlike the thumb technique, in which force is largely directed away from the practitioner's body, in finger treatment the motive force is usually towards the practitioner.
- The arm position therefore alters, and a degree of flexion is necessary to ensure that the pull, or drag, of the finger across the lightly lubricated tissues is smooth.
- Unlike the thumb, which makes a sweep across the palm towards the fingertips, whilst the rest of the hand remains relatively stationary, the whole hand will move when finger technique is applied.
- Certainly some variation in the degree of angle between fingertip and skin is allowable during a stroke, and some slight variation in the degree of 'hooking' of the finger is sometimes also necessary.
- However, the main motive force is applied by pulling the slightly flexed, middle or index, finger towards the practitioner, with the possibility of some lateral emphasis if needed. The treating finger should always be supported by one of its neighbours.

Use of lubricant

The use of a lubricant to facilitate the smooth passage of, for example, the thumb over the surface is an essential aspect of NMT. The lubricant used should not allow too slippery a passage of the thumb or finger, and a suitable balance between lubrication and adherence is found by mixing 2 parts of rapeseed (or almond) oil to 1 part of lime or rose water. At times, the degree of stimulus imparted via this contact can be enhanced by increasing the tensile strain between the thumb or finger and the skin. If a cream is used, standard aqueous ointment, inexpensively available from any pharmacy, is hypoallergenic and offers an appropriate, non-greasy, medium.

If a stimulant effect is required (see notes on Connective tissue massage in Chapters 4 and 5),

possibly in order to achieve a rapid vascular response, then no lubricant should be used.

Clinical experience shows that similar reactions will be achieved (with lubricant) where NMT is applied along the intermuscular septa, or at the origins and insertions of muscles.

It should be clear that whatever underlying tissues are being treated should be visualized. Depending upon the presenting symptoms, and the area involved, any of a number of procedures may be undertaken as the hand moves from one site to another:

- Superficial stroking in the direction of lymphatic flow
- Direct pressure along the line of axis of stress fibres
- Cross-fibre strokes
- Deeper alternating 'make and break' stretching and pressure efforts
- Subtle weaving, insinuating, movements that attempt to melt into the tissues to obtain information or greater access
- Traction on fascial tissue
- Crowding of bunched tissues toward the direction in which they are shortening.

As variable pressure is being applied, the practitioner needs to be constantly aware of diagnostic information that is being received via the contact hands, as this is what should determine the variations in pressure and the direction of force being applied.

Any changes in direction, or degree, of applied pressure should ideally take place without any sudden release, or application, of force, which might irritate the tissues and produce pain or a defensive contraction.

Lief's basic spinal treatment followed the pattern as set out below. The fact that the same pattern is followed at each treatment does not mean that the treatment is necessarily the same each time. The pattern gives a frame-work and a useful starting and ending point, but the degree of emphasis applied to the various areas of dysfunction that manifest themselves is a variable factor based always on what information the palpating hands are picking up: this is what makes each treatment different.

The areas of dysfunction noted during NMT application should be recorded on a case card, together with all relevant material and assessment and diagnostic findings relating to myofascial tissue changes, trigger points and reference zones, areas of sensitivity, restricted motion, fibrotic changes, asymmetrical features, and so on.

 ## Lief's basic spinal treatment

Lief's basic spinal NMT treatment follows a pattern in which the patient is prone, with a pillow of medium thickness under the chest, forehead supported by the patient's hands or, ideally, resting in a split head-piece or face-hole. Alternatively – and more appropriately – a contoured cushion, which supports the entire body, should be used.

1. The whole spine from occiput to sacrum, including the gluteal area, should be lightly oiled or creamed.
2. The practitioner should begin by standing half-facing the head of the couch on the left of the patient, with the hips level with the mid-thoracic area.
3. To facilitate the intermittent application of pressure and the transfer of weight via the arm to the exploring and treating thumb, the practitioner should stand with the left foot forward of the right by 12–18 inches (30–45 cm), weight evenly distributed between them, knees slightly flexed.
4. The first contact, to the left side of the patient's head, is a gliding, light-pressured movement of the medial tip of the right thumb, from the mastoid process along the nuchal line to the external occipital protuberance. This same stroke, or glide, is then repeated with deeper pressure (see Fig. 6.4A,B).

The non-treating hand's role

- The practitioner's left hand should at this time rest on the upper thoracic or shoulder area to act as a stabilizing contact.
- Whichever hand is operating at any given time, the other hand can give assistance by means of gently rocking or stretching tissues to complement the efforts of the treating hand, or it can be useful in distracting tissues that are

'mounding' as the treating hand works on them.
- Whenever the practitioner changes to the other side of the table, it is suggested that one hand always maintains light contact with the patient. Indeed, it is suggested that, once treatment has commenced, no breaks in contact be allowed.
- There is often a noticeable increase in tension in the tissues if the series of strokes, stretching movements and pressure techniques that make up NMT are interrupted by even a few seconds because of a break in contact. Continuity would seem, in itself, to be of therapeutic value, simply as a reassuring and calming feature.

What the treating thumb feels

The movement of the right thumb through the tissue is slow – not uniformly slow, but deliberately seeking and feeling for 'contractions' and 'congestions' (to use two words that will be meaningful to any manual therapist). If and when such localized areas are felt, the degree of pressure can be increased and, in a variably applied manner, this pressure carries the thumb tip across, or through, the restricting tissues, decongesting, stretching and easing them.

The patient will often report a degree of pain but may say that it 'feels good'. This is a contradiction in terms, but constructive pain is usually felt as a 'nice hurt'.

Practitioner's posture (Fig. 6.3)

- When applying thumb strokes, whether facing the head or the foot of the table, the treating arm should not be flexed, because the optimum transmission of weight from the practitioner's shoulder, through the arm to the thumb tip, is best achieved with a relatively straight arm.
- This demands that the practitioner ensures the table height is suitable for his or her own height. The practitioner should not be forced to stand on tiptoe to treat the patient, nor should an unhealthy bent posture have to be adopted.
- The practitioner's weight should be evenly spread between the separated feet, both of which are forward facing at this stage.

Figure 6.3 NMT – practitioner's posture should ensure a straight treating arm for ease of transmission of body weight, as well as leg positions that allow for the easy transfer of weight and centre of gravity. These postures assist in reducing energy expenditure and ease spinal stress.

- In this way, by slightly altering the weight distribution from the front to the back foot, and vice versa, an accurate, controlled degree of pressure can be exerted with minimal arm or hand effort.

The mechanics of NMT – achieving economy of effort

- The hand itself should not be rigid but in a relaxed state, moulding itself to the contours of the neck or back tissues.
- To some extent the fingertips stabilize the hand.

- The thumb's glide is controlled by this support, so that the actual stroke is achieved by the tip of the extended thumb being brought slowly across the palm towards the fingertips.
- The fingers, during this phase of cervical treatment, would be placed on the opposite side of the neck to that being treated.
- The fingers maintain their position as the thumb performs its diagnostic/therapeutic glide. Figure 6.4A,B will aid the reader to a better understanding of this description.

However, were all the effort to be on the part of the thumb, it would soon tire. Consider which parts of the practitioner's arm/hand are involved with the various aspects of the glide/stroke as delivered by the thumb (finger strokes involve completely different mechanics):

1. The transverse movement of the thumb is a hand or forearm effort.
2. The relative straightness, or rigidity, of the last two thumb segments is also a local muscular responsibility.
3. The vast majority of the energy imparted via the thumb results from transmission of body weight, through the straight arm and into the thumb.
4. Any increase in pressure can be speedily achieved by simple weight transfer from back towards front foot, and a slight 'lean' on to the thumb from the shoulders.
5. A lessening of imparted pressure is achieved by reversing this body movement.

Treatment continues

- The first two strokes of the right thumb having been completed – one shallow and almost totally diagnostic, and the second, deeper, imparting therapeutic effort – the next stroke is half a thumb-width caudal to the first.
- Thus a degree of overlap occurs as these strokes, starting on the belly of the sternocleidomastoid, glide across and through the trapezius, splenius capitus and posterior cervical muscles.
- A progressive series of strokes is applied in this way until the level of the cervicothoracic junction is reached.

Figure 6.4A, B   First positions of suggested sequence of applications of NMT, to ensure optimal thumb and/or finger contact with primary trigger point sites and with the origins and insertions of most muscles. Note foot positions.

- Unless serious underlying dysfunction is found, it is seldom necessary to repeat the two superimposed strokes at each level of the cervical region.

Variable pressure – the key to painless pressure

- If underlying fibrotic tissue appears unyielding, a third, or fourth, slow deep glide may be necessary.
- The degree of discomfort felt by the patient is of some importance. The sensitivity of this region is well known and if pressure is too deep, or sustained for too long, the defensive resistance that may be created can make the treatment counterproductive.
- It is possible to achieve deep, penetrating pressure if it is variable in nature and not held for long, without undue pain or discomfort.
- Thus a thinking, intuitive feel for the work is a prerequisite of successful application.

Deactivating trigger points

Should trigger points be located during the NMT assessment/treatment strokes – as indicated by the reproduction, in a target area, of an existing, familiar, pain pattern – then a number of choices are open:

1. The point can be marked and noted (on a chart and if necessary on the body with a skin pencil) for later attention, or treatment can be offered immediately.
2. Sustained pressure, or 'make and break' pressure, can be used (see Chapters 8 & 9 for details and choices).
3. Application of a positional release approach (strain/counterstain) will reduce activity in the hyperreactive tissue, as outlined in Chapter 8 (Simons 2002).
4. Initiation of an isometric contraction followed by local and whole muscle stretching should be used (Lewit 1999).

5. A combination of pressure, positional release and muscle energy technique (MET) (integrated neuromuscular inhibition technique (INIT), as described in Ch. 9) can be introduced (Chaitow 1994).

6. Alternatively, spray and stretch methods can be used (vapocoolant technique, as discussed in Chapter 8) (Kostopoulos D, Rizopoulos K 2008, Sola & Bonica 1990, Travell & Simons 1992).

7. An acupuncture needle or procaine injection can be used (as, it is suggested, can laser or microcurrent application) (Baldry 2001, McMakin 1998).

8. Sustained pressure, if applied, should be variable: deep pressure for 5–7 seconds, followed by a slight easing for a further few seconds, and so on, repeated until the local or reference pain changes (usually diminishing, but sometimes increasing), or until 2 minutes have elapsed. It is suggested that no more than this amount of manual pressure should be applied to a trigger point at any one session.

9. Further ease of the hyper-reactive patterns in a trigger point can be achieved by the application of a hot towel to the area, followed by effleurage (Lowe & Honeyman-Lowe 1999).

10. Whichever approach is used, a trigger point will only be permanently deactivated if the muscle in which it lies is restored to its normal resting length, and MET can assist in achieving this (Travell & Simons 1992).

The neck treatment continues

- Once the right thumb has completed its series of transverse strokes across the long axis of the cervical musculature, the left hand, which has been resting on the patient's left shoulder, now comes into play.
- A series of strokes is applied by the left thumb, upward from the left of the upper thoracic area towards the base of the skull.
- The fingers of the left hand rest (and act as a fulcrum) on the front of the shoulder area at the level of the medial aspect of the clavicle.

- The thumb tip should be angled to allow direct pressure to be exerted against the left lateral aspects of the upper thoracic and the lower cervical spinous processes as the thumb glides cephalad.
- The subsequent strokes of the thumb should be in the same direction, but placed slightly more laterally.
- The fingers should then be placed on the patient's head at about the temporo-occipital articulation. The left thumb then deals in the same way with the mid and upper cervical soft tissues, finishing with a lateral stroke or two across the insertions on the occiput itself.

In travelling from the nuchal line to the level of the cervicothoracic junction, and back again, in a series of overlapping searching/gliding movements, common sites of a number of possible trigger points will have been evaluated.

- The midpoint of the sternomastoid, at the level of the posterior angle of the jaw, can be the source of an intensely painful trigger point, which refers to an area from above the temple in the ear region, to below the angle of the jaw.
- Similar triggers exist in the splenius capitis, upper trapezius, posterior cervical and other muscles of the region, all with different target areas. (See Fig. 3.6 for these and other examples of trigger point distribution patterns.)

Posterior reflex centres

Also in the cervical area are to be found the posterior neurolymphatic reflex centres (Chapman's reflexes), notably those connected with conjunctivitis, cerebellar congestion, and ear, nose and throat problems of an inflammatory or congested type, from sinusitis to tonsillitis.

It is suggested that a study is made of the illustrations of neurolymphatic reflex positions (see Ch. 5). Treatment of these points is via lightly sustained pressure, as described in Chapter 4.

Among the more important *tsubo* or acupressure points in the upper cervical area are:

- Gall bladder 20, which lies bilaterally in a depression midway between the occipital protuberance and the mastoid at the base of the skull.

- Bladder 10, which lies bilaterally just lateral to the large bundle of muscular insertions at the occiput.
- Triple heater 17, which lies bilaterally in the depression between the lobe of ear and the mastoid process.

These points, if sensitive, should receive a sustained or variable pressure, as for the other trigger points. Their influence is felt in a variety of conditions relating to the head, such as migraine, neuralgia, cold symptoms, hypertension and hypotension, and liver dysfunction.

Goodheart (1987) mentions levator scapulae 'weakness' as indicating digestive problems and recommends pressure techniques in the cervicothoracic area and on the medial border of the scapula to help normalize this.

Following NMT treatment of the left side of the cervical area, the same procedures are repeated on the right.

A tall practitioner can probably adapt to treat both sides from one standing position; however, a move to the opposite side makes for a more controlled delivery of the appropriate strokes.

Origins and insertions

During NMT assessment and treatment, special notice should be given to the origins and insertions of the muscles that are being accessed. Where bony landmarks are palpable by the thumb tip, they should be treated by slow, variably applied, pressure.

All bony surfaces within reach of the probing finger or thumb should be searched for undue sensitivity and dysfunction of their attachments – described by Lewit (1999) as 'periosteal pain points' (PPP) – which are amongst the commonest sites of trigger points, according to Travell & Simons (1992). See Table 4.4 in Chapter 4 for a list of the major PPP.

Duration of treatment

Treatment of the left cervical area should take no more than 2–3 minutes and, in the absence of dysfunction, can be comfortably and successfully

dealt with in 90 seconds. Indeed, in its assessment mode, the entire basic spinal NMT treatment can usually be completed in 15 minutes.

 ### Adopting a new position

Once both left and right cervical areas have been treated, the practitioner moves to the head of the table (Fig. 6.5).

- Resting the tips of the fingers on the lower, lateral aspect of the patient's neck, the thumb tips are placed just lateral to the first thoracic–spinal process.
- A degree of downward (toward the floor) pressure is applied via the thumbs, which are then drawn cephalad, alongside the lateral margins of the cervical spinous processes,

Figure 6.5 Third position of suggested sequence of application of NMT.

searching for irregularities, asymmetries (see TART notes in Chapter 3).

- This bilateral stroke culminates at the occiput, where a lateral stretch, or pull, is introduced across the bunched fibres of the muscles inserting into the base of the skull.
- The upward stroke should contain an element of pressure medially, towards the spinous process, so that the pad of the thumb is pressing downward (towards the floor), whilst the lateral thumb tip is directed towards the centre, attempting to contact the bony contours of the spine, all the time being drawn slowly cephalad to end at the occiput.
- This combination stroke is repeated two or three times.
- The fingertips, which have been resting on the sternomastoid, may also be employed at this stage, to lift and stretch the muscle posteriorly and laterally.
- The lateral stretch, via the thumbs, across the occipital protuberance may be likened to 'trying to break open a melon'.
- The thumb tips insinuate themselves deep into the medial fibres of the paraoccipital bundle, and an outward stretch is initiated, using the leverage of the arms, as though attempting to 'open out' the occiput.
- The thumbs are then drawn laterally across the fibres of muscular insertion into the skull, in a series of strokes culminating at the occipito-parietal junction.
- The fingertips, which act as a fulcrum to these movements, rest on the mastoid area of the temporal bone.
- Several strokes are then performed, by one thumb, or the other, running caudally, directly over the spinous processes, from the base of the skull to the upper thoracic area. Pressure should be moderate and slow.
- Standing in the same position, the left thumb should then be placed on the right lateral aspect of the first thoracic vertebra, and a series of strokes performed caudally, and laterally, as well as diagonally towards the scapula.
- The fingers should be splayed out ahead of the thumb in whichever direction it is travelling,

so that the force transmitted via the extended arm can be controlled.

- The fingers act as a fulcrum, with the thumb tip being drawn across the palm, towards the the tip of the middle or little finger.
- The thumb should never lead the hand, nor be solely 'digging' or pressing, without the stabilizing and controlling action of the hand, or fingertips, also being in operation.
- A series of strokes, shallow and then deep, is therefore applied from T1 to about T4 or T5, and outwards towards the scapula, and along and across the upper trapezius fibres and the rhomboids.
- The left hand treats the right side, and vice versa, with the non-operative hand resting on the neck or head, stabilizing it.
- Weight transfer to the thumb is achieved, as described previously, by leaning forward.

Trapezius and sternomastoid muscles

Standing at the head of the table, facing caudally, allows the practitioner to access the region of the upper trapezius from above, so to speak. By lowering the angle at which the hand contacts the muscle, perhaps by kneeling or at least by lowering the centre of gravity significantly, and by standing a little to one side of the centre, it is possible to apply a series of sensitively searching contacts into the area of the thoracic outlet (see Fig. 6.5).

- Strokes that start in this triangular depression would move towards the trapezius fibres and through them towards the upper margins of the scapula. A treasure-house of trigger points awaits this searching digit.
- As it is often difficult to apply pressure to the trapezius or sternocleidomastoid muscles in such a way as to involve underlying bony structures, it may be necessary lightly to pinch (flat pincer grip), or squeeze, the more sensitive areas of dysfunction to assess trigger points and their related target areas of pain.
- Several strokes should also be applied directly over the spinous processes, caudally as far down as the mid-thoracic area. Trigger points sometimes lie on the attachments to the spinous processes, or between them.

By referring to the illustrations of trigger points (see Ch. 3, Fig. 3.6), the location of some of the commonest trigger points in this area can be predicted, and their presence rapidly established.

When it is not possible to apply thumb pressure onto such a point, a flat pincer compression (using pads of fingers) of the involved muscle area, instead of direct pressure, using varying pressure as described earlier in this chapter, will usually induce a reduction of the referred pain. Once pain reduces, the pressure should be released. If no success is achieved by these means, one of the other trigger point treatment approaches, as previously outlined in Chapter 3 (see Box 3.5), should be used.

 ### Left-side trunk treatment

- The practitioner then moves to the patient's left side and stands in the same manner as at the commencement of the treatment, but at the level of the patient's waist (see Fig. 6.6A).
- With the right hand now resting at the level of the lower thoracic spine, the left thumb commences a series of strokes in a cephalad direction, from the mid-thoracic area.
- Each stroke covers two or three spinal segments, and runs immediately lateral to the spinous processes, so that the angle of pressure imparted via the medial tip of the thumb is roughly towards the contralateral nipple.
- Again, light assessment and deep therapeutic strokes are employed, and a degree of overlap occurs on successive strokes.
- In this way the first two strokes might run from T8 to T5, followed by two strokes (one light, one deeper) from T6 to T3, and finally two strokes from T4 to T1.
- Deeper and more sustained pressure can be exerted if marked congestion, or resistance to the gliding, probing thumb, is noted.
- In the thoracic area a second line of cephalad strokes may be employed, to include the spinal border of the scapula, as well as one or two searching lateral probes along the inferior spine of the scapula, and across the musculature inferior to, and inserting into, the scapula.

 ### Right-side treatment

Treatment of the right side of the mid and upper thoracic region may be carried out without necessarily changing position, other than to lean across the patient. However, the shorter practitioner should change sides so that, standing half-facing the head of the patient, the right thumb can perform the strokes discussed above.

- Apart from trigger points in the lower trapezius fibres, others may be sought in levator scapulae, supraspinatus and infraspinatus, and subscapularis (by accessing via the axilla).
- The connective tissue zones affecting the arm, stomach, heart, liver and gall bladder are apparent in this region, and neurolymphatic reflexes relating to the arm, thyroid, lungs, throat and heart occur in the upper thoracic spine, including the scapular area (see Chapter 5).
- The intercostal spaces are rich sites of soft tissue dysfunction. The thumb tip, or a fingertip, should be run along both surfaces of the rib margin, as well as in the intercostal space itself.
- In this way the fibres of the small muscles involved will be treated adequately.
- If there is over-approximation of the ribs, a simple stroke along the space may be all that is possible until a degree of normalization has taken place.
- These intercostal areas are extremely sensitive, and care should be taken not to distress the patient.
- In most instances the intercostal spaces on the side opposite that on which the practitioner is standing will be treated using the finger stroke, as illustrated (see Figs 6.2 & 6.6A, B).
- The tip of a finger should be placed in the intercostal space, and gently but firmly brought upwards and around the curve of the trunk towards the spine, feeling for contracted or congested tissues in which trigger points might be located.

Change of position

- The practitioner now half turns so that, instead of facing the patient's head, he or she faces the patient's feet. The pattern of strokes is now

Figure 6.6A, B Fourth (A) and fifth (B) positions of suggested sequence of applications of NMT.

carried out on the patient's left side by the practitioner's right hand (see Fig. 6.7A & B).

- A series of strokes, starting from T8 to T11, followed by T11 to L1 and then L1 to L4, is carried out, as previously described.
- Two or more gliding strokes, with the pressure downwards but angled so that the medial aspect of the thumb is in contact with the lateral margin of the spinous processes, are performed at each level.
- The lower intercostal areas are treated in much the same way as described above.
- The practitioner then steps back from the table and glides the thumb, to allow access to a stroke that runs along the superior iliac crest, from just above the hip to the sacroiliac joint.
- Several such strokes may be applied into the heavy musculature above the crest of ilium.
- To treat the opposite side, the practitioner changes sides, so that he or she is facing the patient's waist and half-turned towards the feet; the left hand can deal with the lower

thoracic and upper lumbar area, and the iliac crest, in the manner described above.

- One or two strokes should then be applied, running caudad over the tips of the spinous processes from the mid-thoracic area to the sacrum, searching for attachment trigger points.

The area we have been describing contains a network of reflex areas and points:

1. The *tsubo* or acupressure points lying symmetrically on either side of the spine and along the midline have great reflex importance. Associated points (see Fig. 4.3) are located alongside the spine.
2. These points are virtually identical to those described in Thai Yoga Massage as Sen back points (or lines). Evans (2009, p58) describes accessing them as follows: 'To locate these lines we allow the thumbs to feel for the spinous processes of the vertebrae and then let them fall into the two channels either side of

Figure 6.7A, B Sixth and seventh positions of suggested sequence of applications of NMT.

the spine. We can follow these channels with our thumbs from the pelvis to the seventh cervical vertebrae, although in practice we usually stop at the lower edge of the scapulae. In general we are following the medial borders of the erector spinae muscles.'

3. The so-called 'Bladder meridian' acupuncture points lie in two lines running parallel with the spine, one level with the medial border of the scapula, and the other midway between it and the lateral border of the spinous processes.

4. Goodheart's work (1987) suggests that rhomboid weakness indicates liver problems and that pressure on C7 spinous process, and a point on the right of the interspace between the 5th and 6th thoracic spinous process, assists its normalization. Latissimus dorsi weakness apparently indicates pancreatic dysfunction. Lateral to 7th and 8th thoracic interspace is the posterior pressure reflex to normalize this. These and other reflexes would appear to derive from Chapman's reflex theories, and may deserve further study.

5. In general terms, dysfunction of the erector spinae group of muscles, between 6th and 12th thoracic, suggests liver involvement. Similarly 4th, 5th and 6th thoracic area congestion or sensitivity usually involves stomach reflexes and gastric disturbance, whereas T12 and L2 indicate possible kidney dysfunction.

6. Connective tissue zones (see Ch. 5) relating to the stomach, head and lower limb circulation, are located in this region.

7. Jones' tender points (see Ch. 4, Fig. 4.5B in particular) in this region may relate to extension strains.

 Left hip position

The next treatment position requires the practitioner to stand at the level of the patient's left hip, half-facing the head of the couch:

- The left hand and thumb describe a series of cephalad strokes from the sacral apex towards the sacroiliac area, and then laterally along the superior and inferior margins of the iliac crest to the insertion of the tensor fascia lata at the anterior, superior iliac spine (see Fig. 6.8A,B).

- A further series of short strokes of the thumb upwards and laterally in the lumbar area may be described as attempting to stretch the paraspinal muscles away from the spine, notably the sacrospinal group.
- Having treated both left and right sides of the lumbar spine, as above, the practitioner uses a series of two-handed gliding manoeuvres, in which the hands are spread over the upper gluteal area laterally, the thumb tips are placed at the level of the second sacral foramen with a downward (towards the floor) pressure; they glide in a cephalad direction, and slowly laterally, to pass over and through the fibres over the sacroiliac joint. This gliding stroke is repeated several times. (*Note*: the arrow directions on the figures are not meant to be definitive; for example, these strokes could be

performed with the thumbs moving caudad, rather than cephalad, as illustrated).

- Still standing on the left, the practitioner leans across the patient's upper thigh and engages the right thumb on to the ischial tuberosity.
- A series of gliding movements is carried out from that point, laterally to the hip and caudally, towards the gluteal fold.
- A further series of strokes, always applying deep, probing but variable pressure, is then carried out from the sacral border, across the gluteal area, to the hip margins. The fingertips during these strokes are splayed out so that they can guide and balance the hand and thumb movement.
- In these deep muscles the line of the thumb's direction is more towards the tip of the index finger, or middle finger, rather than to the little fingertip, as it was in the cervical area.
- In deep, tense gluteal muscle, the thumb may be inadequate to the task of prolonged

(A)   (B)

Figure 6.8A, B   Eighth and ninth positions of suggested sequence of applications of NMT.

pressure application, and the elbow may be used to sustain deep pressure, for minutes at a time if necessary (see notes on the use of elbow in Ch. 8). Care should be taken, however, as the degree of pressure possible via the elbow is very great, and tissue damage and bruising can result from its careless use.

The practitioner then moves to the right side, repeating the strokes as described. Alternatively, rather than changing sides, the practitioner may lean across the patient, using hooked finger strokes to access the tissues above the hip, and around the curve of the iliac crest effectively.

Trigger points, connective tissue zones and neurolymphatic reflexes that may be involved in the lower lumbar and gluteal areas are shown in Box 6.2.

Box 6.2   Trigger points, connective tissue zones and neurolymphatic reflexes of the lower lumbar, gluteal and lateral thigh areas

- The trigger points that are found in the lower lumbar and gluteal areas include those in the following muscle groups: iliocostal, multifidus, longissimus, gluteus medius and gluteus minimus (see Fig. 3.6 for illustrations of many of these).
- The connective tissue zones that may be involved include those that involve arterial and venous disturbance to the legs, constipation, liver, gall bladder, heart and bladder (see Fig. 5.3).
- The neurolymphatic reflexes, located in this area, include those involving the following areas and conditions: the appendix, haemorrhoids, female generative organs, vasculitis, sciatic nerve, abdominal tension and constipation, prostate, colitis, kidneys, adrenal glands, digestive system, pancreas, liver, spleen and gall bladder. The TFL contains neurolymphatic reflexes to the groin glands, the broad ligaments, spastic constipation and colitis, and the prostate (see Ch. 5).

Lateral thigh and gluteal structures

Having treated the low lumbar area and the gluteals, the practitioner might usefully include a series of strokes across the fibres of the tensor fascia lata (TFL), from the hip area to the lateral knee area.

The tensor fascia lata contains neurolymphatic reflexes to the groin glands, the broad ligaments, spastic constipation and colitis, prostate, etc., and is itself a major contributor to knee, pelvic and low back problems via its influence on the mechanics of the region. It is commonly extremely sensitive to pressure, and care is needed to prevent patient distress in treating it. (See also Alternative methods for treating TFL in Chapter 8.)

Completion of treatment

This completes the basic spinal NMT treatment, apart from any manipulative, mobilization or additional soft tissue procedures that might be indicated or thought desirable.

- Boris Chaitow completed the spinal treatment by standing at the head of the table, leaning over the patient's upper thoracic area, with the palms of both hands totally in contact with the upper lumbar region so that the thenar eminences were resting on the paraspinal musculature, and the fingers pointing laterally.
- The heel of the hand imparted the main contact, laterally.
- A series of gliding strokes was performed, with the hands rhythmically alternating with each other, so that, as the right hand stroked downwards towards the end of its movement on the gluteals, the left was being brought back to the lower thoracic area.
- After the right hand reached the gluteal region, it was brought back to the start.
- In this way a series of 10 to 20 deep, rhythmic, strokes was carried out, in order to stimulate local circulation and drainage, as well as to help relax the patient, who may well have tensed during the NMT treatment of the lumbar and gluteal areas.
- As stated previously, the basic 'assessment' treatment should take no more than 15–20

minutes; however, far longer may be needed if whatever is found, of a dysfunctional nature, were to be treated.

The patient should have a sense of release from tension, and a sense of well-being lasting for some days. Many feel a sense of tiredness, and a great desire to sleep; this should be encouraged. Pain may result in those areas that have borne the brunt of the deeper pressure application, and this should be explained to the patient, who should be encouraged to note any changes in his or her condition, and to report these at the subsequent visit, or by phone/email.

The frequency of application of NMT will vary with the condition. In chronic conditions, one or two treatments weekly are all that is required, for several weeks, or until progress dictates that the interval be lengthened. In acute conditions, treatment may be much more frequent (but almost always less invasive): daily if possible until ease is achieved. Of necessity, this must depend upon what other modalities are employed.

References

Baldry P: *Myofascial pain and fibromyalgia syndromes*, Edinburgh, 2001, Churchill Livingstone.

Chaitow L: Integrated neuromuscular inhibition technique, *British Journal of Osteopathy* 13:17–20, 1994.

Chaitow L: *Muscle energy techniques*, ed 2, Edinburgh, 2001, Churchill Livingstone.

Chaitow L: *Muscle energy techniques*, ed 3, Edinburgh, 2006, Churchill Livingstone.

Dowling D: Progressive neuromuscular inhibition technique (PINS), *J Am Osteopath Assoc* 100(5):285–298, 2000.

Dvorak J, Dvorak V, Schneider W: *Manual medicine therapy*, Stuttgart, 1988, Georg Thieme.

Evans H: *A Myofascial Approach to Thai Massage*, Edinburgh, 2009, Churchill Livingstone.

Goodheart G: *Applied kinesiology workshop procedure manuals 1976–1987*, Detroit, 1987, Published privately.

Kostopoulos D, Rizopoulos K: Effect of topical aerosol skin refrigerant (Spray and Stretch technique) on passive and active stretching, *Journal of Bodywork and Movement Therapies* 12(2):96–104, 2008.

Lewit K: *Manipulation in rehabilitation of the motor system*, ed 3, London, 1999, Butterworths.

Lowe J-C, Honeyman-Lowe G: Ultrasound treatment of trigger points: differences in technique for myofascial pain syndrome and fibromyalgia patients, *Medecine du Sud-est* April–May–June, no. 2:12–15, 1999.

McMakin C: Microcurrent treatment of myofascial pain in head, neck and face, *Topics in Clinical Chiropractic* 5(1):29–35, 1998.

Rolf I: *Rolfing – integration of human structures*, New York, 1977, Harper & Row.

Simons D: Understanding effective treatments of myofascial trigger points, *Journal of Bodywork and Movement Therapies* 6(2):81–88, 2002.

Sola A, Bonica J: Myofascial pain syndromes, ed 2. In Bonica JJ, editor: *The Management of Pain 1*, Philadelphia, 1990, Lea and Febiger, p 354.

Travell J, Simons D: *Myofascial pain and dysfunction: the trigger point manual*, vol 2: *the lower extremities*, Baltimore, 1992, Williams & Wilkins.

Basic abdominal and pelvic NMT application

7

CHAPTER CONTENTS

Objectives 141
Somaticovisceral symptoms 142
Junctional tissues 142
Assisting organ dysfunction 143
More on abdominal reflex areas 143
Abdominal NMT application 148
Intercostal treatment 148
Rectal sheath 150
Symphysis pubis 151
Positional release implications of abdominal tender points 151
Lateral rectus sheath 151
Umbilicus 152
Linea alba 153
Specific release 153
NMT and chronic pelvic pain dysfunction 153

Objectives

The objectives for the use of NMT – and associated methods – in the treatment of abdomino-pelvic tissues vary considerably and may include:

1. To attempt to normalize local soft tissue dysfunction and pain (including symptoms produced by myofascial trigger points) resulting from postural or overuse strain (occupational or leisure activities, patterns of use, overload, repetition of movement, lifting, etc.), breathing pattern disorders, obesity, visceroptosis (causing drag of supporting structures, and associated congestion).
2. To enhance relaxation and reduction in symptoms relating to emotional or stress influences, particularly long-held psychological distress.
3. To improve function when the area has been traumatized (accidents, blows, surgery, etc.).
4. To influence internal organ function via reflex stimulation, for example using neurolymphatic (Chapman) reflexes and/or acupuncture points (see Ch. 4).
5. To modify painful and distressing symptoms such as those associated with chronic pelvic pain (CPP), interstitial cystitis and urgency (Weiss 2001). See Box 7.1 for details of research into such influences.
6. To attempt to improve function of the abdomino-pelvic organs by directly influencing circulatory and drainage functions (including lymphatic function) of the region (Wallace et al 1997).

7. To modify the negative local effects of viscerosomatic influences (see Ch. 3).
8. To improve diaphragmatic and respiratory function.

Somaticovisceral symptoms

In Chapter 3 there was discussion of the phenomenon in which organ dysfunction reflects reflexogenically to the soma particularly as areas of segmental facilitation (sensitization) in the spinal region. These are, of course, the viscerosomatic reflexes. Later in this chapter possible variations on causes of viscerosomatic reflex pain will be outlined.

Simons et al (1999) reverse the consideration when they report details of somatovisceral responses, particularly arising from abdominal musculature, influencing internal visceral organs and functions.

They note that injection of the trigger affecting an organ may offer symptomatic relief. This is not meant to suggest that local changes (such as trigger points) in the soma, muscles, etc. are necessarily the cause of such dysfunctions and diseases (see list below), but that there exists a strong possibility, in any given case, that the

conditions/disease processes may be aggravated and/or maintained by reflexogenic activity associated with myofascial trigger points:

- projectile vomiting
- anorexia
- nausea
- intestinal colic
- diarrhoea
- urinary bladder and sphincter spasm
- dysmenorrhoea
- pain symptoms mimicking those of appendicitis and cholelithiasis
- symptoms of burning, fullness, bloating, swelling or gas (Gutstein 1944)
- heartburn and other symptoms of hiatal hernia
- urinary frequency
- groin pain
- chronic diarrhoea
- pain when coughing
- belching
- chest pain that is not cardiac in origin
- abdominal cramping
- colic in infants as well as adults.

Junctional tissues

Simons et al (1999) have discussed the sites of trigger points as falling largely into two categories:
1. close to attachments
2. close to motor end-points near the bellies of muscles.

These guidelines also apply when treating abdominopelvic, and related areas, where, in addition, the author's clinical experience suggests that particular attention should be given to specific junctional tissues, such as:

- The central tendon
- Lateral aspect of the rectal muscle sheaths
- Attachments of the recti muscles and external oblique muscles to the ribs
- The xiphisternal ligament, as well as the lower attachments of the internal and external oblique muscles
- Intercostal areas from 5th to 12th ribs are equally important

- Scars from previous operations may be the site of formation of connective tissue trigger points (Simons et al 1999). After sufficient healing has taken place, these incision sites can be examined by gently pinching, compressing and rolling the scar tissue between the thumb and finger to examine for evidence of trigger points, as discussed in earlier chapters (Chaitow & DeLany 2000).

Assisting organ dysfunction

Specific general areas are worthy of consideration in treating conditions that affect particular organs or functions, based on the evidence of the different reflex systems described in Chapter 4 (see also notes on percussive methods, such as spondylotherapy, in Chapter 8) (Baldry 1993, Chaitow & DeLany 2000, Fitzgerald et al 2009, Kuchera & Kuchera 1994, Wallace et al 1997):

- Liver dysfunction and portal circulatory dysfunction calls for special attention to the right-side intercostal musculature, from the 5th to the 12th ribs. Especially important are the various muscular insertions into all these ribs.
- Gall bladder dysfunction involves similar areas, with extra attention to the area on the costal margin, roughly midway between the xiphisternal notch and the lateral rib margins.
- Spleen function may be stimulated by attention to the intercostal spaces between the 7th and 12th ribs on the left side.
- Digestive disorders in general may benefit from NMT applied to the central tendon, between the recti, and directly to the rectal sheaths.
- Stomach pain is treated via its reflex area to the left of the xiphisternal notch and to the tendon and rectal sheaths.
- Colonic problems and ovarian dysfunction may benefit from reflex NMT application to both iliac fossae as well as to the midline structures.
- Dysfunction of the kidneys, ureters and bladder requires attention to the inguinal borders of the internal and external oblique insertions, the suprapubic insertions of the

recti, the overlying muscles and sheaths of the area, and the internal aspects of the upper thigh.
- In pelvic congestion relating to gynaecological dysfunction, NMT should be applied to the hypogastrium and both iliac fossae. This appears to relieve congestion and stimulates pelvic circulation.
- Ileitis and other functional disturbances of the transverse colon and small intestine may benefit from NMT applied to the umbilical area.
- Prostatic dysfunction may benefit from NMT to the central hypogastric region. Internal drainage massage of the prostate should also be considered.

The above brief indications should be considered in conjunction with other reflex systems and points (see below), as well as attention to the appropriate spinal areas (see notes on facilitation in Ch. 3), which may also benefit from NMT.

More on abdominal reflex areas

Gutstein (1944) noted 'trigger areas' in the sternal, parasternal and epigastric regions, and in the upper portions of the recti muscles, all relating to varying degrees of retroperistalsis. He also noted that colonic dysfunction related to triggers in the mid and lower recti muscles. These were all predominantly left-sided.

Other symptoms that improved or disappeared with the obliteration of these triggers include excessive appetite, poor appetite, flatulence, nervous vomiting, nervous diarrhoea, etc.

The triggers were always 'tender spots', easily found by palpation, and situated mainly in the upper, mid and lower portions of the recti muscles, over the lower portion of the sternum and the epigastrium, including the xyphoid process and the parasternal region. The parasternal region corresponds to the attachments of the rectus muscles into the 5th, 6th and 7th ribs.

Fielder & Pyott (1955) described a number of reflexes occurring on the large bowel itself. These could be localized by deep palpation and treated by specific release techniques (see Chapter 8, and Figure 8.21). These reflexes palpate as areas of tenderness, and may include a degree of swelling and congestion resulting from adhesions, spasticity, diverticuli, chemical or bacterial irritation, etc.

In considering the reflexes available for therapeutic intervention, in the thoracic and abdominal regions, the neurolymphatic points of Chapman are worthy of close attention (see Chapter 4 for more detail). When applying NMT in its evaluative mode, to the anterior thorax and abdomen (as described later in this chapter), an awareness of the reflexes described by Chapman (Owen 1980) is a distinct advantage, especially if there is a need to take account of visceral or thoracic organ dysfunction.

Kuchera (1997) notes:

Palpate for tender anterior Chapman's [neurolymphatic] points as an indication to specific visceral irritation ... Abdominal viscera, because of their innervations, have their first Chapman's [neurolymphatic] points at the level of the fifth intercostal spaces. If an anterior Chapman's [neurolymphatic] point is tender, ask the patient questions relating to dysfunction of the organ most likely to produce the tender point.

Anterior neurolymphatic reflexes for the upper lungs are found between the 3rd and 4th ribs, and between the 4th and 5th ribs (lower lung), close to the costal cartilage and the sternum.

See Figure 7.1 for the location of common abdominally related reflexes noted in this region (and also Figs 5.8A,B).

Discussion

To what extent Gutstein's myodysneuric points are interchangeable with Chapman's, or Fielder's, reflexes, or other systems of reflex study (e.g. acupuncture or *tsubo* points or Travell's trigger points), and to what extent these involve Mackenzie's work (Mackenzie 1909) as illustrated in Figure 5.4, is a matter for further research.

What is certain is that, within the soft tissues of this region, there abound palpable, sensitive, discrete areas of dysfunction that, on a local basis, interfere with or modify functional integrity to a greater or lesser degree, and reflexively are capable of massive interference with normal

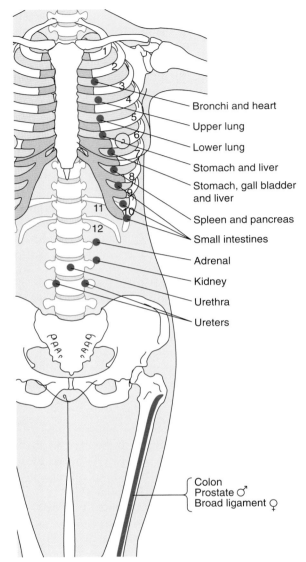

Figure 7.1 Common neurolymphatic points. From Ward (1997), with permission.

physiological function on a neural, circulatory and lymphatic level, to the extent of producing or mimicking serious pathological conditions. As these areas of dysfunction often yield to the simple, soft tissue manipulative techniques that are incorporated into Lief's NMT, the value of these techniques becomes apparent.

Many of Jones' (positional release/strain/counterstrain) tender points (see Figure 4.5A) are located in the abdominal region, specifically relating to those strains that occur in a flexed position (Jones 1981).

Bennett's neurovascular points (see Chapter 4 and Figure 5.9A) are located mainly on the anterior aspect of the body, and may be located during abdominal NMT work. This may be a link with the work of Mackenzie and others, who have demonstrated a clear relationship between the abdominal wall and the viscera. This and other reflex patterns provide the rationale for NMT application to the abdominal and sternal regions.

These reflex patterns vary in individual cases, but it is clear that the majority of the organs are able to protect themselves by producing contraction, spasm and hyperaesthesia of the overlying, reflexively related, muscle wall – the myotome – which is also often augmented by hyperaesthesia of the overlying skin – the dermatome.

Baldry (1993) details a huge amount of research that validates the link (a somatovisceral reflex) between abdominal trigger points, and symptoms as diverse as anorexia, flatulence, nausea, vomiting, diarrhoea, colic, dysmenorrhoea and dysuria.

Pain of a deep aching nature, or sometimes of a sharp or burning type, is reported as being associated with this range of symptoms, which mimic organ disease or dysfunction (Fitzgerald et al 2009, Melnick 1954, Ranger et al 1971, Travell & Simons 1983).

Baldry (1993) has further summarized the importance of this region as a source of considerable pain and distress involving pelvic, abdominal and gynaecological symptoms. He says:

Pain in the abdomen and pelvis most likely to be helped by acupuncture is that which occurs as a result of activation of trigger points in the muscles, fascia, tendons and ligaments of the anterior and lateral abdominal wall, the lower back, the floor of the pelvis and the upper anterior part of the thigh. Such pain, however, is all too often erroneously assumed to be due to some intra-abdominal lesion, and as a consequence of being inappropriately treated is often allowed to persist for much longer than is necessary.

If we replace the word acupuncture with the term 'appropriate manual methods', we can appreciate that a large amount of abdominal and pelvic distress may be remediable via the methods outlined in this book.

What activates these triggers? – similar factors that produce 'stress' anywhere else in the musculoskeletal system: postural faults, trauma, environmental stressors such as cold and damp, surgery (another form of trauma) and so on.

Differential diagnosis is obviously important in a region housing so many vital organs, and attention to the overall pattern of symptom presentation is critical.

If in doubt, obtain expert opinion.

 Is the pain in the muscle or an organ?

As there is no underlying osseous structure available to allow compression of the musculature of many of the soft tissues of the abdomen, there is a need for a particular strategy that helps to screen palpated pain occurring at depth from that being produced in surface tissues.

When a local area of pain is noted, using NMT or any other palpation method, it should be firmly compressed by the palpating digit, sufficient to produce pain/referred pain (if a trigger is involved) but not enough to cause distress.

- The supine patient is then asked to raise both (straight) legs from the table (heels must be raised by several inches).
- As this happens there will be a contraction of the abdominal muscles, which produces a compression of the trigger point between the muscle and the finger/thumb, and pain should increase.
- If pain decreases on the raising of the legs, the site of the pain is beneath the muscle and probably involves a visceral problem (Thomson & Francis 1977).

It is, of course, possible for there to be a problem in the viscera as well as in the abdominal wall (see item 3 in the discussion immediately below), in which case this test would be in error in ascribing all symptoms of pain to a muscle wall lesion.

The superficial musculature may be receiving distress sensations from an inflamed or irritated organ. The test described above therefore gives a clue, but not an absolute finding, as to the locality of the problem causing the pain.

Pain variables in abdominal somatic tissues

Kuchera (1997) points to three different manifestations of pain and discomfort arising from irritation or inflammation in the pelvic and abdominal viscera:

1. A 'vague, gnawing, deep, poorly localized, and mid-abdominal' pain, derives from afferent impulses from the organs of the region travelling towards the spinal cord.
2. Organs are supplied with their sympathetic input from specific spinal levels. Afferent messages also travel towards the spine, from the organs, along the same pathways, and when the organ is dysfunctional (inflamed, irritated, etc.) paraspinal changes (including tenderness, asymmetry, tissue changes and altered range of movement) will be noted at the level from which sympathetic innervation emerges for particular organs. (See notes on facilitation and viscerosomatic reflexes in Chapter 3, connective tissue massage in Chapter 4, and also zones of dysfunction in Chapter 5.) Beal (1985) has summarized the levels as:
   - T1–T5 = heart and lungs
   - T5–T10 = oesophagus, stomach, small intestine, liver, gall bladder, spleen, pancreas and adrenal cortex
   - T10–L2 = large bowel, appendix, kidney, ureter, adrenal medulla, testes, ovaries, urinary bladder, prostate gland and uterus. (See also notes under heading 'Assisting organ dysfunction' above).
3. Pain may be noted in the soft tissues superficial to the organ. Kuchera (1997) describes these as being due to irritation of contiguous peritoneal tissues and the abdominal wall, and as being 'responsible for rebound tenderness and abdominal guarding, associated with severe abdominal pain.' (See also Fig. 5.4 showing abdominal reflexes, as described by Mackenzie in 1909).

Treatment of attachment stress in the mesentery (e.g. visceroptosis effects)

The mesentery (literally 'the middle intestine') is the name given to the double layer of peritoneal membrane that supports the small intestine. It is shaped like a fan, with its shorter edge attaching to the back of the abdomen, and the longer edge attaching to the small intestine for a length of around 20 feet (6 metres). The main mesenteric attachment is located in a line running from approximately 1 inch (2.5 cm) above and 1 inch (2.5 cm) to the left of the umbilicus, downward and to the right lower quadrant of the abdomen, just anterior to the sacroiliac joint (see Fig. 7.2).

If the organs of the abdomen sag, as occurs in obesity and visceroptosis, enormous degrees of drag occur on the mesenteric attachment tissues, with resulting congestion. Kuchera (1997) reports:

> '[Appropriate] treatment improves organ function, and can decrease many functional visceral symptoms, including bloating, constipation, and pelvic or abdominal pain.

Kuchera acknowledges the clinical research and teachings of the French osteopath Barral, whose work in visceral manipulation has opened this area to improved therapeutic intervention (Barral & Mercier 1988).

The mesenteric structures carry the sympathetic and parasympathetic fibres (as well as arteries) to the viscera, and also afferent fibres, lymphatic and venous vessels, away from the viscera.

Kuchera (1997) suggests that tenderness and tension in the mesentery can be palpated for tension and treated as follows:

> By placing the extended fingers flat over the lateral margin of the ascending or descending colon and moving the viscera toward the midline of the body. The [practitioner] monitors continuously for changes in resistance to this movement.

- The mesentery of the sigmoid colon is moved toward the umbilicus (see Fig. 7.3A, B).
- The 6-inch (15 cm) mesentery, along with the 30 feet (9 metres) of small intestines, is palpated by placing the extended fingers carefully into the lower left abdominal quadrant to obtain as much of the small intestines as possible, and

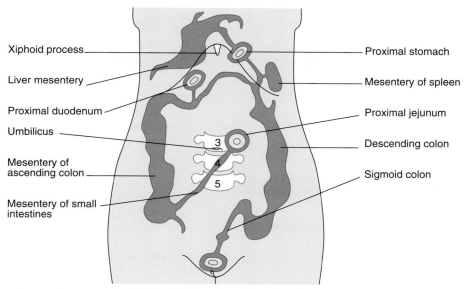

Figure 7.2   Mesenteric attachments as described by Kuchera. From Ward (1997), with permission.

moving this towards the upper right quadrant of the abdomen (see Fig. 7.4).

To treat restrictions noted in such palpation:

- The patient lies supine, with knees flexed and feet flat on the table.
- The fingers are extended and placed flat over the lateral margin of the mesentery (to be treated).

- Medial pressure is then placed over the section of bowel, at right angles to its posterior, mesenteric, abdominal wall attachment.
- The tension is held as the patient takes a half-breath and holds it.

Wallace et al (1997) caution against causing any pain during these procedures, and further

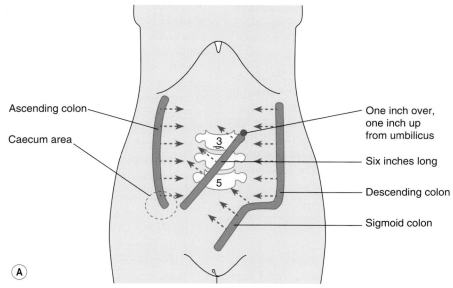

Figure 7.3A   Suggested directions of movement in treating intestinal mesentery (after Kuchera). From Ward (1997), with permission.

Figure 7.3B   Lifting the small intestine/sigmoid colon to ease mesenteric drag (after Wallace et al). From Ward (1997), with permission.

Figure 7.4   Lifting the caecum to ease mesenteric drag (after Wallace et al). From Ward (1997), with permission.

suggest that the tissues being held should be gently 'turned' clockwise and anticlockwise, to sense their position of greatest tissue freedom. The tissues are then held for not less than 90 seconds, or until a sense of relaxation is noted.

When breathing resumes, after this positional release approach, the tissues should be repalpated.

Abdominal NMT application

(Boxes 7.2 & 7.3)

In treating the abdominal and thoracic regions, the patient should be supine with the head supported by a medium-sized pillow and the knees

---

Box 7.2   Caution: pulsations

If, during palpation or treatment, any large pulsating mass is noted in the midline between the xyphoid and the umbilicus, caution should be exercised.

Kuchera (1997) notes: 'A normal abdominal aorta in an adult should not be wider than an inch (2.5 cm). Pulsations occurring anteriorly are normal, but lateral pulsations from the aorta suggest a weak vessel wall or aneurysm. Palpate [also] the inguinal area for a good pulse and compare the right and left sides. If a decreased pulse is found on one or both sides, ask the patient about claudication and then palpate and evaluate the pulse at the popliteal, posterior tibial, and dorsal pedis arteries in that leg, and compare to pulses in the opposite leg.'

---

flexed, either with a bolster under them or drawn right up so that the feet approximate the buttocks. Generous application of lubricant should be made to the area being treated.

Intercostal treatment

Abdominal and anterior intercostal NMT (see Fig. 7.5)

The initial objective of the treatment strokes described below is to evaluate for soft tissue changes (active or latent trigger points, tissue texture changes, asymmetry, tenderness, etc.) with a contact that 'meets and matches' tissue tension.

Only when a decision has been made to use subsequent strokes to attempt to alter the status of the tissues should pressure be increased to overcome tension, fibrotic resistance, etc., so stretching, inhibiting, draining – and in other ways modifying – structural features. (See Chapter 3, particularly Box 3.5, for notes on the effects of compressive force.)

- The practitioner should be facing the patient, and be half-turned towards the head, with legs apart for an even distribution of weight, and with knees flexed to facilitate the transfer of pressure through the arms. As many of the manoeuvres in the intercostal area, and on the abdomen itself, involve finger and thumb

Box 7.3   Differential abdominal symptoms (Grieve 1994)

Most abdominal disorders can produce pain in the back (e.g. peptic ulcer, colonic cancer, abdominal arterial disease). Therefore, all other symptoms should be evaluated alongside the musculoskeletal assessment.

- A hiatus hernia is usually associated with bilateral thoracic and shoulder pain. Anginal pain classically presents with chest, anterior cervical and (usually left) arm pain.
- Thoracic facet or disc conditions can mimic angina, as can active trigger point activity. Aggravating and ameliorating factors usually offer clues as to whether the condition is cardiac related, or whether it is aggravated or eased by biomechanical influences.
- A dysfunctional gall bladder commonly refers pain to the mid-thoracic area, unilaterally or bilaterally. Aggravating and ameliorating factors can usually offer clues as to whether the condition is related to digestive function or is biomechanically influenced.
- Sacroiliac and right buttock pain may be produced by perforation of the ileum in regional ileitis (Crohn's disease).
- Pronounced low back pain (possibly referring to the testicles in men) may be associated with an aneurysm that is about to rupture. Grieve (1994) reports that 'the onset of dissection of the ascending aorta or aortic arch is characterized by a sudden, tearing chest pain', which may radiate to the neck, thorax, abdomen and legs. The distinction between such symptoms and an acute musculoskeletal problem may be discerned by the 'suddenness, severity and spread' of the pain.
- If a patient has a background of coronary, pulmonary or bronchial disease, the vertebral veins may have become varicosed, leading to an ill-defined backache. Grieve (1994) discusses the widespread nature of venous drainage from the vertebral column. These veins, as well as associated arteries and arterioles, are 'supplied with a dense plexiform arrangement of unmyelinated nerve fibers which constitute an important part of the vertebral column, and which may be irritated in a variety of ways to give rise to pain.'

Figure 7.5   Neuromuscular abdominal technique. Suggested lines of application to access primary trigger point and attachment sites, and interfaces between different muscle groups. Note that the lines of application on this chart show one side only, and a full assessment/ treatment involves these thumb or finger strokes being applied on each side of the body.

movements of a lighter nature than those applied through the heavy spinal musculature, the elbows need not be kept as straight as possible for spinal NMT (see Ch. 6).
- However, when deep pressure is called for, and especially when this is applied via the thumb, the same criterion of weight transference, from the shoulder through the thumb, applies, and the straight arm is then an advantage for the economic and efficient use of energy.
- The practitioner should be positioned to be level with the patient's waist, and a series of strokes would be applied with the tip of the thumb, along the course of the intercostal spaces from the sternum, laterally.
- It is important that the attachments of the internal and external muscles receive attention.

- The margins of the ribs, both inferior and superior aspects, should receive firm gliding pressure from the distal phalanx of the thumb or middle finger.
- If there is too little space to allow such a degree of differentiated pressure, then a simple stroke along the available intercostal space has to suffice.
- If the thumb cannot be insinuated between the ribs, a finger (side of finger) contact can be used (see description of NMT finger technique in Chapter 6), in which this is drawn towards the practitioner, from the side contralateral to that being treated, towards the sternum.
- The intercostals, from the 5th rib to the costal margin below the 12th rib, should receive a series of two or three deep, slow-moving, gliding, sensitive strokes on each side, with special reference to points of particular congestion or sensitivity. These areas may also benefit from sustained or variable pressure techniques, depending on the objective. It is useful to note the possible presence, in the intercostal spaces, close to the sternum of neurolymphatic (Chapman) reflex points.
- These points require only light circular pressure when being treated (see Chapter 5 for more detail). The practitioner should bear in mind other reflex patterns in the region, including those related to acupuncture alarm points and neurovascular points.
- If a localized area of dysfunction is located, which refers pain or other symptoms that are familiar to the patient, an active trigger point will have been located (see Ch. 3).
- Gentle probing on the sternum itself may elicit sensitivity in the rudimentary sternalis muscle, which has been found to house trigger points. If this is found to be sensitive, any of the various trigger point treatments recommended in Chapter 8 may be used.
- It is not necessary for the practitioner to change sides during treatment of the intercostals, unless it is found to be more comfortable to do so.
- Having treated the intercostal musculature and connective tissue, and having charted and/or treated any trigger points located during assessment, the practitioner, using either a deep thumb pressure, or a contact with the pads of the fingertips, applies a series of short strokes in a combination of oblique lateral and inferior directions from the xyphoid process.

Rectal sheath

- Thumbs or fingers may then be used to apply a series of deep slow strokes, along and under the costal margins. Whether diaphragmatic attachments can be located is questionable; however, sustained, firm (but not invasively aggressive) pressure allows for gradual access to an area that may reveal trigger points of exquisite sensitivity, with often surprising areas of referral. Many seem to produce sensations internally, while others create sensations in the lower extremities or in the throat, upper chest and shoulders.
- Deactivation of such triggers needs to be carried out slowly, carefully and with sensitivity.
- A series of short strokes using fairly deep, but not painful, pressure should then be applied by the thumb, from the midline up to the lateral rectal sheath.
- This series of strokes starts just inferior to the xyphoid and concludes at the pubic promontory where trigger points are common.
- The series may be repeated on each side several times, depending on the degree of tension, congestion and sensitivity noted. It is useful during these applications to be aware of the mesenteric attachments as described by Wallace et al (1997) and Kuchera (1997) (see Figs. 7.2 & 7.3).
- A similar pattern of assessment/treatment is followed (using the thumb if working ipsilaterally, and the fingers if working contralaterally) across the lateral border of the rectal sheath, a series of short, deep, slow-moving (usually thumb) strokes being applied from just inferior to the costal margin of the rectal sheath, until the inguinal ligament is reached. Both sides are treated in this way (Fig. 7.5).
- A series of similar strokes is then applied on one side and then the other laterally, from the lateral border of the rectal sheath (see Fig. 7.5).

- These strokes follow the contour of the trunk, so that the upper strokes travel in a slightly inferior curve whilst moving laterally (following the curve of the lower ribs), and the lower strokes have a superior inclination (following the curve of the crest of the pelvis) as the hand moves laterally.
- A total of five or six strokes should be adequate to complete these movements, and this could be repeated, before performing the same strokes on the opposite side.
- Evidence is being sought of local soft tissue changes, as well as any underlying sense of tension or 'drag' on supporting tissues.

When treating the side on which the practitioner is standing, it may be more comfortable to apply the therapeutic stroke via the flexed fingertips, which are drawn towards the practitioner, or the usual thumb stroke may be used (see Ch. 6).

In treating the opposite side, thumb pressure can be applied more easily, as in spinal technique, with the fingers acting as a fulcrum and the thumb weaving towards them in a series of 2 to 3 inch (3 to 5 cm) strokes.

The sensing of contracted localized areas of dysfunction is more difficult in abdominal work, and requires great sensitivity of touch, and great concentration on the part of the practitioner.

Symphysis pubis

The sheaths of the rectus abdominis muscles, from the costal margins downwards to the pubic bones, are evaluated by finger or thumb strokes. Attention should be given to the soft tissue component of, as well as the insertions into, the iliac fossa, the pubic bones and the symphysis pubis, including the inguinal ligaments (see Fig. 7.5).

- Strokes should be made, commencing at the anterior superior iliac spine (ASIS), while attempting to assess the attachments of internal and external obliques as well as transversus abdominis, which can be contacted.
- A deep but not painful stroke, employing the pad of a thumb, should be applied to the superior aspect of the pubic crest. This should start at the symphysis pubis and move

laterally, first in one direction and, then after repeating it once or twice, in the other.
- A similar series, starting at the centre and moving laterally, should then be applied over the anterior aspect of the pubic bone. Great care should be taken not to use undue pressure as the area is sensitive at the best of times, and may be acutely so if there is dysfunction associated with the insertions into these structures (as well as in relation to sacral torsions, sacroiliac dysfunction or chronic pelvic pain – which is discussed briefly later in this chapter).
- A series of deep slow movements should then be performed, via the thumb, along the superior and inferior aspects of the inguinal ligament, starting at the pubic bone and running up to and beyond the iliac crest.

Positional release implications of abdominal tender points

In this lower abdominal area, close to the ASIS, and towards the umbilicus, many of the tender points (see Chapter 4 on Jones' points, and Figure 4.5A) associated with flexion strains of the lumbar and lower thoracic spine may be located.

Positional release methods should be employed to relieve the dysfunctional patterns associated with these (see notes on strain/counterstrain in Chapter 8 and also Box 7.4).

Lateral rectus sheath

- The thumbs, or fingertips, may then be insinuated beneath the lateral rectus border at its lower margins, and deep pressure applied towards the midline.
- The hand or thumb should then slowly move cephalad, in short stages, whilst maintaining this medial pressure.
- This is thought to lift the connective tissue from its underlying attachments, so helping to normalize localized contractures and fibrous infiltrations.
- Additionally, when working on the right the ascending colon, and on the left the descending colon, will be receiving the 'lift' appropriate for release of mesenteric drag symptoms (see Fig. 7.3B).

Box 7.4 Positional release technique for abdominal muscles

Tender points (which may or may not also be trigger points) located in the abdominal musculature often represent dysfunction of the lumbothoracic region; they result from strain or stress, and occurred in flexion.

Tender points are almost always located in tissues shortened at the time of strain. For a greater understanding of the strain/counterstrain theory, which supports this assertion (see Chaitow 2007, Chaitow & DeLany 2000, Deig 2001, Jones 1981).

Gross positioning to relieve lumbar flexion stresses and strains takes the (usually supine) patient painlessly into flexion (by raising the flexed lower limbs to induce lumbar flexion), with the final position of ease being held for at least 90 seconds.

The 'position of ease' is determined by means of palpation of the tender point, with the patient reporting on the change in 'score' as the

positioning is 'fine tuned'. A score of 3 or less is the objective, having commenced from a score of 10 before the repositioning starts.

- Jones (1981) reports that L1 has two tender points: one at the tip of the anterior superior iliac spine and the other on the medial surface of the ilium, just medial to ASIS.
- The tender point for 2nd lumbar anterior strain is found lateral to the anterior inferior iliac spine.
- The tender point for L3 lies 1 inch (2.5 cm) below a line connecting L1 and L2 points.
- L4 tender point is found at the attachment of the inguinal ligament on the ilium.
- L5 points are on the body of the pubes, just to the side of the symphysis.
- In bilateral strains, both sides should be treated. L3 and L4 usually require greater side-bending in fine-tuning than the other lumbar points.

Umbilicus

A series of strokes should then be applied around the umbilicus.

- Using thumb or flexed fingertips, a number of movements of a stretching nature should be performed, in which the non-treating hand stabilizes the tissue at the start of the stroke, which first runs from approximately 1 inch (2.5 cm) superior and lateral to the umbilicus on the right side, to the same level on the left side.
- The non-treating hand then stabilizes the tissues at this end-point of the stroke and a further stretching and probing stroke is applied inferiorly to a point about 1 inch (2.5 cm) inferior and lateral to the umbilicus, on the left side. This area is then stabilized, and the stroke is applied to a similar point on the right. (See circular arrows around umbilicus on Figure 7.5.)
- The circle is completed by a further stroke upwards, to end at the point at which the cicular exploration of these tissues began.
- This series of movements should have a rhythmical pattern so that, as the treating hand reaches the end of its stroke, the non-treating hand comes to that same point and replaces the contact with a stabilizing pressure, whilst the treating hand begins its next stroke.

- A series of three or four such circuits of the umbilicus should be performed.
- Note that the superior mesenteric attachment, which supports the small intestine, is located approximately 1 inch (2.5 cm) superior and 1 inch (2.5 cm) laterally, to the left of the umbilicus.
- Additional strokes may be applied along the midline and the sheaths of the recti muscles from the costal margins downwards.

A soothing culmination to the foregoing (which should take approximately 10–15 minutes) may be applied by a circular clockwise series of movements in which the palm of one hand and the heel of the other alternately circle the whole abdominal area.

Thus, with the practitioner standing to the right of the patient, the palm and fingers of the left hand stroke deeply but gently down the left abdominal structures and then across the lower abdomen towards the practitioner where, using the heel and palm, the right hand takes over the stroke and proceeds up the right side to the costal margin. At this point it changes direction to run across the upper abdomen, where the left hand takes over to repeat this pattern several times. Alternatively, the positional release methods, as described by Wallace et al (1997) and Kuchera (1997) (see Figs 7.3 & 7.4), may be performed.

Linea alba

Additional strokes should be applied along the midline, on the linea alba itself, while searching for evidence of contractions, adhesions, fibrotic nodules, oedema and sensitivity.

Caution is always required to avoid deep pressure on the linea alba, especially if the patient has weakened this muscular/fascial interface as a result of pregnancy, surgery or trauma (*diastasis recti*). It should also be recalled that the linea alba is a place of attachment of the external obliques as well as transversus abdominis (Braggins 2000).

Specific release

Specific release techniques may be applied during, or after, this general NMT treatment (see Figure 8.21A,B and accompanying notes in Chapter 8). This might be particularly appropriate in cases where there are abdominal scars, or internal adhesions.

The general NMT abdominal treatment (including specific release methods) can be repeated several times weekly, if indicated, but normally once a week should prove adequate, until improvement in function is achieved.

In chronic conditions of abdominal or pelvic dysfunction (see below), the NMT approach as described, together with specific release movements, and appropriate spinal and whole body treatment, is capable of having a profound effect on function in the area.

With an improvement in circulation and drainage, and a reduction in tensions, contractions and reflex activities, homeostatic mechanisms are automatically enhanced.

NMT and chronic pelvic pain dysfunction

Chronic pelvic pain (CPP) is a widespread and distressing condition that accounts for between 10% and 15% of all gynaecological referrals. Zondervan et al (2001) report that the estimated lifetime occurrence of CPP is 33%, affecting primarily, but not exclusively, females. The main symptoms – apart from chronic pain – are:

- Interstitial (non-bacterial) cystitis (IC) – frequency, urgency discomfort/pain on urination
- Vulvar vestibulitis syndrome – a subset of urinary and genital pain disorders or 'painful bladder' syndromes
- Dyspareunia – painful intercourse.

There are numerous potential causes – however one in particular is relevant to this book.

The European Association of Urology (Fall et al 2008) note that trigger points can be located within the pelvic floor muscle, as well as external pelvic and abdominal muscles (Slocumb 1984, Anderson et al 2005, Srinivasan 2007).

The pelvic floor trigger points can develop for a variety of reasons, one of which involves excessive tone in the muscles of the pelvic floor – something commonly noted in female (mainly) athletes, gymnasts, dancers, or individuals who excessively perform Pilates-style exercises (Chaitow 2007). For example Bo & Borgen (2001) found that 41% of elite female athletes experience stress urinary incontinence, a common feature of CPP.

Pain deriving from pelvic floor trigger points is usually aggravated by specific movements and alleviated by certain positions – for example a patient may sit down cautiously, often on one buttock, and standing up again will commonly be painful. CPP may also be aggravated by sustained or repeated contractions (during urination and/or defecation for example).

Trigger points that reproduce pelvic pain, as well as urgency and other symptoms, can often be identified and treated by deactivating active triggers, both internally, as well as externally in the abdominal, gluteal and piriformis muscles.

Weiss (2001) has noted that in his experience the majority of patients with IC report an early history that resulted in pelvic floor muscle dysfunction, suggestive of increased pelvic floor tension. Weiss reports that he has found that an integral part of the treatment regimen, in such patients, involves normalization of these muscles via manual deactivation of trigger points, while also reducing the pelvic floor hypertonicity by means of stretching and strengthening exercises. See Box 7.1.

Connective tissue manipulation (CTM) as described earlier, has also been used to alleviate the symptoms of CPP, as has deep relaxation and biofeedback (Fitzgerald et al 2009).

Trigger point release, involving NMT methods – as discussed throughout the book, is an effective therapeutic approach, as is stretching of the muscle housing the trigger points.

Note: Internal examination, palpation and treatment of pelvic floor trigger points requires:

- A legal status that allows such procedures
- Signed informed consent from the patient
- A suitable chaperone
- Adequate training.

References

Anderson R, Wise D, Sawyer T, Chan C: Integration of myofascial trigger point release and paradoxical relaxation training treatment of chronic pelvic pain in men, *J Urol* 174(1):155–160, 2005.

Baldry P: *Acupuncture, trigger points and musculoskeletal pain*, Edinburgh, 1993, Churchill Livingstone.

Barral JP, Mercier P: *Visceral manipulation*, Seattle, 1988, Eastland Press.

Beal M: Viscerosomatic reflexes: a review, *J Am Osteopath Assoc* 85(12):786–801, 1985.

Bo K, Borgen J: Prevalence of stress and urge urinary incontinence in elite athletes and controls, *Med Sci Sports Exerc* 33(11):1797–1802, 2001.

Braggins S: *Back care: a clinical approach*, Edinburgh, 2000, Churchill Livingstone.

Chaitow L: *Positional release techniques*, ed 3, Edinburgh, 2007, Churchill Livingstone.

Chaitow L, DeLany J: *Clinical applications of neuromuscular technique*, Edinburgh, 2000, Churchill Livingstone.

Chaitow L: Chronic pelvic pain: Pelvic floor problems, sacroiliac dysfunction and the trigger point connection, *Journal of Bodywork and Movement Therapies* 11:327–339, 2007.

Deig D: *Positional release technique*, Boston, 2001, Butterworth Heinemann.

Fall M, et al: Guidelines on Chronic Pelvic Pain, *European Association of Urology*, 2008.

Fielder S, Pyott W: *The science and art of manipulative surgery*, American Institute of Manipulative Surgery, Salt Lake City, Utah, 1955.

Fitzgerald et al. Randomized feasability trial of myofascial physical therapy for the treatment of urological chronic pelvic pain syndromes. *J of Urol*. Aug(182) 570–580, 2009.

Grieve G: The masqueraders. In Boyling JD, Palastanga N, editors: *Grieve's modern manual therapy*, ed 2, Edinburgh, 1994, Churchill Livingstone.

Gutstein R: The role of abdominal fibrositis in functional indigestion, *Miss Valley Med J* 66–114, 1944.

Jones L: *Strain and counterstrain*, Colorado Springs, 1981, Academy of Applied Osteopathy.

Kuchera M, Kuchera W: *Considerations in systemic dysfunction*, Columbus, Ohio, 1994, Greyden Press.

Kuchera W: Lumbar and abdominal region. In Ward R, editor: *Foundations for osteopathic medicine*, Baltimore, 1997, Williams & Wilkins.

Mackenzie J: 1909, *Symptoms and their interpretation*, London.

Melnick J: Treatment of trigger mechanisms in gastrointestinal disease, *N Y State J Med* 54:1324–1330, 1954.

Owen C: *An endocrine interpretation of Chapman's reflexes*, Newark, Ohio, 1980, American Academy of Osteopathy.

Ranger I, et al: Abdominal wall pain due to nerve entrapment, *Practitioner* 206:791–792, 1971.

Simons D, Travell J, Simons L: *Myofascial pain and dysfunction: the trigger point manual*, vol 1, *Upper half of body*, ed 2, Baltimore, 1999, Williams & Wilkins.

Slocumb J: Neurological factors in chronic pelvic pain: trigger points and the abdominal pelvic pain syndrome, *Am J Obstet Gynaecol* 149(5):536–543, 1984.

Srinivasan A, Kaye J, Moldwin R: Myofascial dysfunction associated with chronic pelvic floor pain: management strategies, *Curr Pain Headache Rep* 11(5):359–364, 2007.

Theobald G: Relief and prevention of referred pain, *J Obstet Gynaecol Br Commonw* 56:447–460, 1949.

Thomson H, Francis D: Abdominal wall tenderness: a useful sign in the acute abdomen, *The Lancet* i:1053, 1977.

Travell J, Simons D: *Myofascial pain and dysfunction – trigger point manual*, Baltimore, 1983, Williams & Wilkins.

Wallace E, McPartland J, Jones J, et al: Lymphatic system. In Ward R, editor: *Foundations for osteopathic medicine*, Baltimore, 1997, Williams & Wilkins.

Ward R, editor: *Foundations for osteopathic medicine*, Baltimore, 1997, Williams & Wilkins.

Weiss J: Pelvic floor myofascial trigger points: manual therapy for interstitial cystitis and the urgency–frequency syndrome, *J Urol* 166:2226–2231, 2001.

Zondervan K, Yudkin P, Vessey M, et al: The community prevalence of chronic pelvic pain in women and associated illness behavior, *Br J Gen Pract* 51:541–547, 2001.

8

Associated techniques

CHAPTER CONTENTS

Soft tissue approaches   **155**
Active release technique® (ART)   155
Elbow (and forearm) technique   156
Sacrospinalis   156
Chronic shoulder restriction   156
Chill-and-stretch (spray-and-stretch) technique   157
Ice as an alternative   158
Deep tissue release   160
Induration technique   161
Integrated neuromuscular inhibition technique (INIT)   162
Ischaemic compression and trigger point release   162
Massage   163
Muscle energy techniques (MET) – including isolytic stretch   166
Neuromuscular therapy (soft tissue manipulation)   **171**
Percussion technique or spondylotherapy   172
Piriformis muscle technique   175
Proprioceptive adjustment (applied kinesiology)   177
Psoas techniques   178
Pectoralis minor release   179
Pump techniques – lymphatics, liver/spleen, pedal   181
Skin techniques   **184**
Skin rolling   184
'S' and 'C' bends: myofascial release methods for lengthening soft tissues   186
Stretching fascia – myofascial release   188
Specific (abdominal) release techniques   189
Strain–conterstrain – and positional release techniques   193
Tensor fascia lata (iliotibial band) techniques   196

Soft tissue approaches

In Chapter 6 a detailed description was given of NMT in spinal, cervical, pelvic and intercostal structures, and abdominal techniques were described in Chapter 7.

In this chapter a number of additional soft tissue approaches/modalities/methods that are frequently employed alongside NMT (listed in Box 8.1) will be outlined in alphabetical order, rather than any other sequence.

Active release technique® (ART)

Active release technique is a registered modality, that is in many ways similar to traditional 'pin and stretch' techniques. ART is a soft tissue approach that at its most basic involves the practitioner isolating a contact point close to the region of soft tissue dysfunction, after which the patient is directed to move in a way that produces a longitudinal sliding motion of soft tissues (nerves, ligaments, muscles) beneath the anchored contact point. Alternatively the movements may be initiated by the practitioner, or may be combined with active movements, whichever achieves the best outcome.

There have been relatively few studies to evaluate efficacy, however one pilot study demonstrated no benefit to quadriceps function in athletes with anterior knee pain where ART was applied (Drover et al 2004). While in different pilot studies:

1. Hamstring length was shown to have increased subsequent to treatment (George 2006).
2. Active release technique was found to be beneficial in management of carpal tunnel syndrome patients (George et al 2006).

Box 8.1 Additional soft tissue approaches

- Active release technique (ART)
- Elbow and forearm technique
- Chill-and-stretch technique
- Deep tissue release
- Induration technique
- Integrated neuromuscular inhibition technique (INIT)
- Ischaemic compression/trigger point release
- Massage
- Muscle energy techniques
- Neuromuscular therapy/soft tissue manipulation discussion
- Percussion technique
- Piriformis muscle technique
- Proprioceptive adjustment
- Psoas technique
- Pectoralis minor release
- Pump techniques (liver, lymphatics, spleen, pedal)
- Skin techniques
- S & C bends
- Stretching fascia – myofascial release
- Specific (abdominal) release techniques
- Strain/counterstrain
- Tensor fascia lata techniques

Elbow (and forearm) technique

Caution – Direct elbow pressure should be avoided, or should be performed with great care:

1. if tissues are inflamed or during the remodelling phase, following trauma, is incomplete
2. in cases of malignancy
3. close to blood vessels and nerves
4. close to attachment sites
5. if pain (local or referred) is excessive.

In treating certain muscle groups, notably the gluteals and the sacrospinalis group, it is sometimes difficult, or even impossible, to impart adequate force via the thumb or fingers, owing to the degree of resistance in the tissues involved. Where it is considered appropriate, elbow and/or forearm technique should be applied preparatory to NMT, on a number of occasions, so that NMT can subsequently be applied more effectively.

Sacrospinalis

In treating sacrospinalis, for example, the entire spine should be lubricated, and the practitioner should stand on the patient's left side (patient supine, pillow under thorax) (Fig. 8.1).

- The right elbow tip should be placed just superior to the sacral base, with the forearm at right angles to the patient's body, as in Fig. 8.1A (and also Figs 10.13B,C)
- By flexing the knees slightly and allowing weight to be transferred via the elbow, the practitioner can apply controlled pressure to the paraspinal muscles with the broad contact of the forearm, or by raising the hand slightly, more precisely by the elbow itself.
- The more the hand is elevated, the sharper the angle of contact of the elbow, and the more precise strokes will be, at the point of contact.
- The elbow/forearm should be allowed to glide slowly cephalad.
- If pain is reported, pressure should be reduced.
- Several glides or strokes along the full length of the spine will greatly relax even marked contractions.
- Similar techniques can be applied to the gluteal area.

Chronic shoulder restriction

An example of more focused use of elbow technique involves work on the lateral border of the scapula in cases of chronic shoulder restriction (see Fig. 8.1B).

In order to encourage more normal movement of the humerus in the glenoid fossa, as well as the free glide of the scapula on the rib-cage:

- The patient is side-lying with the side to be treated uppermost, and with the arm abducted, elevated, extended and externally rotated, so that the patient's hand is close to her head.
- The practitioner should be behind the patient, standing sideways on to the table, facing her head.
- With his non-tableside hand the practitioner grasps the patient's upper arm, close to the elbow, reinforcing the external rotation, abduction, etc.

Figure 8.1A   Elbow technique applied to paraspinal musculature. **B.** Elbow technique to lateral scapula border.

- The practitioner's tableside arm is flexed at the elbow, which should be carefully placed in the patient's exposed axilla, as close to the lateral border of the scapula as possible.
- Short, slow-moving strokes should be applied along the scapula border, as well as anteriorly and posteriorly, following the curve of the ribs below the axilla.
- If localized contracted tissue is sensed it may be helpful to simply apply sustained, tolerably comfortable, pressure – and wait for a softening to occur.
- The non-treating hand should use any release resulting from the elbow treatment to gradually increase the range of rotation and abduction at the shoulder, to improve humeroglenoid movement.

Treatment of piriformis muscle, and its central trigger points, can usefully be achieved by means of direct elbow pressure, applied to the main trigger point area in the belly of the muscle, while the side-lying patient's leg is rotated to internally rotate the hip, in order to achieve a lengthening of the muscle. (See illustrated details of the use of the elbow in this way, later in this chapter under the heading Piriformis Technique (see Fig. 8.11)).

Chill-and-stretch (spray-and-stretch) technique

Chilling and stretching a muscle housing a trigger point rapidly assists in deactivation of the abnormal neurological behavior of the site. Travell & Mennell have described these effects in detail (Mennell 1969, 1975, Simons et al 1999, Travell 1952, Travell & Simons 1992).

Travell & Simons (1992) and Simons et al (1999) have discouraged the use of vapocoolants to chill the area, because of environmental considerations relating to ozone depletion, and have instead urged the use of stroking with ice in a similar manner to the spray stream to achieve the same effect. The objective is to chill the surface tissues while the underlying muscle housing the trigger is simultaneously stretched. They also point out that the spray is applied before or during the stretch and not after the muscle has already been elongated.

However recently, Gebauer's *Spray and Stretch* (prescription) and *Instant Ice* (non-prescription), both non-flammable, nonozone-depleting vapo-coolants, have emerged into a market that has until recently been devoid of environmentally friendly sprays. Spray and stretch techniques can therefore now not only be applied in the treatment room, but also in home care with the patient's use of the non-prescription version – without environmental risk.

A container of vapocoolant spray with a cali-brated nozzle which delivers a moderately fine jet stream, or a source of ice, is needed. The jet stream should have sufficient force to carry in the air for at least 3 feet. Experience suggests that a mist-like spray is less effective. (See Figs 8.2A,B.)

Simons & Mense (2003) report that the vapo-coolant spray appears to inhibit pain and reflex motor, and autonomic responses in the central nervous system. When the pain stimuli subside a degree of relaxation takes place allowing stretching and lengthening of the muscle to be more effective and less uncomfortable (Lupandin & Kuz'mina 1985). (See Fig. 8.2C).

Ice as an alternative

Ice used to achieve the same effects as the cold spray discussed above, can comprise a cylinder of ice formed by freezing water in a paper cup and then peeling this off the ice. A wooden han-dle will have been frozen into the ice to allow for its ease of application, as it is rolled from the trigger towards the referred area in a series of sweeps.

The author has found that a cold soft-drink-can, that has been partially filled with water and then frozen, is more suitable, because ice applied directly onto skin melts rapidly and, as Travell & Simons (1992) have pointed out, the skin must remain dry for this method to be successful, because dampness slows the rate of cooling of the skin and may also delay rewarming.

An ice-cold, metal container, can however be rolled over the skin, and will retain its chilling potential for long enough to achieve the ends desired.

Method

Whichever source of cold is chosen, the patient should be comfortably supported to promote muscular relaxation.

- If a spray is used, the container should be held approximately 2 feet (60 cm) away, in such a manner that the jet stream meets the body surface at an acute angle or at a tangent, not perpendicularly (Figs 8.2A,B).
- This lessens the shock of the impact. For the same reason, the stream is sometimes started in air, or on the practitioner's hand, and is gradually brought into contact with the skin overlying the trigger point.
- The stream/ice massage/frozen canister should be applied in one direction only, not back and forth.
- Each sweep should commence in the tissues overlying the trigger point and be moved slowly and evenly outward over towards reference zone (where pain is reported as being experienced by the patient). The direction of movement of the spray/ice should follow the fibre direction of the muscle.
- It appears that it is advantageous to spray, or ice-chill, both trigger and reference areas, because secondary trigger points are likely to have developed within reference zones when pain is very strong.
- Clinical experience suggests that the optimum speed of movement of the sweep/roll over the skin, is approximately about 4 inches (10 cm) per second.
- Each sweep should be started slightly proximal to the trigger point, and be moved slowly and evenly through the reference zone, to cover it and extend slightly beyond it.
- These sweeps should be repeated in a rhythm of a few seconds on, and a few seconds off, until all the skin over trigger and reference areas has been covered once or twice.
- If aching or 'cold pain' develops, or if the application of the spray/ice/canister sets off a reference of new pain, the interval between applications should be lengthened.
- Care should be taken not to frost or blanch the skin.

Figure 8.2A,B   Anterior and posterior view of application of vapocoolant spray to trigger point (quadratus lumborum in this illustration). Muscles housing trigger points are placed at stretch while a coolant spray is utilized to chill the point and the area between it and the target reference area.

Continued

Figure 8.2C Schematic illustration of the proposed effects of cold spray application.

- During the application of cold the taut fibres should be placed at light stretch, and after the chilling should be further stretched passively.
- Steady, gentle stretching is usually essential if a satisfactory result is to be achieved.
- As relaxation of the muscle occurs, continued stretch should be maintained for 20–30 seconds, and after each series of cold applications active motion should be tested.
- The patient should be asked to move in the directions that were restricted before spraying/chilling, or that were painful to activate.
- An attempt should be made to restore the full range of motion, but always within the limits of discomfort, as sudden overstretching can increase existing muscle spasm.
- The treatment is continued in this manner until the trigger points (often several are present) and their respective pain reference zones have been treated.
- The entire procedure may occupy 15–20 minutes and should not be rushed.

The importance of re-establishing normal motion in conjunction with the use of the chilling is well founded. It may be that the brief interruption of pain impulses is insufficient and that input of normal impulses must also occur for the obliteration of trigger points to be successfully achieved by these means.

Simple exercises that use the principle of passive or active stretch should be outlined to the patient, to be carried out several times daily, after the application of gentle heat (hot packs, etc.) at home. Usual precautions should be mentioned, such as avoiding the use of heat if symptoms worsen or if there is evidence of inflammation.

Deep tissue release

(Fielder & Pyott 1955)

In using NMT it is often helpful to apply a local 'tissue release' technique to areas of marked contraction or spasticity. In areas overlying bone, the techniques suitable for use in the abdominal region (see Specific (abdominal) release techniques, later in this chapter) are not applicable.

The method recommended is as follows:

- The contact on the tissues involved is made by extending the digits of either hand and making firm contact with the area between the first and second metacarpophalangeal joints, taking out the slack of the tissues and engaging a resistance barrier.
- This contact is rotated clockwise or anticlockwise in order to increase the tension in the underlying tissues, until the tissues with the greatest resistance are noted and combined barrier is engaged – downwards and in a torsional manner.

- The other hand is then placed over the contact hand so that the downward pressure and rotation are reinforced.
- In addition, a further direction of stretch should be introduced by the second hand – directed laterally/medially or superiorly/inferiorly, whichever offers the greatest resistance.
- The tissues would therefore be receiving a direct downward pressure, a rotational stretch, and a further degree of stretch in another direction, all maintained by the two treating hands.
- The overlying hand should have been placed in such a way that the radial border of the metacarpal base of the thumb is directly over the contact point of the first hand's contact (i.e. over the second metacarpal joint area). (See Fig. 8.3.)

Figure 8.3 Deep tissue release technique applied, in this example, close to the temporomandibular joint area. The soft tissue slack will have been removed (i.e. barriers engaged) by a precise contact from the right hand (the area between the first and second metacarpophalangeal joints) in directions of greatest resistance (a) into the soft tissues, (b) into rotation (counterclockwise in this example) and (c) inferiorly. This contact is supported by the left hand, which then completes the release by means of either a sharp contraction of the contact or a short sharp thrust (see text for further detail). Redrawn from Fielder & Pyott (1955).

- The fingers of the overlying hand should be tightly in contact with the lateral border of the contact hand.

The last stage of the release technique may be performed in one of two ways:

1. The overlying hand executes a short sharp squeeze by flexing the middle finger against the metacarpals of the contact hand. The resulting pressure in the intermetacarpal area provides the 'thrust' or release force. The line of force of this squeeze is towards the practitioner.
2. The second method of release, which is more suitable for deeper contractions of tissue, is applied via short sharp thrust by the overlying hand against the contact hand, with a simultaneous medial rotation of the contact hand. The line of force in this technique is away from the practitioner.

This soft tissue approach, which emerged from American naprapathy (a form of soft tissue manipulation popular primarily in Sweden, and the Chicago area of the United States), and an adhesion releasing method (known as 'bloodless surgery' between the two World Wars), has been adapted for use in the UK by McTimoney chiropractic practitioners.

Induration technique

(Morrison 1969)

Note: This method is suitable even in cases of great fragility (osteoporosis) because pressure is not meant to exceed an ounce or two (30 to 60 grams), at most.

As many patients are too frail, or too ill, to allow the full NMT treatment to be applied, a useful technique exists to aid in normalizing reflex and local areas of the paraspinal musculature. Stoddard (1969) has pointed out that protective spasm in muscle can often indicate underlying pathology (osteoporosis, etc.) and, clearly, deep pressure techniques would be contraindicated in such conditions.

- With the patient sitting or lying, the practitioner, using a very light 'skin-on-skin' contact which evaluates 'drag' or hills/valleys (see Ch. 5), runs the fingertips longitudinally down the side of the spine (side of spine opposite that on which practitioner is standing) over the transverse processes.

- Any spot or area of 'hardened' or indurated tissue, that also palpates as tender to the patient is marked for attention.
- Treatment is applied by palpating the sensitive area with the tip of the thumb (or a finger), of one hand, while applying light pressure towards the painful spot with the soft thenar or hyperthenar eminence of the other hand, which is resting on the spinous process of the vertebra, adjacent to the indurated tissue (Fig. 8.4).
- Direct pressure (extremely light – ounces/ grams only) towards the pain should lessen the degree of tissue contraction, and the sensitivity.
- If it does not do so, the angle of light pressure on the spinous process, towards the painful point, should be varied slightly, so that, somewhere within an arc embracing a half circle, an angle of push towards the pain will be found to abolish the pain totally, and will lessen the palpated feeling of tension.
- This 'position of ease' is held for around 20 seconds, before moving on to the next sensitive area.

This technique, which has strong echoes of 'strain/counterstrain' (described later in this chapter) can be used with NMT or instead of

Figure 8.4   Hand positions for induration technique. Pressure used on the spinous process is measured in ounces (grams) at most.

deeper probing measures, that, for practical reasons, may be contraindicated (for example if the patient's condition involves extreme sensitivity, inflammation or pathology).

Integrated neuromuscular inhibition technique (INIT)

(see Fig. 9.1 and Ch. 9) (Chaitow 1994)

INIT, when used to deactivate a trigger point, involves the application of a sequence that includes:

- Inhibitory (ischaemic) compression (either sustained or intermittent: 5 seconds pressure/ 2 seconds release/repeated) until a change is reported or noted.
- Place the tissues into a position of ease, to encourage a muscle spindle release of excessive tone (see descriptions of 'positional release' below).
- The patient introduces an isometric contraction involving the precise tissues housing the trigger point.
- This is followed by passive stretching of the local tissues.
- Followed by active and passive stretching of the entire muscle (subsequent to another isometric contraction) (see notes on muscle energy technique (MET) below).
- After this activation of antagonists to muscle housing the trigger point may be used to complete the sequence.

This approach achieves a triple effect: inhibition/ ischaemic compression, positional release, followed by an isometrically enhanced stretch. The sequence represents a significant advance in deactivating trigger points and the tissues that house them. The initial pressure application (and subsequent positional release and MET) may follow on from identification of the trigger point during NMT evaluation.

Ischaemic compression and trigger point release

Direct inhibitory pressure has a long history of use in many forms of bodywork, including osteopathy, in order to achieve a release of hypertonic, tense tissues, spasm, cramp, etc.

Hou et al (2002) report: 'Ischemic compression therapy provides alternative treatments using either low pressure (pain threshold) and a long duration (90 s) or high pressure (the average of pain threshold and pain tolerance) and short duration (30 s), for immediate pain relief and myofascial trigger point sensitivity suppression.'

Caution – Direct pressure should be avoided, or performed with great care:

1. If tissues are inflamed, or are in the remodelling phase, following trauma
2. In cases of malignancy
3. Close to blood vessels and nerves
4. Close to attachment sites (to avoid provoking enthesitis)
5. If pain (local or referred) is excessive.

Travell & Simons (1983, 1992) have suggested that in treatment of trigger points, these should receive ischaemic compression ('sustained digital pressure') for a period of between 20 seconds and 1 minute. The pressure should be gradually increased as the trigger point's sensitivity (referred sensation, as well as the local discomfort) reduces, and the tension of the tissues housing the trigger ('taut band') eases. Stretching techniques should be applied following the compression; see integrated neuromuscular inhibition technique (INIT) described later in this chapter.

Fernández-De-Las-Peñas et al (2006) report on a study that verified these suggestions. 'Ischemic compression technique and transverse friction massage were equally effective in reducing tenderness in myofascial trigger points.'

The mechanisms involved, as seen from a Western perspective, would include 'neurological overload', the release of endogenous morphine-like products (endorphins, enkephalins, endocannabinoids) (McPartland & Simons 2007) as well as 'flushing' of tissues with fresh oxygenated blood following the compression. Oriental interpretations would include modulation of energy transmission.

See Chapter 3, Box 3.5, for more detail on compression effects.

Massage

Using standard massage protocols, Field (2000) and others have demonstrated, in hundreds of research projects, that significant benefits occur in the following conditions and patient populations: enhanced growth in preterm infants, cocaine and human immunodeficiency virus (HIV)-exposed infants, pain reduction, during labour, pre-debridement for burn patients, juvenile rheumatoid arthritis, fibromyalgia, premenstrual syndrome, migraine, children with autism, adolescents with attention deficit hyperactivity disorder (enhanced attentiveness), anxiety (e.g. exam settings), depression, post-traumatic stress, adolescent psychiatric patients, adolescent mothers, bulaemia and anorexia, chronic fatigue syndrome, autoimmune and immune disorders, diabetes mellitus (reduced glucose levels), asthma, cystic fibrosis, atopic dermatitis, HIV-positive adults, oncology patients.

Some of Field's explanations for the benefits of massage are summarized later in this section.

We should also not lose sight of the tried and tested effects of massage on the soft tissues. The degree of that effect will vary with the type of soft tissue manipulation employed, and the nature of the patient and the problem. Soft tissue techniques, apart from those specifically associated with NMT, may include the following.

Safety

There are few modalities that are more universally useful than massage. In its most generic form massage is non-invasive, almost totally safe, and with few contraindications. When massage incorporates techniques based on soft tissue manipulation, or when it becomes 'deeper' and has specific therapeutic goals (such as deactivation of trigger points, reduction of fibrosis) universal suitability is reduced and cautions are required – for example when serious pathology (cancer, arthritis), active inflammation and/or vulnerability (osteoporosis for example) are current.

Massage methodology

The various modes of application of massage (e.g. gliding, effleurage, kneading, petrissage, compression) provide the most efficient means of applying variations of therapeutic load to tissues. Each method can be modified, depending on the desired outcome, by adjusting depth of pressure, drag (amount of tensile force applied), direction, speed, rhythm, frequency and duration of contact.

The strokes that make up massage strokes include:

- *Petrissage* – wringing and stretching movements, across the fibre direction of muscles.
- *Kneading* – where the hands shape themselves to the contours of the area being treated. The tissues between the hands are lifted and pressed downwards and together.
- *Inhibition* – which involves application of pressure directly to the belly or origins or insertions of contracted muscles or to local soft tissue dysfunction for a variable amount of time or in a 'make-and-break' (pressure applied and then released) manner to reduce hypertonic contraction or for reflexive effects.
- *Effleurage* – this is a relaxing technique that is used, as appropriate, to initiate or terminate other manipulative methods. Pressure is usually even throughout the strokes, which are applied with the whole hand in contact.
- *Vibration and friction* – such contacts are used near origins and insertions and near bony attachments for relaxing effects on the muscle as a whole and to reach layers deep to the superficial tissues. It is performed by small circular or vibratory movements, with the tips of fingers or thumb. The heel of the hand may also be used.
- *Roulement* – this involves skin lifting and rolling, which, as with most massage methods, can be used diagnostically as well as therapeutically (see earlier in this chapter for discussion of skin rolling).
- *Transverse or cross-fibre friction* – this is performed along or across the belly of muscles using the heel of the hand, thumb or fingers applied slowly and rhythmically or vigorously, depending upon the objectives.
- *Tapotement* – involves percussive tapping, clapping, drumming and vibrating activities, involving fingertips or the ulnar borders of the hands.

Massage cautions (Wittlinger & Wittlinger 1982)

- In areas that have been recently traumatized (2–3 weeks) and which are in the remodelling phase (including surgery).
- When a person is fatigued the duration and depth of the application should be reduced.
- If a patient has a fragile bone structure, the depth of pressure should be modified.
- When the patient is agitated the rhythm should be modified to create a calming effect.
- Acute infections and acute inflammation (generalized and local)
- Thrombosis
- Cardiac conditions
- Hemorrhage
- Malignant cancers
- Thyroid problems
- Acute phlebitis
- Prominent varicosities.

Physiological effects of massage

The biochemical influences of massage include altered stress hormone (cortisol) production (Field 2000). Perhaps surprisingly, massage fails to increase blood flow through muscle unless it is exceptionally vigorous (Shoemaker et al 1997); however, drainage efficiency is improved when light techniques are employed (Ikimi et al 1996).

- Pain perception is reduced by massage, possibly due to gating of impulses (Clelland et al 1987).
- Massage mechanically modifies soft tissue status (stretching, mobilizing, etc.) depending on the variations in load application (sustained pressure, shearing load, etc.).
- The colloids in fasciae that surround, support and invest all soft tissues respond to appropriately applied pressure and vibration by changing state from a gel-type consistency to a solute, which increases internal hydration and assists in the removal of toxins from the tissue (Oschman 1997).
- Psychological effects include reduced arousal, calmer mood and modified perception of anxiety (Rich 2002).
- Neurological influences include a transient reduction in motor neuron excitability during and following massage (Goldberg 1992).
- Massage also produces a decrease in the sensitivity of the gamma efferent control of the muscle spindles and thereby reduces any shortening tendency of the muscles (Puustjarvi 1990).

Other methods that we would associate with the above techniques of traditional massage might include the various applications of NMT, as described in this text, as well as connective tissue massage techniques, which are used primarily for reflex effects.

Massage effects explained

How are the various effects of massage and soft tissue manipulation explained? Field (2000), discussing her many research findings, states:

In all these studies depression, anxiety, and stress hormones significantly decreased following massage therapy. Because depression, anxiety and stress hormones (particularly cortisol) are notably elevated in autoimmune and immune disorders, we hypothesized that massage therapy might also help these problems.

Field further suggests that the evidence from her studies points to enhanced homeostatic function, in both infants and adults, following massage therapy, as evidenced by improved sleep patterns (and therefore higher levels of somatostatin), as well as increased serotonin levels. These thoughts are supported by the work of other researchers (Ironson et al 1993).

Apart from the undoubted anxiety and stress-reducing influences of massage, a combination of physical effects also occurs (Sandler 1983):

1. Pressure, as applied in deep kneading or stroking along the length of a muscle, tends to displace its fluid content.
2. Venous, lymphatic and tissue drainage is thereby encouraged.
3. The replacement of this with fresh oxygenated blood aids in normalization via increased capillary filtration and venous capillary pressure.
4. This reduces oedema and the effects of pain-inducing substances that may be present (Hovind & Nielson 1974, Xujian 1990).
5. Massage also produces a decrease in the sensitivity of the *g*-efferent control of the muscle spindles, and thereby reduces any shortening tendency of the muscles (Puustjarvi et al 1990).
6. Pressure techniques, such as are used in NMT, and the methods employed in MET have a direct effect on the Golgi tendon organs, which detect the load applied to the tendon or muscle.
7. These have an inhibitory capability, which can cause the entire muscle to relax.
8. The Golgi tendon organs are set in series in the muscle, and are affected by both active and passive contraction of the tissues. The effect of any system that applies longitudinal pressure or stretch to the muscle will be to evoke this reflex relaxation. The degree of stretch has, however, to be great, as there is little response from a small degree of stretch.
9. The effects of MET, articulation techniques and various functional balance techniques depend to a large extent on these tendon reflexes (Sandler 1983).

Soft tissues at centre stage

We are in the midst of a change in the concepts of manual therapy that has far-reaching implications. One of the major changes is the restoration of the soft tissue component to centre stage, rather than the peripheral role to which it has been assigned in the past as ever more general health problems are found to involve musculoskeletal dysfunction, for example chronic fatigue conditions (Chaitow 1990).

Lewit (1985) discusses aspects of what he describes as the 'no man's land' that lies between neurology, orthopaedics and rheumatology, which, he says, is the home of the vast majority of patients with pain derived from the locomotor system, and in whom no definite pathomorphological changes are found. He makes the suggestion that these be termed cases of *'functional pathology of the locomotor system'*. These include most of the patients attending osteopathic, chiropractic and physiotherapy practitioners.

The most frequent symptom of individuals involved in this area of dysfunction is pain, which may be reflected clinically by reflex changes such as muscle spasm, myofascial trigger points, hyperalgesic skin zones, periosteal pain points, or a wide variety of other sensitive areas that have no obvious pathological origin. As the musculoskeletal system is the largest energy user in the body by far, it is no surprise that fatigue is a feature of chronic changes in the musculature. It is a major part of the role of NMT to help in identifying such areas, and also in offering some help in differential diagnosis. NMT and other soft tissue methods are then capable of positively influencing many of the causative aspects of these myriad sources of pain and disability.

Muscle energy techniques (MET) – including isolytic stretch

Muscle energy technique (MET) involves the use of isometric contractions (Mitchell et al 1998) to assist in modification of muscle and joint behavior. Variations on this basic theme involve the use of isotonic concentric, or eccentric, contractions (Schmitt 1999), or a series of rhythmically pulsating contractions (Ruddy 1961) instead of, or as well as, basic isometric variations.

Definition of MET

MET involves a muscle, or group of muscles, being voluntarily contracted, in a specified direction, for a defined length of time (commonly 5 to 7 seconds), involving submaximal effort, with the contraction being matched by the practitioner/therapist's effort, so that no movement occurs (Mitchell & Mitchell 1995, Mitchell 1976).

- MET has been shown to improve joint range of motion, including spinal joints (Kamani & Walters 2000, Lenehan et al 2003).
- MET has been shown to improve muscle extensibility more effectively than passive, static stretching – both in the short and long term (Mehta & Hatton 2002, Feland et al 2004, Ferber et al 2002).
- In addition studies offer support for the hypoalgesic effects of MET – for example in relation to spinal pain (Brodin 1962, Cassidy et al 1992, Wilson et al 2003).
- Myofascial trigger point deactivation has been shown to be enhanced by use of MET (Chaitow 1994, Fernández-de-las-Peñas 2005, Simons et al 1992, 1999).

MET origins

Much of the research from which conclusions regarding MET efficacy and mechanisms are taken, relates to studies involving proprioceptive neuromuscular facilitation (PNF) stretching. (Fryer 2006, Schmitt et al 1999) PNF (and MET) application may involve one of 3 variations:

- *Contract–relax (CR)*, in which the muscle being stretched (the agonist) is contracted and then relaxed, before stretching. (See Fig. 8.5A and 8.5B).
- *Agonist contract–relax (ACR)*, in which contraction is of the antagonist, rather than the muscle to be stretched (the agonist). It is suggested that the confusing title of *Agonist contract-relax (ACR)* should be ignored. The approach relies, it is suggested (see below), on reciprocal inhibition.
- *Contract–relax agonist–contract (CRAC)*, involves a combination of the two methods (CR and ACR) listed above.

Proposed MET mechanisms

Kuchera & Kuchera (1992) as well as Denslow et al (1993) have speculated on the neurological

(A)

Figure 8.5A   MET treatment of left rectus femoris muscle. Note the practitioner's right hand stabilizes the sacrum and pelvis to prevent undue spinal stress during the stretching phase of the treatment.

(B)

Figure 8.5B   MET treatment of tensor fascia lata. If a standard MET method is being used, the stretch will follow the isometric contraction in which the patient will attempt to move the right leg to the right, against sustained resistance. It is important for the practitioner to maintain stability of the pelvis during the procedure.

mechanisms that may follow use of MET (contract/relax version).

• They hypothesize that the effects may result from the inhibitory Golgi tendon reflex, activated during the isometric contraction that leads to reflex relaxation of the muscle, as a result of *post isometric relaxation (PIR)* (see Fig. 8.6A).
• An alternative reflex effect has been suggested in which an isometric contraction of the antagonist(s) of affected muscle(s) induce relaxation via *reciprocal inhibition (RI)* (ACR version) (see Fig. 8.6B).

Some studies support the concept of neurological muscle inhibition, following MET isometric contraction. For example Moore & Kukulka (1991) found that a strong brief depression of the soleus H-reflex occurred, for about 10 seconds, following sub-maximal isometric plantar flexion contractions, probably as a result of pre-synaptic inhibition.

However simultaneous monitoring of the tibialis anterior muscle's EMG activity revealed minimal activity, so excluding the possibility of reciprocal inhibition operating (Moore & Kukulka 1991).

Since many studies have demonstrated that active motor activity plays a minimal role in producing resistance to stretch (Magnusson et al 1996b) the question remains as to whether low-level motor activity plays a role in limiting the passive stretch of a muscle.

Self-evidently, in order for it to be accepted that MET produces increased muscle length, by means of reflex muscle relaxation, low-level motor activity needs to be shown to play a role in limiting passive stretching of muscle, and this has not been possible (Fryer 2006).

• Ballentyne et al (2003) suggest that the PIR theory is poorly supported by research. Citing EMG evidence they note that 'various studies have shown that passive stretch does not influence the electrical activity of the hamstring muscle (Klinge et al 1997, McHugh et al 1998) demonstrating that low level muscle contraction does not limit muscle flexibility, disputing the proposal of [such] a neurological mechanism.[i.e. PIR]'
• Lederman (1995) states that the PIR model ignores the complex and dominant influence of the central nervous system.
• Fryer (2000) points to the lack of evidence supporting muscle contraction as a factor in restricted joint ROM, or in spinal dysfunction.
• Magnusson et al (1995) found that low-level EMG activity was unchanged following isometric contractions, or passive stretching.
• Magnusson et al (1996a) have demonstrated that increases in muscle length, following 90 seconds of passive stretching, occurs without any change to the low-level EMG activity of that muscle.
• Fryer (2006) has speculated that although the exact mechanism by which increased muscle extensibility occurs, remains unclear, it probably involves both neurophysiological and mechanical factors, possibly including viscoelastic and plastic changes in the connective tissue elements of the muscle. In fact Fryer maintains that although MET techniques produce greater ROM changes than static stretching, they also produce greater EMG activity in the muscle undergoing the stretch.

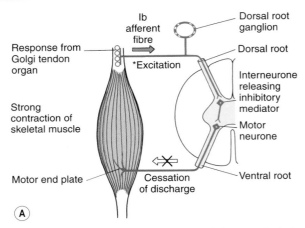

Figure 8.6A   Schematic representation of the neurological effects of the loading of the Golgi tendon organs of a skeletal muscle by means of an isometric contraction, which produces a post-isometric relaxation effect in that muscle.

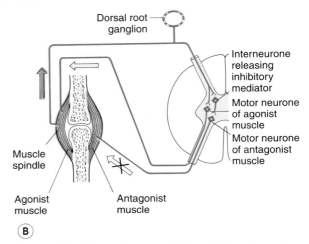

Figure 8.6B   Schematic representation of the reciprocal effect of an isometric contraction of a skeletal muscle, resulting in an inhibitory influence on its antagonist.

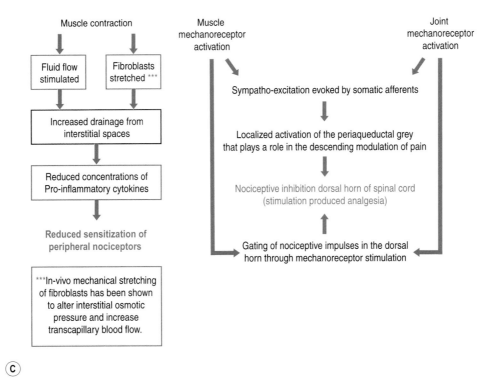

Figure 8.6C   Schematic diagram of hypoalgesic effects of MET. Modified from Fryer G., Fossum C. 2009. Therapeutic Mechanisms Underlying Muscle Energy Approaches. In: Physical Therapy for tension type and cervicogenic headache. Fernández de las Peñas C., Arendt-Nielsen L., Gerwin R. (Eds): Jones & Bartlett, Boston.

- Fryer & Fossum (2008) have hypothesized a neurological explanation for the analgesic effects of MET. A sequence is suggested in which activation of muscle mechanoreceptors and joint mechanoreceptors occur, during an isometric contraction. This leads to sympatho-excitation evoked by somatic efferents and localized activation of the periaqueductal grey that plays a role in descending modulation of pain. Nociceptive inhibition then occurs at the dorsal horn of the spinal cord, as simultaneous gating takes place of nociceptive impulses in the dorsal horn, due to mechano-receptor stimulation (see Fig. 8.6C).

Alternative explanations

So if PIR and RI are not the neurophysiological mechanisms that lead to the effectiveness of MET, in increasing joint ROM, or extensibility of soft tissues, and analgesia, what does produce these results?

The phrase *'increased tolerance to stretch'* has emerged to describe *what* happens, although it does not explain *how* it happens.

- At its simplest this explanation observes that if, after an isometric contraction, the same degree of effort is used, as was employed to take the muscle or joint to its end of range, before the contraction, no increase in range or extensibility occurs.
- Magnusson et al (1998, 1996b) measured the degree of applied effort used during passive knee extension, before and after the hamstrings were stretched to the point of pain. They found that both ROM and passive torque were increased following the contraction – *because subjects were able to tolerate a stronger stretch.*
- Ballantyne et al (2003) confirmed these findings by showing that when the degree of post-test force applied to the muscle remained constant (i.e. the same as used in pre-testing), no change in length took place, suggesting that a single application of MET created a change in tolerance to stretch.
- Fryer (2006) explains: 'The application of MET would appear to decrease an individual's perception of muscle pain, and is greater than that which occurs with passive stretching. Stretching and isometric contraction stimulate muscle and joint mechanoreceptors and proprioceptors, and it is possible that this may attenuate the sensation of pain. ... MET and stretching appear to produce lasting changes in stretch tolerance, and so the mechanism is likely to be more complex than just gating at the spinal cord, and may also involve changes in the higher centres of the CNS.'
- Hamilton et al (2007) suggest that techniques – such as MET – that stimulate joint proprioceptors, via the production of joint movement, or the stretching of a joint capsule, may be capable of reducing pain by inhibiting the smaller diameter nociceptive neuronal input at the spinal cord level.

What else might produce MET's analgesic effects?

Brodin (1982), Cassidy et al (1992) and Wilson et al (2003) have all reported that there is a reduction in spinal pain, following application of MET. These reports therefore support the evidence described above, of an increased tolerance to stretch, of muscles treated by MET.

- Degenhardt et al (2007) report that concentrations of several circulatory pain biomarkers (including endocannabinoids and endorphins) were altered following osteopathic manipulative treatment incorporating muscle energy, and other soft tissue techniques. The degree and duration of these changes were greater in subjects with chronic LBP than in control subjects.
- McPartland (2008) and others (Pertwee 2005, Agarwal & Pacher 2007) note that the endocannabinoid (eCB) system, like the better-known endorphin system, consists of cell membrane receptors, endogenous ligands and ligand metabolizing enzymes. Two cannabinoid receptors are known:

1. CB1 is principally located in the nervous system
2. CB2 is primarily associated with the immune system.

Two of the eCB ligands, anandamide (AEA) and 2-AG, are mimicked by cannabis plant compounds. McPartland reports that: 'AEA and 2-AG are not stored in vesicles like classic neurotransmitters. Rather they are synthesized "on demand" from precursor phospholipids in the neuron cell membrane and immediately released into the neural synapse. (Pertwee 2005). The eCB system dampens nociception and pain, and decreases inflammation in myofascial tissues.'

- Agarwal & Pacher (2007) suggest that cannabinoids mediate analgesia largely via peripheral type 1 cannabinoid receptors (CB1), in pain receptors.

Alternatives to standard isometric contraction versions of MET

- An *isotonic eccentric stretch* is one in which the practitioner overcomes the effort of the contracting muscle, stretching and simultaneously toning it (Liebenson 2006, Norris 1999, Kolar 1999).
- A *rapid isotonic eccentric contraction*, the origin and insertion of the muscles involved are taken further apart while the muscle is contracting, due to the greater effort of the practitioner's counterforce overcoming the muscular effort. When such a manoeuvre is performed rapidly, it is known as an *isolytic contraction*. Isolytic stretches are useful in cases where a marked degree of fibrotic change is present in the soft tissues. The effect is to create microtrauma during the rapid stretch, subsequently allowing an improvement in elasticity and circulation. To achieve an isolytic contraction (eccentric isotonic), the patient should be instructed to use no more than 20% of possible strength on the first contraction, which is resisted and overcome by the practitioner, in a contraction lasting 2–3 seconds. This is then repeated, but with an increased degree of effort on the part of the patient (assuming the first effort was relatively painless). This continuing increase in the amount of force employed in the contracting musculature may be continued until, hopefully, a fairly strong but painless

contraction effort is possible, again to be resisted and overcome by the practitioner. In some muscles, of course, this may require a heroic degree of effort on the part of the practitioner, and alternative methods would need to be found. NMT would seem to offer one such alternative. The isolytic manoeuvre should have as its ultimate aim a fully relaxed muscle, able to reach its normal resting length. This will seldom be possible in one treatment session.

- A *slow isotonic eccentric contraction* offers various important clinical benefits (Lewit 1999, Liebenson 2001, Norris 1999): To tone postural (type I) muscles that may have lost their endurance potential, a slow isotonic eccentric contraction should be performed, involving increasing degrees of effort. For example, slowly overcome flexion of the wrist forcing it into extension (i.e. the arm flexors, which are postural type I muscles, are stretched while contracting). To relax hypertonic postural (type I) muscles, a slow isotonic eccentric stretch should be performed of their inhibited antagonists (using 40–80% strength). For example, slowly overcome the extended wrist, forcing it into flexion (i.e. the arm extensors, which are phasic type II muscles, are contracting but their effort is overcome).
- A concentric isotonic contraction tones the muscle that is active.
- Ruddy (1961) suggested that the effects of what he termed rapid resisted duction (i.e. *pulsed isometric contractions*) include improved local oxygenation, enhanced venous and lymphatic circulation, as well as an improved static and kinetic posture, due to the effects on proprioceptive and interoceptive afferent pathways.
- These variations, along with their particular influences, appear to produce *identical benefits in terms of increased ROM and extensibility of soft tissues* irrespective of which form of MET methodology is employed. For example, in a study of the use of MET in treatment of piriformis dysfunction, it was found that the same results emerged whether the agonist or the antagonist was used in the contraction phase of ME usage (Wright & Drysdale 2008). (See Figs 8.7A,B.)

Figure 8.7   Fig. 8.7A shows MET treatment of piriformis using an antagonist contraction. Fig. 8.7B shows MET treatment of piriformis using a stretch following an antagonist contraction.

Caution – Stretching of tissues should be avoided:

1. During the recovery and remodelling phase after injury (3 weeks)
2. If acutely painful before treatment
3. If pain is noted during stretching or contraction
4. If a joint is involved ('slack' should be taken out until new barrier(s) are engaged – defined as the 'first sign of resistance')
5. If tissues are inflamed.

Update on stretching time in MET

Smith & Fryer (2008) tested the usefulness of extending a hamstring muscle stretch, following a MET Contraction, from 5 seconds (Greenman 1996) to 30 seconds (Chaitow 2002):

Both techniques appeared to be equally effective in increasing hamstring extensibility, and there appeared to be sustained improvement 1 week following the initial treatment. The findings suggest that altering the duration of the passive stretch component does not have a significant impact on the efficacy of MET for short-term increases in muscle extensibility…. both these post-isometric techniques were superior to passive stretching in this group of subjects.

Comment: The study referred to above involved healthy individuals. It may still be the case that sustained (up to 30 second) stretches would be clinically more useful, when treating chronically shortened tissues.

Neuromuscular therapy (soft tissue manipulation)

The term 'soft tissue manipulation' (STM) is frequently used to incorporate all manual methods (including massage) that address tissues other than bone, and this phrase (STM) appears to be interchangeable with the term *Neuromuscular Therapy*, as described by DeLany, in Chapter 10 (as distinct from *Neuromuscular Technique* – which describes Lief's approach, explained in detail in Chapter 6).

Neuromuscular therapy therefore incorporates Neuromuscular technique, myofascial release, connective tissue massage, muscle energy techniques and positional release methods (e.g. strain/counterstrain).

These can (with other modalities such as chilling agents), all be used as effective measures to detect, and help normalize, dysfunctional soft tissues, including areas housing noxious trigger points, which can themselves be associated with, and at times be responsible for, the promotion or maintenance of muscular weakness, muscular contraction, pain, vasodilatation, vasoconstriction, tissue degeneration, gastrointestinal, respiratory and a myriad other disorders, including emotional and 'psychological' disorders (Baldry 1993, Lewit 1999, Simons et al 1999).

The logical approach to correction of dysfunction involving shortened tight musculature, or weak inhibited musculature, is to identify the reasons for the dysfunction, and to address these. Local application of STM methods then become palliative, as well as creating an environment where more constitutional approaches (postural re-education, for example) can be more effectively achieved.

Is there a 'correct' sequence of therapy?

Treatment of dysfunction associated with muscles that have become weakened could involve initial attention to their overtight antagonists, which may be inhibiting them, as well as to isotonic concentric MET methods applied to the weakened muscles, plus exercises specific to the area.

Possible joint influences on dysfunctional soft tissues should be addressed, either through mobilization or, in instances where true joint blockage exists, by active (high-velocity thrust) manipulation.

It is a contention of many practitioners who work with somatic dysfunction that in most instances soft tissue normalization leads to joint normalization; however, the reverse is not a rarity, and at times the joint restriction is the primary feature in an area involving soft tissue dysfunction (Lewit 1996, 1999, Chaitow 2008). General postural re-education and body-toning exercises could follow.

Before such exercise is initiated, however, it is important to discover and treat local dysfunction within shortened or weakened muscles – such as trigger points – and NMT will usefully help towards achieving this.

It is often useful to allow the results of normalization of shortened muscles to unfold without confusing the issue by focusing on the weakened antagonists too soon, as a natural toning effect will occur when inhibitory influences are removed.

If, after several weeks of treatment (and possibly home stretching) of the shortened, contracted, postural muscles and their trigger points, there is not an observable and measurable improvement in the weak antagonists, then MET and exercise could usefully be introduced to these as well.

The use of gentle functional techniques, such as strain/counterstrain, is suitable for combining with NMT and MET methods.

By using MET to help to lengthen shortened structures, and NMT to aid in this, as well as in identifying localized areas of soft tissue dysfunction (myofascial trigger points or other forms of soft tissue dysfunction), the practitioner has a wide range of diagnostic and therapeutic methods, literally at his or her fingertips. Correct sequencing will be individual, but requires a correct (or at least reasonable) understanding of the causes of the dysfunction, so that treatment takes account of local and bodywide biomechanical influences (posture, breathing patterns, etc.), as well as psychosocial and lifestyle features (nutrition, exercise, sleep, etc.).

Percussion technique or spondylotherapy

For soft tissue treatment

Trigger points can be treated effectively using a series of percussive strokes according to Travell & Simons (1992):

1. The muscle is lengthened to the point of onset of passive resistance.
2. The clinician or patient uses a hard rubber mallet or reflex hammer to hit the trigger point at exactly the same place approximately 10 times.
3. This should be done at a slow rate of no more than one impact per second, but at least one impact every 5 seconds; slower rates are likely to be more effective.

Travell & Simons suggest that this enhances, or substitutes for, intermittent cold with stretch ('spray and stretch') methods, as described above.

The muscles that they list as benefitting most from percussion techniques include quadratus, brachioradialis, long finger extensors and peroneus longus and brevis.

Caution – It is specifically suggested that anterior and posterior compartment leg muscle should not be treated by percussion, owing to the risk of compartment syndrome, should bleeding occur in the muscle.

TCM percussion

Contraindications:

- acute disease
- severe heart disease
- tuberculosis
- malignant tumours
- haemorrhagic disease
- skin disease in area to be treated
- poor constitutional states such as malnutrition or asthenia.

In recent years, Chinese methods involving percussion have added dramatically to our knowledge of the potential of these methods (Zhao-Pu 1991). In traditional Chinese medicine (TCM), percussion methods are incorporated into a broad heading of 'acupressure'.

Zhao-Pu states:

Acupressure is based on the same theory as acupuncture and uses the same points and meridians ... the therapeutic effect of acupressure technique lies in the way in which it regulates and normalises blocked functions.

Included in these functions (as well as hypothesized energy transmission) are, 'stimulating circulation of blood ... and improving conductivity of nerves.'

In TCM, percussion techniques involve one of three variations (Fig. 8.8):

1. One-finger percussion, using the middle finger braced by the thumb and index finger.
2. Three-finger percussion, using the thumb, index and middle fingers.
3. Five-finger percussion, using the thumb and all fingers.

The degree of force applied during percussion is also of three types:

1. Light, which involves a movement of the hand from the wrist joint
2. Medium, which involves a movement from the elbow joint with wrist fairly rigid
3. Strong, which involves a movement of the upper arm, from the shoulder, with a rigid wrist.

Figure 8.8A   One-finger percussion uses middle finger braced by thumb and index finger. Redrawn from Zhao-Pu (1991), with permission.

Figure 8.8B   Three-finger percussion uses thumb, index and middle finger. Redrawn from Zhao-Pu (1991), with permission.

Figure 8.8C   Five-finger percussion uses thumb and all fingers. Redrawn from Zhao-Pu (1991), with permission.

Treatment is offered daily, on alternate days or once every 3 days, and a course would involve 20 sessions. Patients often receive three courses or more.

Professor Wang Zhao-Pu (whose work using this approach was based on his extensive experience as an orthopaedic surgeon) describes remarkable clinical results involving patients with paralysis and cerebral birth injuries.

He states (Zhao-Pu 1991):

Research was carried out on the cerebral haemodynamics of patients with cerebral birth injury before and after acupressure (percussion and pressure techniques) therapy. Scanning techniques were used in monitoring the short half-life radioactive materials through the cerebral circulation; in almost one-third of the patients the regional cerebral blood flow was increased after acupressure therapy ranging from 28 to 60 sessions.

In an introduction to Zhao-Pu's book, Graeme Schofield states:

After cerebral birth injury, significant though the damage may be, there are large areas of the brain and many millions of nerve cells which are still intact. These areas and the cells they contain are the targets of education for future living.

This approach is, therefore, not one that produces instant results, but that influences and gradually harnesses the potential for recovery and improvement that is latent in the tissues of the patient. For more information on oriental bodywork approaches, a complete manual of Chinese therapeutic massage (with many aspects that echo NMT methodology) edited by Sun Chengnan is highly recommended (Chengnan 1990).

Western percussion

Contraindications:

- osteoporosis
- malignancy
- inflammation in the area to be treated
- recent trauma in the area to be treated
- pain during application of percussive treatment.

In order to stimulate organs via spinal pathways, direct percussion techniques have long been employed by osteopathic and chiropractic practitioners.

Over the past century in the USA, a number of mechanical methods of percussion has evolved (Abrams 1922), as have effective manual systems in which the middle finger is placed on the appropriate spinous process(es) while the other hand concusses the finger with a series of rapidly rebounding blows. This approach is known as spondylotherapy (Johnson 1939) (see Fig. 8.9). One or two percussive repetitions are applied per second. Spondylotherapy percussion is usually applied to a series of three or four (or more) adjacent vertebrae.

Examples

- An example of this is the treatment, as above, of the 5th thoracic spinous process, proceeding downwards to the 9th, in the case of liver dysfunction. Treatment would be applied only if the area were painful to palpating pressure.
- Similarly, concussion over the 10th, 11th and 12th thoracic spinous processes would stimulate kidney function.

In order to stimulate an organ, or tissues, using the spinal reflexes, percussion can involve only a

Figure 8.9   Percussion technique (spondylotherapy) for reflexive effects or treatment of trigger points (slow percussion).

short amount of time: 15–30-second applications repeated three or four times, over approximately 4–5 minutes. A mild 'flare up' of symptoms and increased sensitivity in the area treated suggests that the desired degree of stimulation had been achieved. In order to inhibit function or to produce dilatation of local blood vessels, Johnson (1939) suggested that percussive repetitions be repeated for prolonged periods, to fatigue the reflex.

Manual spondylotherapy complements NMT because of its reflex influences and its ease of application. A sound knowledge of spinal mechanics and neurological connections is a prerequisite to its usage, which is based on anecdotal and experiential data, rather than any research validation.

Piriformis muscle technique (Retzlaff et al 1974, Wright & Drysdale 2008)

Contraindications:

- severe pain on application of pressure
- pain on rotation of hip joint as described
- sciatic inflammation.

The piriformis muscle syndrome results from contraction of the muscle either due to trauma or repetitive mechanical or postural stress, or due to the presence in the muscle of active trigger points. The effects of piriformis shortening can be circulatory, neurological, reflex or functional, inducing pain and paraesthesia of the affected limb as well as alterations to pelvic and lumbar function, as the muscle anchors the sacrum to the femur. Diagnosis usually hinges on the absence of spinal causative factors for the symptoms.

Piriformis muscle syndrome is frequently characterized by such bizarre symptoms that they may seem to be unrelated. One characteristic complaint is a persistent, severe, radiating low-back pain extending from the sacrum to the hip joint, over the gluteal region and the posterior portion of the upper leg and down to the popliteal space. In the most severe cases the patient will be unable to lie or stand comfortably, and changes in position will not relieve the pain. Intense pain will occur when the patient sits or squats.

A common sign of the piriformis syndrome is a persistent external rotation of the upper leg. This indication, which is known as the positive piriformis sign, is easily detected when the patient is examined in the supine position.

The buttock on the same side as the piriformis lesion is usually sensitive to touch or palpation. Severe pain may occur when pressure is applied to the area over the piriformis muscle and its tendinous insertion on the head of the greater trochanter.

Another diagnostic sign may be the shortening of the leg on the affected side due to contraction of the piriformis muscle. In cases where the leg on the opposite side appears shortened, it is probable that some other dysfunction exists, and that the condition is not directly related to the piriformis syndrome.

The patient may also mention pain that follows the distribution pattern of the sciatic nerve to the level of the popliteal space and sometimes to the more distal branches of this nerve. When the common perineal nerve is involved, there may be a paraesthesia of the posterior surface of the upper leg and some portions of the lower leg.

One of the most perplexing problems arising from the piriformis syndrome is the involvement of the pudendal nerve and blood vessels. This nerve, with its branches, provides the major sensory innervation of the perineal skin and the somatic motor innervation of much of the external genitalia and related perineal musculature in both women and men, with the pudendal blood vessels supplying essentially the same areas.

The pudendal nerve, after passing through the greater sciatic foramen, re-enters the pelvis by way of the lesser sciatic foramen. In a significant proportion of people, the perineal and tibial components of the sciatic nerve actually pass through the piriformis muscle, giving rise in these individuals to a greater likelihood of severe symptoms if the muscle shortens or is stressed (Polstein 1991). Compression of the pudendal nerve and blood vessels can result in serious problems involving the functioning of the genitalia in both sexes. Since external rotation of the upper legs is required for women during coitus, if there is interference with the blood supply and innervation of the genitalia, it is understandable that a female patient might complain of pain during sexual intercourse. This could also be a basis for impotency in men. Ischaemic compression, applied by thumb or elbow, together with stretching of the muscle to its normal resting length (with or without MET), is usually sufficient to remedy the problem.

Precise localization of piriformis trigger points/landmarks

The patient is side-lying, tested side uppermost. The practitioner stands at the level of the pelvis in front of, and facing, the patient and, in order to contact the femoral attachment of piriformis, draws imaginary lines between:

- ASIS and the ischial tuberosity, and
- PSIS and the most prominent point of trochanter.

Where these reference lines cross, just posterior to the trochanter, is the insertion of the muscle, and pressure here will produce marked discomfort if the structure is short or irritated.

If the most common piriformis trigger point site, in the belly of the muscle, is sought, then the line from the ASIS should be taken to the tip of the coccyx rather than to the ischial tuberosity.

Pressure where this line crosses the other will access the midpoint of the belly of piriformis, where triggers are common. Light compression here, that produces a painful response, is indicative of a stressed muscle and possibly an active myofascial trigger point (Fig. 8.10).

Piriformis treatment

 Piriformis method 1

1. The patient is side-lying, close to the edge of the table, affected side uppermost, both legs flexed at hip and knee.
2. The practitioner stands facing the patient at hip level.
3. The practitioner places his or her cephalad elbow tip gently over the point behind trochanter, where piriformis inserts, or on to the central area of the muscle belly, where an active trigger point is common.
4. The patient should be close enough to the edge of the table for the practitioner to

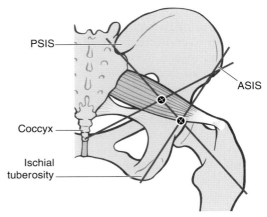

Figure 8.10   Using bony landmarks as coordinates, the commonest tender points are located in piriformis, in the belly and at the attachment or the muscle. From Chaitow (2001), with permission.

stabilize the pelvis against his or her trunk (see Fig. 8.11).
5. At the same time, the practitioner's caudad hand grasps the ankle and uses this to bring the upper leg/hip into internal rotation, taking out all the slack in piriformis.
6. A degree of inhibitory pressure (sufficient to cause discomfort but not pain) is applied via the elbow for 5–7 seconds while the muscle is kept at a reasonable but not excessive degree of stretch.

Figure 8.11   Combined ischaemic compression (elbow or thumb) and MET applied to piriformis muscle.

7. The practitioner maintains contact on the point, but eases pressure, and asks the patient to introduce an isometric contraction (25% of strength, for 5–7 seconds) to piriformis by bringing the lower leg towards the table against resistance, attempting to rotate the hip externally.

8. After the contraction ceases, and the patient relaxes, the lower limb is taken to its new resistance barrier, and elbow pressure is reapplied.

9. This process is repeated until no further gain is achieved (usually 5 to 7 repetitions of the sequence).

This method is a variation on the method advocated by Te Poorten (1969), which calls for longer and heavier compression, and no intermediate isometric contractions.

Piriformis method 2

1. In the first stage of this alternative method, the patient lies on the non-affected side with knees flexed and hip joints flexed to 90°.

2. The practitioner places his or her elbow on the piriformis musculotendinous junction and a steady pressure of 20–30 lb (9–13 kg) is applied.

3. With the other hand, the practitioner abducts the foot so that it will force an internal rotation of the upper leg.

4. The leg is held in this rotated position, at its elastic barrier, for periods of up to 2 minutes.

5. This procedure is repeated two or three times.

6. The patient is then placed in the supine position and the affected leg is tested for freedom of both external and internal rotation.
Note: See also, earlier in this chapter, Figs 8.7A and B for alternative piriformis treatments, using MET.

Proprioceptive adjustment (applied kinesiology)

(Figs. 8.12 & 8.13) (Walther 1988)

Kinesiological muscle tone correction utilizes two key receptors in muscles to achieve its effects. These are the muscle's spindles responsible for reporting on muscle length and changes in length, and the Golgi tendon organs that report on the load on, or tension of, the muscle (see Fig. 8.13).

STRENGTHEN

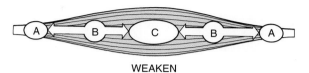
WEAKEN

A = Golgi tendon organs

B = belly of muscle

C = muscle spindle

Figure 8.12 Proprioceptive manipulation of muscles (see text).

A muscle in spasm may be helped to relax by the application of direct pressure (using 1–7 kg (2–15 lb) of pressure:

• away from the belly of the muscle, in the area of the Golgi tendon organs – and/or
• application of the same amount of pressure towards the belly of the muscle, in the area of the muscle spindle cells (see Fig. 8.12).

The precisely opposite effects (i.e. toning or strengthening the muscle) are said to be achieved by applying pressure:

• away from the belly of the muscle, in the muscle spindle region and/or
• towards the belly of the muscle in the Golgi tendon organ region.

Note that Janda (1990, 1992), in particular, has taught that weakness in a muscle can best be addressed by dealing with hypertonicity in its antagonist(s) – as a primary goal (via stretching, etc.).

• Strength can also be restored to a muscle by slowly stretching it during an isotonic eccentric contraction (which will simultaneously reduce tone in hypertonic antagonist).
• Or, strength can be restored to a muscle by slowly contracting it concentrically against resistance.

(See section on Muscle energy techniques, earlier in this chapter.)

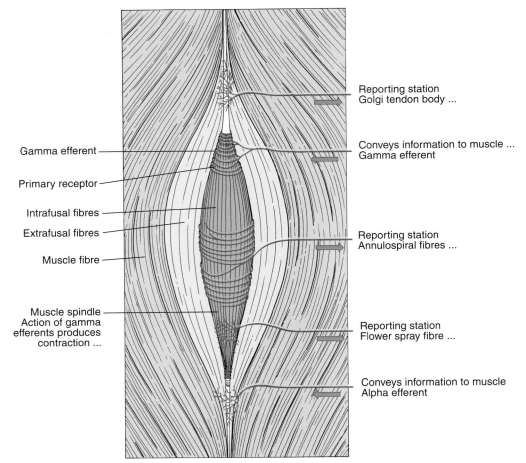

Gamma efferent

Primary receptor

Intrafusal fibres

Extrafusal fibres

Muscle fibre

Muscle spindle
Action of gamma
efferents produces
contraction ...

Reporting station
Golgi tendon body ...

Conveys information to muscle ...
Gamma efferent

Reporting station
Annulospiral fibres ...

Reporting station
Flower spray fibre ...

Conveys information to muscle
Alpha efferent

Figure 8.13   Illustration of muscle spindles, showing Golgi tendon organ and neural pathways to and from these reporting stations.

Psoas techniques

In postural distortion, such as scoliosis, or marked lumbar lordosis, as well as in many acute low back and sciatic cases, the iliopsoas muscle is found to be involved (Lewit 1996, 1999).

Contraindications to methods listed below:

- aortic disease (e.g. aneurism, calcification)
- inflammatory bowel or pelvic disease
- pain on application of palpatory pressure, as described below.

Test for psoas shortness

A simple test involves the patient lying at the end of the bed with the unaffected (non-tested) side leg in full flexion at hip and knee, and the tested leg hanging freely.

- If the thigh is parallel with the floor/table, and has sufficient flexibility to allow for an easy depression into slight extension (10° or so), the iliopsoas is considered normal.
- However, if it is elevated, or is parallel with the floor but has no 'give' when pushed lightly into extension, shortness is presumed.

Psoas technique – direct inhibitory pressure

Method (a)

1. The patient lies supine with knees flexed, hands at side.
2. The practitioner stands on the side opposite the contracted psoas.
3. One hand presses down firmly through the linea alba, 3–4 inches (7–10 cm) below the umbilicus, until the gently probing

fingers contact the body of the 4th to 5th lumbars.

4. The practitioner then eases fingers over the curved anterior surface of the lumbar body, towards the contralateral side, until the attachment of psoas is located.
5. Firm but gentle pressure is maintained for about 1 minute (Fig. 8.14A,B).

Method (b)

1. Same as method (a), practitioner is standing on opposite side to contraction.
2. Same contact with fingers through linea alba but with the other hand bringing the flexed leg towards the opposite shoulder and rotating the pelvis against probing fingers.

Method (c)

1. Same as method (a), except practitioner places flexed leg on the table to support the patient's leg on contracted psoas side.
2. In this way both hands are free to support each other as they penetrate heavier abdomens (Fig. 8.14C).

Method (d)

1. Same as method (a), except practitioner's flexed leg supports both of the patient's legs.
2. This is especially useful when there is a contraction of both psoas muscles (Fig. 8.14D).

Instead of accessing psoas directly through the linea alba, an oblique contact to the belly of the muscle can be made by applying fingertip pressure towards the spine from the lateral border of rectus abdominis (not illustrated).

In addition, during any of the methods described above, MET may be used by having the patient briefly contract the muscle against resistance ('bring your knee gently toward your face'), after which easier access, and a more relaxed muscle, should be noted. Additional tactics include having the patient slowly lengthen (extend) and flex the hip, while direct pressure is maintained on the attachment, or the belly, or psoas ('pin and stretch').

Note: To apply the methods, as described, the practitioner should stand contralaterally when using the linea alba access, and ipsilaterally when applying the oblique access contact.

A number of additional MET and strain/counterstrain approaches exist for safely treating psoas, and appropriate texts should be consulted for details of these (Chaitow 2006, 2008).

Pectoralis minor release for general upper thoracic mobilization

Release of pectoralis minor by the means described below has been clinically shown to produce an increased range of movement for the upper ribs, and a consequent increase in thoracic volume (Wallace et al 1997).

This allows subsequent pump techniques (see below) to be applied more effectively.

Kuchera & Kuchera (1994) note that 'a one centimeter increase in the diameter of the chest increases air intake by 200 to 400cc'.

The effect on lymphatic drainage is profound, because the pumping action involved in the breathing process impacts directly on lymph motion. Kuchera & Kuchera (1994) also note:

This is an efficacious technique that can be used with relative ease with patients with brittle bones, with patients in the intensive care unit, where multiple tubes and monitoring devices may be in place, and with post-surgical patients.

In other words, it is a safe procedure!

Method for pectoralis minor release

- The patient is supine with the arms comfortably at the side.
- The practitioner, while standing at the head of the table, places the palms of the hands (having ensured nails are well clipped) into the axilla, palms touching the medial humerus, thumb side of index fingers touching the axilla.
- In this way the dorsa of the fingers are located under the lateral border of each pectoralis minor.
- The practitioner then slowly externally rotates the arms and, using gentle pressure, insinuates fingertips under the lateral border of the muscle.
- The hands, the palms of which are now facing medially, are then drawn lightly toward each other (medially) until all the slack in pectoralis minor has been removed (Fig. 8.15).

Figure 8.14A Direct finger pressure applied to left side of psoas attachment to spinal structures.

Figure 8.14C Two-handed contact to reinforce psoas contact, with use of practitioner's leg to support patient's contralateral leg in order to modify overlying muscle and psoas tension (left).

Figure 8.14B Use of altered knee positions to enhance access to left side of psoas attachments.

Figure 8.14 Psoas techniques.

Figure 8.14D Both patient's legs supported by practitioner's leg as a means of modifying psoas tension in cases of bilateral psoas dysfunction.

- The practitioner's hands then slowly, deliberately and painlessly lift the tissues towards the ceiling, to their elastic barrier, easing the muscle away from its attachments, until all slack has been removed (i.e. no actual stretching is taking place at this stage, merely a removal of all slack).
- The practitioner should then transfer body weight backwards to introduce a lean, which removes the slack further, by tractioning the

Figure 8.15 Direct myofascial stretch for pectoralis minor.

muscles in a superior direction (toward the head).

- The muscle fibres will now have been eased medially, anteriorly and superiorly, and should be held at these combined barriers as they slowly release over the next few minutes.
- During this period the patient should be requested to breathe deeply and slowly.
- If correctly applied, this procedure should not be painful.

Hruby & Hoffman (2007) note: 'The combination of traction and respiratory motion releases the upper anterior thoracic muscle tension.'

Pump techniques – lymphatics, liver/spleen, pedal

(Arbuckle 1977, Fielding 1983, Hruby & Hoffman 2007)

Indications for the use of lymphatic pump techniques include all conditions that involve congestion, lymphatic stasis and infection (apart from those listed under 'Contraindications').

Wallace et al (1997) report:

Lymphatic pump techniques are designed to augment the pressure gradients that develop between the thoracic and abdominal regions during normal respirations.

The benefits of enhanced lymphatic movement – encouraged by the various techniques described in this section – include (Wallace et al 1997, Knott et al 2005, Sleszynski and Kelso 1993, Hruby & Hoffman 2008):

- increased resorption of fluids
- increased circulation and respiration
- decreased proteins in the interstitium
- facilitation from a more beneficial pH balance
- increase of white blood cell count in peripheral blood (spleen pump)
- increase of lymph flow through the thoracic duct – without changes in mean arterial pressure, heart rate or cardiac output.

Caution – It is important to make sure that the patient has no food, chewing gum or loose dentures in the mouth when these procedures are being applied.

Contraindications to pump techniques:

- malignant or other serious diseases of the lungs, liver, spleen or associated organs
- recent abdominal or thoracic surgery
- hepatitis
- infectious mononucleosis
- osteoporosis
- fracture, dislocation or other painful dysfunction involving the joints of the thoracic cage or spine
- avoid thoracic pump techniques where the patient has a reduced cough reflex.

Lymphatic pump method (a) – prone
1. Patient is prone, pillow under chest, arms over the side, with the practitioner standing at the head of the table, facing caudad.
2. The practitioner's thumbs are pressed, bilaterally, onto the intertransverse spaces, starting at the base of the neck (Fig. 8.16A).
3. Pressure is exerted towards the floor as the patient swings the arms slowly forwards (so that arms lie alongside the head at the end of the swing), and simultaneously inhales deeply.
4. On exhalation (slow) the arms are swung slowly down until they lie alongside the trunk.
5. This process of arm movements, linked to inhalation/exhalation, is repeated as the thumbs move down one intervertebral space.
6. This will have a stimulating effect on the lymphatic drainage of the body as a whole.

Figure 8.16   Lymphatic pump techniques. (A) Patient prone.
(B) Patient supine. (C) Liver pump technique.

Figure 8.16D   Hand position for side-lying spleen pump
technique (side-lying liver pump is performed in precisely the
same position on the right).

Figure 8.16E   Start position for pedal lymphatic pump
method.

**Lymphatic pump method (b) – supine
(Sleszynski & Kelso 1993, Wallace et al 1997,
Hruby & Hoffman 2008)**

1. The patient lies supine, knees and hips flexed.
2. The practitioner is at the head of the table with
   hands spread across the patient's chest, with
   thenar eminences just inferior to the clavicles,
   with thumbs resting next to each other on the
   sternum, fingers spread laterally. The arms
   should be more or less straight for ease of

transmission of force from the shoulder to the hands.

3. Rhythmic pumping pressure is introduced by the practitioner, in a downward and caudad direction, which is just sufficient to overcome resistance, by means of a repetitive, minimal, flexion and extension of the elbows.

4. The patient should breathe through the mouth during the treatment and should not resist the repetitive pressure applied by the practitioner, at a rate of 100 and 120 per minute (Fig. 8.16B).

5. This should continue for at least 3 minutes, and for up to 5 minutes.

In babies, the method can be used with one hand over the sternum, the other under the spine, with the baby cradled or seated on the practitioner's lap. The effect of this is to improve lymphatic drainage markedly.

This method is useful in all cases of oedema and infection. It also has a beneficial effect on immune function (Hoag 1969).

Treatment using Chapman's reflexes (see Ch. 4) provides additional localized drainage, which supports the general drainage and stimulation of lymphatic function (Washington et al 2003, Owen 1977).

These methods are particularly useful in children.

Note: None of the procedures described should be painful.

Lymphatic pump method with activating breath (c) – supine

1. The patient, practitioner and the hand positions are as in method (b) above.

2. The patient inhales and exhales fully through an open mouth.

3. As the patient exhales, the practitioner, elbows straight, encourages exhalation by applying pressure to the upper thorax, and maintains the degree of compression achieved at the full exhalation.

4. This process is repeated three or four times, with the degree of sustained compression increasing slightly after each exhalation (i.e. the patient commences each subsequent breath with the upper chest held in compression).

5. Approximately a third to a half of the way through the fourth or fifth *inhalation*, as pressure builds up against the restraining

hands following a request to 'breathe deeply', the hands should be removed extremely rapidly, releasing pressure from the chest. A vacuum will have been created and a sound of in-rushing air should be heard. A byproduct of this should be a major shift in lymphatic movement.

Note: Liver and spleen pump techniques are identical, apart from the fact that the spleen is located on the left side of the body and the liver on the right.

Liver/spleen pump method (a) – supine

1. A simple measure, via which function of either the liver or the spleen may be enhanced, involves the practitioner standing on the side opposite the organ that is being stimulated (left side of patient, reaching across for the liver, and vice versa for the spleen).

2. The patient is supine, knees and hips flexed, and the practitioner's caudad hand is placed under the lower ribs, and the other is placed anteriorly, just medial to the costal cartilages of the lower five ribs (Fig. 8.16C).

3. Bimanual compression should initially be carried out in a direct anterior–posterior direction, in a rhythmic manner in which the hands squeeze the tissues together approximately 20 times per minute, for 1–2 minutes.

4. After this, the direction of the pumping action should be in a more anterolateral direction, for a further minute.

5. The effect, when this is applied to the spleen rather than the liver, is to increase the leucocyte count by an average of 2200 cells per cubic millimetre (Castlio 1955, Wallace et al 1997).

Liver/spleen pump method (b) – side-lying

1. The patient is sidelying with the practitioner standing at hip level, facing the head.

2. The practitioner places both hands on the lower thoracic cage, one hand anterior and the other posterior, thumbs meeting on the axillary line.

3. The patient inhales deeply, and as she exhales the practitioner applies a cephalad directed pressure, combined with a

vibratory action, with both hands, to induce a pumping action on the liver (see Fig. 8.16D).

4. This is repeated for several minutes.

Pedal lymphatic pump method

1. The physician stands at the feet of the supine or prone patient.
2. The practitioner introduces a force that dorsiflexes the feet past neutral, and then releases the pressure, while still holding the feet as they return to neutral.
3. Use the umbilicus to gain a sense of the wave-like motion that develops via the rebound (see Fig. 8.16E).
4. As the rebound wave reaches the feet, a dorsiflexion force is reapplied, repeating the process, and creating an oscillatory pump-action.
5. This sequence should continue for several minutes.

Skin techniques

Skin rolling

Skin rolling (see Figs 8.17 and 5.5) is a useful all-purpose approach that involves the use of either or both hands. It can be used for assessment (Jay 1995), as well as for treatment. For example in assessment, Taylor et al 1990) report that: 'The skin roll technique provides an accurate indication of local areas of decreased pain threshold, along the dorsal spine ... [as] ... a correlation

Figure 8.17 Skin rolling method.

between tender skin roll areas and spinal joint dysfunction (fixations) does exist'

Therapeutically skin rolling is used as a companion approach to Connective Tissue Massage/Manipulation, as described in Chapter 5.

Method

The fingers draw tissue towards the practitioner, whilst the ball(s) of the thumb(s) roll over the gathered mound of tissue. In this way the tissue is effectively lifted, stretched and squeezed.

The most useful areas of application occur where the tissues lie tight to the underlying structures, such as directly over the shoulder joint and on the lateral aspect of the thigh. The squeezing pressure imparted by the roll of the thumb can be extremely uncomfortable, and care should be exercised during its application.

The angle of stretch, pull and roll may be varied and repeated several times to impart maximum stimulus to the reflex effects and to stimulate circulation and drainage.

The degree of stretch and/or pinch employed during rolling of the tissues is a variable factor that the practitioner may decide upon, depending upon the amount of stimulus called for. Either skin alone, or skin and underlying tissue, may be lifted, stretched and stimulated (pinched) in this way.

Stanley Lief and Boris Chaitow employed this simple, yet effective, manoeuvre as part of their general treatment. The latter described its usefulness as follows (Boris Chaitow ND DC, personal communication, 1983):

> One of my favourite techniques to enhance nerve and blood circulation is 'skin rolling'. Between the skin and the muscular and bony structures it covers, is a veritable network of blood and nerve structures and functions which can, and often do, fail to achieve their full, effective circulation for high efficiency and health because the skin is often so adhered to its lower structures (fascia) that circulation and function is appreciably reduced. This of course adversely affects the efficiency and health of the patient. There is probably no formula that will enhance this aspect of function more effectively than 'skin rolling'. A specific example of its effective benefit is to

skin-roll a major joint such as a shoulder in conditions of articular rheumatism, arthritis, neuritis or frozen shoulder.

Note: Traditional Chinese medicine calls for this procedure to be undertaken, working from the base of the spine upwards, for a tonifying effect, and from the neck downwards, for a sedating effect.

Hyperalgesic skin zones

As noted in earlier chapters, the skin overlying regions or points of reflex activity (such as myofascial trigger points and their referral areas) will frequently be found to have markedly reduced elasticity and to adhere to underlying structures (see Fig. 5.6 and the text that discusses assessment of these areas – including those associated with scars – in Chapter 5) and to be areas of increased sensitivity – hyperalgesic skin zones (HSZs).

Such zones are common in many musculoskeletal conditions, and in chronic pain syndromes. In cases of recurrent headache, HSZs may be found medially below the mastoid process, at the temples and eyebrows, and/or on the forehead above the eyebrows, and on both sides of the nose. These areas correlate with many of Bennett's neurovascular reflexes, as discussed in earlier chapters.

Some confirmation of the possible neurovascular nature of these areas comes from Ali et al (2000). They conducted studies to evaluate some of the mechanisms associated with HSZs, by injecting norepinephrin (NE), into tissues of individuals with characteristic sympathetically mediated pain (SMP), and concluded that:

NE injections produce pain in SMP patients at doses that are at the threshold for producing vasoconstriction. These studies support a role for cutaneous adrenoceptors in the mechanisms of sympathetically maintained pain.

By altering the degree of hypertonicity, and enhancing local circulation, by methods such as skin rolling (above), or the methods discussed below, hyperalgesia can be modulated by manual therapy. Underlying aetiological factors, of course, also require attention to prevent recurrence.

Stretching, to release overlying tissues of HSZs (Lewit 1992)

1. To treat a hyperalgesic area, the fingertips (for a small area) or the ulnar aspects of the crossed hands (for a larger area) are placed together on the skin surface overlying the affected area.
2. The tissues should then be gently stretched apart, to their easy resistance barrier, as the fingers, or hands, separate.
3. To establish the presence, or lack of, physiological elasticity, the skin would be stretched in various directions.
4. When restriction is noted, the tissues are held in a painlessly stretched position until a degree of release is noted. This commonly takes 10–20 seconds.
5. The same area may be stretched in this manner in various directions, each time being held at its barrier of resistance until a release occurs (see Fig. 5.7A,B).
6. The release of the tissues is itself the therapeutic effort, providing reflex stimulus to underlying structures.
7. The subsequent maintenance of the free elastic state of the tissues is evidence of an improvement in the causative factors. Naturally, if underlying factors maintain the reflex activity, whether this be musculoskeletal or visceral dysfunction, the improvement will be short-lived.

In this way HSZs are used both diagnostically, and prognostically.

Lewit (1992) states:

If pain is due to the HSZ, this method is quite as effective as needling, electrostimulation, and other similar methods. Moreover, it is entirely painless, and can be applied by the patient himself.

Treating overlying tissues of HSZs – positional release

1. The practitioner places a contact (finger pad(s) or whole hand) onto the skin, which appears less pliable, more adherent (to underlying fascia; see Ch. 5), or palpates as 'different' to, or more sensitive than, surrounding tissues, suggesting that it is a HSZ.

2. The contact hand or finger pad(s) should slide the skin superiorly and inferiorly, medially and laterally, and should turn in a clockwise and then an anticlockwise direction, and with each of these movements should seek the direction of most comfort and least tension/bind.
3. The motion of the contact fingers or whole hand on the tissues is asking: 'In which direction do the tissues move most easily?' (Fig. 8.18).
4. When the various positions of ease, evaluated in this way, are 'stacked' together, this produces the combined 'preference pattern' – the skin and fascia will have been taken in their respective directions of motion away from whatever restriction barriers they currently exhibit.
5. Normal, unstressed, tissues exhibit an equal excursion in all directions of rotation, although this is seldom found in adults, even if surgical trauma has not been a factor (Zink & Lawson 1979).
6. The final position of ease should be held until tension releases spontaneously, usually a period of 30–90 seconds. This will commonly

Figure 8.18   Achieving positional release of tissues – skin and fascia – by holding them in their preferred 'ease' directions. From Chaitow (2002), with permission.

release recently acquired stress patterns in the fascia, possibly revealing older patterns, which can then be treated.

'S' and 'C' bends: myofascial release methods for lengthening soft tissues

Lederman (1997) has described the relatively few ways in which tissues can be modified by forms of direct therapeutic pressure. These involve:

- Tension loading – including traction, stretching and other lengthening approaches are involved, resulting in changes in connective tissue status (see 'C' bends below).
- Compression loading, on the other hand, shortens and widens tissues. See Chapter 3, Box 3.5, for a summary of these effects, which include fluid changes as well (possibly) as changes in length.
- Rotation loading elongates some fibres while compressing others (see 'S' bend description below).
- Bending loading combines compression loading (on the concave side) and tension loading on the convex side (see 'C' bend description below).
- Shearing loading involves shift or translation movements, and is used primarily in joint mobilization, while elongating and compressing associated soft tissues.
- Combined loading incorporates a variety of the models listed above (see Fig. 8.21).

Other variables to be considered when evaluating therapeutic 'pressure' include:

- The degree of pressure (see Box 3.6).
- How great an area of contact is involved and/or how large an area is receiving one or other form of loading.
- How great an amplitude is involved – in other words, how far are the tissues being moved, stretched? (The degree of force largely determines the amplitude.)
- How rapid is the application of force – does it involve high velocity or low velocity?
- For how long are the tissues loaded?
- Is the application of force static or rhythmic, and, if rhythmic, is it rapid or slow, perhaps coinciding with the breathing cycle?

- How steady is the force application, static or moving (gliding)?
- Is the patient participating in the process, actively moving, or resisting the force application?

Examples of the application of force include the 'C' and 'S' bend techniques.

 ### 'C' bend technique

In order to lengthen local areas of muscle and/or connective tissue, the tissues may be 'bent' (into a 'C' shape), to a first barrier of resistance, so that the thumbs engage the barrier, waiting for this to release and retreat, over a period of 5–30 seconds.

Lewit (1996) points out that:

Shortness of the connective tissue is most characteristic for short (taut) muscles, usually overactive muscles. Producing a tissue fold and stretching it is the most effective way to obtain lengthening, because the stretch reflex can be avoided.

See Figures 8.19A and 8.23A for examples of a 'C' bend fold. Figure 8.19A shows this being slowly applied to paraspinal muscles, allowing a gentle lengthening to occur. (Lewit 1996). Figure 8.23A (see later in this chapter, under the heading Tensor fascia lata techniques), involves the distal aspects of the iliotibial band, where the method involves a series of rapid, high-velocity, low-amplitude 'snapping' bends of the tissues.

'S' bend technique

To achieve a relaxation of a specific area of muscle tension using an 'S' bend, the hands should be positioned in such a way as to allow thumb or hand pressure to be applied across the fibres of a contracted or indurated muscle, so that the contacts are travelling in opposite directions to each other (Lewit 1992).

As pressure is applied simultaneously with each thumb or hand (see Figs 8.19B and 8.23B), the tissues between the two contacts will progressively have the slack removed, and be placed in a slightly lengthened situation, in which they can be held until release occurs (or 'springing' is introduced).

Figure 8.19A   Application of 'C' bend to paraspinal musculature.

Figure 8.19B   'S' bend pressure applied to tense or fibrotic musculature.

This technique can be applied along the course of particularly spastic, and hard unyielding, tissues, in addition to the basic NMT thumb technique (see Chapters 6 & 7).

Additionally, the 'S' bend may be used with a flicking action of the thumb to complete the stroke, once effective tension has been created in the tissues by the opposing thumbs. This 'springing' has the effect of stimulating local circulation most effectively and, if the tissues are not too sensitive, may assist in breaking down infiltrated or indurated tissues.

The 'S' contact is so named because the tissues being treated form that shape, as the strokes are performed. If used in its 'slow' mode, the tissues are held in this opposition lengthening state for upwards of 30 seconds, before slightly different fibres are selected to receive the same procedure. Alternatively a rapid, heel of hand, thrust, across the tissues (see Fig. 8.23B), may be used on particularly rigid structures, such as the iliotibial band. That approach is described later in the chapter.

Stretching fascia – myofascial release

Indications for use of MFR include a need to improve movement potential, and/or for the stretching/lengthening of shortened, contracted or fibrosed soft tissues, or for reducing tone in hypertonic muscles. See Fig 8.20.

Fascia is a tough fibroelastic body-wide web of tissue that performs both structural and proprioceptive functions. Because of its contiguous nature, and its virtually universal presence in association with every muscle, vessel and organ, the potential influences of fascia are profound if shortening, adhesions, scarring or distortion occurs as a result of either slow adaptation (microtrauma) or trauma.

Figure 8.20   Cross handed myofascial release. © 2007 Elsevier Ltd. Chaitow & Fritz. A Massage Therapists guide to Lower Back & Pelvic Pain.

Barnes (1997a, 1997b), a leading MFR expert, has said:

Myofascial release is a hands-on soft tissue technique that facilitates a stretch into the restricted fascia. A sustained pressure is applied into the tissue barrier; after 90 to 120 seconds the tissue will undergo histological length changes allowing the first release to be felt. The therapist follows the release into a new tissue barrier and holds. After a few releases the tissues will become softer and more pliable.

Mock (1997) has described a hierarchy of MFR stages or 'levels':

1. Level 1 involves treatment of tissues without introducing tension. The practitioner's contact (which could involve thumb, finger, knuckle or elbow) moves longitudinally along muscle fibres, distal to proximal, with the patient passive.
2. Level 2 is precisely the same as the previous description but in this instance, the glide is applied to muscle which is in tension (at stretch).
3. Level 3 involves the introduction to the process of passively induced motion, as an area of restriction is compressed while the tissues being compressed are taken passively through their fullest possible range of motion.
4. Level 4 is the same as the previous description but the patient actively moves the tissues through the fullest possible range of motion, from shortest to longest, while the practitioner/therapist offers resistance.

For example, the practitioner might apply moderate digital pressure to the involved tissue, in a direction proximal to distal, while the patient actively moves the muscle through its range of motion in both eccentric and concentric contraction phases. This modification of basic MFR has been called Active Release Technique (ART) (Leahy 1999).

Methodology

The basic methodology of MFR requires that it should be applied slowly. Barriers of resistance are engaged, and these are forced to retreat by means of steadily applied load. In this way physiological responses of creep and hysteresis are produced, leading to lengthening. This is a non-violent, direct, approach that has little potential for causing damage (however, see cautions below).

When active or passive movements are combined with the basic methodology, caution is required depending on the status of the patient and the tissues, to avoid excessive irritation. For example enthesitis could occur if localized repetitive stretching combined with compression were applied close to an attachment (Simons et al 1999).

Cautions

- Acute arthritis and other inflammatory conditions (contraindicated during acute stages)
- Aneurysm
- Bone fractures or acute soft tissue injuries: wait for full healing (6 weeks – 3 months)
- Haemophilia
- Hodgkin's disease
- Leukaemia
- Malignancy with metastasis (or TB) involving bone
- Osteoporosis
- Pain production during procedure
- Patients on cortisone (wait 2–3 months)
- Patients with high fever
- Phlebitis
- Recent scar tissue
- Syphilitic articular or peri-articular lesions
- Uncontrolled diabetic neuropathy.

Note: The skin stretching methods described above under the heading 'Hyperalgesic skin zones' are, in effect, examples of miniature myofascial releases. Whenever skin, or other soft tissues, fails to present symmetrical freedom of movement, either in terms of lengthening potential, range of motion, or ability to glide on underlying tissues, a degree of dysfunction can be assumed (Lewit 1996). Lewit (1996) also describes releasing these tightened, often fascial, tissues as 'shifting', rather than stretching. Tissues are taken to their painless elastic barrier, by application of a separation force between the hands or fingers, and held until a lengthening occurs.

Specific (abdominal) release techniques

Boris Chaitow, who worked closely with Stanley Lief, wrote the following about Lief's 'adhesion breaking', 'bloodless surgery', techniques (personal communication, 1983):

Using these 'bloodless surgery' [specific release technique] methods, Stanley Lief achieved dramatic changes in tissue structure and functional improvements in many types of abdominal stresses, including digestive problems, gall bladder blockage, constipation, spastic colon, colic, uterine fibroids, dysmenorrhoea, postoperative adhesions etc. This was designed to break up deep-seated adhesions and contractions. It also enables the practitioner to improve function and circulation [of the region].

Lief used methods (outlined below) derived from an American system of manipulative or 'bloodless' surgery to amplify his abdominal techniques. These 'release' techniques can be applied to soft areas of the body, e.g. the throat, as well as to the abdomen. The original concept of 'bloodless surgery' was that adhesions were being 'peeled' away from their anchorage by the technique, and in some cases this might have been so. However, its current application is to any area of tight, fibrosed, spastic, contracted or adhering soft tissue in the abdominal region, or elsewhere – for example, on the lateral thigh in tense and contracted fascial tissues (Fig. 8.21A,B).

Precisely what takes place after abdominal release technique is open to conjecture. An improvement in tone and circulation, and usually of general function, is the most obvious result. Whether this is because of a release of a long-held contracted state in the soft tissues, or because of an actual breaking of adhesions, or because of some other mechanism, is open to debate.

- A general abdominal neuromuscular treatment (see Ch. 7) should precede application of specific release technique (technique A below).
- This serves both to relax and to tone the abdomen in a general manner, while enabling the practitioner to identify areas that feel indurated or contracted, as well as noting all

(A)

Figure 8.21A   Both hands release tissue that has been taken to its elastic barrier in various directions: compressed, stretched apart, counter-rotated and finally 'sprung'.

(B)

Figure 8.21B   The right hand springs the restricted tissues after all slack has been removed and some stretch applied, while the left hand acts mainly to produce a stabilizing contact against which a precisely controlled force is applied.

Figure 8.21   Specific release technique as used in treatment of adhesions and tensor fascia lata restrictions.

areas of subjective sensitivity as reported by the patient.

- It is these (a) tight, contracted and (b) sensitive areas that receive the release technique.

Localizing dysfunction

The ability of the practitioner to localize such areas accurately is important, and needs to be practised until the hands and fingers feel such abnormalities as a matter of course. It is suggested that the middle finger of the right hand (in a right-handed practitioner) should be trained to seek and mark those areas where specific release technique is to be applied.

The patient should be supine, with knees flexed, and feet as close to the buttocks as possible, for maximum abdominal relaxation, and with the head on a small pillow. The practitioner should stand facing the patient, on the side opposite that being treated, i.e. to treat the left inguinal area the practitioner stands, knees

flexed, leaning across from the patient's right side. This allows the tissues being manipulated to be drawn towards the practitioner in a controlled manner.

Technique A

1. Having located an area of contracted (often sensitive) tissue, the middle finger locates the point of maximum resistance and the tissues are drawn towards the practitioner, to the limit of pain-free movement. In this description there will be a right hand initial contact, as illustrated in Fig. 8.21A, when working on a left lower abdominal area, while standing on the right).

2. The middle finger (right hand) and its neighbours should be flexed and fairly rigid, and be imparting force in two directions at this stage, i.e. downwards (towards the floor) and towards the practitioner. (In 'bloodless surgery' techniques, the right hand is always in contact with the 'adhesion'/taut area, with

the other contact on the organ/tissues to which the adhesion is attached.)

3. With the fingers maintaining the above position, the thumb of the left hand is placed almost immediately – no more than $^1/_4$ inch (6 mm) away – adjacent to the middle finger of the right hand, in such a way that a downward pressure (towards the floor) will provide a fulcrum point, against which force can be applied via the right hand, in order to stretch, or reduce the degree of contraction in, the tissue (or indeed to break or 'peel' adhesions).

4. The thumb should also be flexed, and the contact can be via its tip or its lateral border, or a combination of both.

5. The idea of a fulcrum is important because the two points of contact are both on soft tissue structures, and the effect of the manipulation is achieved, not by pulling or twisting these apart, but by a combination of movements that impart force in several directions at the same time.

6. This is accomplished – after all slack has been removed, by a rapid clockwise movement of the right hand (middle finger contact) against the stabilizing anchorage of the left thumb (see Fig. 8.21A).

7. Synchronous movement of the thumb, during this release, is not essential or necessary. However, when using this method Boris Chaitow would impart a degree of additional torsional force, by releasing the thumb contact in an anticlockwise direction, at the moment of manipulation.

8. With both hands in contact, as described, and the contact digits flexed and rigid, the practitioner should be so positioned that he or she is leaning over the affected area, knees flexed with the legs separated for stability, and elbows flexed and separated to 180° separation. The forces operating at the point of contact will be downward, as well as a slight separation of the hands to the soft tissue barrier. The manipulative force is imparted by *a very rapid clockwise flick of the right contact*, while maintaining the left thumb contact rigid (or simultaneously,

rapidly, taking it in an anticlockwise direction).

9. The effect of the right hand movement would be to snap the right elbow towards the practitioner's side. If a double release is performed, then both elbows come rapidly to the sides.

10. The amount of force imparted should be controlled so that no pain is felt by the patient.

The essence of this technique is the speed with which it is applied. This very high velocity release involves tissues that have been 'wound up', by being taken in three directions of distraction – i.e. compression, separation and a degree of torsion. Its success depends upon this speed, as much as on the correct positioning of the hands, and the precise location of the area of tissue restriction.

The same procedure can be repeated several times on the same area, and the release of a number of such areas of contracted or indurated tissue, at any one treatment is usual. The same thumb contact is often maintained whilst variations in the direction of tissue tension are dealt with by slightly altering the angle of the right hand contact and manipulative effort.

If, after manipulation, no objective improvement is noted on palpation, the angle of the contacts should be varied. Nothing will be gained, however, by attempting to use excessive force in order to achieve results. As the degree of soft tissue trauma to the patient is minimal, the after-effects should not include bruising or much discomfort. Any such after-effect would indicate undue pressure or force being used.

Boris Chaitow (personal communication, 1983) described this method as follows:

For the technique of NMT on the abdomen referred to as 'bloodless surgery', palpate with the tips of the fingers of the right hand, and having located the area of abnormal feel, place those four fingers as a group at the distal border of the lesioned area, and place the thumb of the left hand alongside the nails of the right fingers. Give a sharp flick with both hands simultaneously, the left hand thumb being twisted anticlockwise, and the fingers of the right hand clockwise (difficult if not impossible to describe on paper). This achieves an appreciable breaking-up, without trauma or hurt to the patient, of tensions, adhesions, congestions etc., both on the wall of the abdomen and structures within the cavity. Obviously these flicks with the hands have to be repeated a number of times to feel a discernible difference in the lesioned tissue.

Technique B.   A second method for the release of tense, contracted, indurated connective and muscular tissue is sometimes employed. This requires the same positioning of the patient and the practitioner, as in method A.

It is worth recalling that thickening will occur in fascia in accordance with the degree of stress imposed upon it. As enormous gravitational stress occurs in the abdominal region, as a result of postural embarrassment, it is frequently the case that tight 'stress bands' will be felt inferior, superior or lateral to internal organs (e.g. intestinal structures) that have sagged and become displaced. Such contracted tissue is often the source of reflex trigger activity, and is often, in itself, the cause of mechanical interference with normal venous and lymphatic drainage, as well as being a possible source of pain.

Any procedure that helps to normalize such tension should be accompanied by a programme of postural re-education and exercise, if it is to have any lasting beneficial effects.

1. The practitioner's right hand, fingers flexed and middle finger slightly in the lead, probes through the surface abdominal musculature and attempts to 'lift' the structures.
2. In this way, areas of abnormal resistance will be traced, quite easily, by the tip of the middle finger of the right hand. The most inferior point of attachment of such a band is located and held firmly by this flexed digit.
3. The tip and lateral border of the thumb of the left hand is then placed adjacent to this contact, so that the right hand contact is on the tension band and the left contact is on the structure to which it attaches.
4. The manipulative force is achieved by a rapid anticlockwise movement of the right contact, whilst firm, stabilizing pressure is maintained by the left thumb (Fig. 8.21B).

5. The closer the two contacts are to each other at the moment of release, the less force is required and the less danger of injury to the tissues there will be.
6. It is suggested that, by visualizing an attempt to tear an envelope held between thumbs and forefingers, this concept will be better understood. The closer the holding digits are to each other, the easier such an operation would be. As the manipulative effort is attempting to, at least, stretch and, at most, separate the fibres involved, it is necessary to deliver a high-velocity, low-amplitude torsional force, and not a vague stretching effort imparted over a large area of unyielding tissue.
7. The actual manipulative force is imparted by the tip of the middle finger of the right hand, but is, of course, the result of the movement of the whole hand. The wrist snaps medially and the elbow outwards, at the moment of release.
8. This speedy 'flicking' action is one that should be practised many times, so that its execution is a matter of routine. A release of contracted tissue will be followed by an immediate freedom of mobility of tissues, or of organs formerly 'bound' and immobile.

Such 'release' procedures (technique A or B) should be performed throughout the abdominal area and preceded by the general neuromuscular treatment (see Chapters 6 & 7), and be followed by a general procedure to 'lift' the abdominal contents back to a physiologically correct position.

Instructions should be given of abdominal and postural exercises, to be performed by the patient, as should improved postural and breathing rehabilitation techniques.

A series of six to ten such 'specific release' treatments, over a period of a month or so, is suggested in chronic conditions involving visceroptosis and abdominal congestion. The application of these techniques to the hypogastric and inguinal regions may be of benefit to patients suffering from menstrual irregularities. Local function can often be improved as a result of the structural and circulatory improvements following specific release techniques.

Strain–counterstrain – and other positional release techniques (Fig. 8.22)

We have already seen examples of positional release in the section on treatment of hyperalgesic skin zones, earlier in this chapter (Fig. 8.18). Positional release techniques belong to that class of modalities that invite change, rather than forcing change, when treating dysfunctional tissues. By their nature they are *indirect*, i.e. the process almost always involves a disengagement from restriction barriers, rather than any direct attempt to engage and overcome such restrictions, as would be the case in HVLA, myofascial release or stretch methodology (Deig 2001). As such, PRT methods are best suited to acute and sub-acute settings, although they are considered a useful aid in chronic conditions.

Simplistically, PRT methods attempt to create 'positions of ease' or 'comfort' for shortened and distressed tissues, commonly by taking already shortened (spasm, contracture, fibrosis, etc.) tissues into a supported degree of greater shortness, in the belief that a beneficial change will result, by means of mechanisms including a neurological resetting involving the muscle spindles, and a circulatory 'flushing' of previously ischaemic tissues. These and other possible mechanisms are discussed in the 'Physiological effects' section below (Chaitow 2002, D'Ambrogio & Roth 1997, Deig 2001, Rathbun & MacNab 1970).

Methodology

The art of applying positional release methods lies in identifying the direction(s) in which a painful joint, or soft tissues, should be moved, so that

Figure 8.22A A tender point is identified by the operator's left hand.

Figure 8.22B A degree of ease is produced from that point by the initial positioning of the arm.

Figure 8.22C A final position of ease is found by fine tuning to relieve pain in the tender point, and the position is held for 20–90 seconds.

Figure 8.22 Application of positional release (strain/counterstrain) to the supraspinatus muscle.

a spontaneous release occurs (i.e. the position of 'ease' or 'comfort'). When passively placed in such a position, inhibition of painful stimuli results, and the range of motion of the area will usually be significantly enhanced afterwards.

There are two main PRT methods, with a number of variations, that have emerged out of osteopathic methodology.

1. **Strain-counterstrain** (SCS) utilizes a painful area in dysfunctional tissues (a 'tender point') as a monitor to guide the practitioner, as tissues are positioned and fine tuned, until the initial tenderness reduces from a pain score of 10, to 3 or less. The tissues are then held in this position for variable periods (90 seconds is a common recommendation) before being gently released to their resting state (Chaitow 2007, Jones 1981). Jones has compiled lists of specific tender point areas relating to every imaginable strain of most joints, and many muscles, of the body. These are his 'proven' (by clinical experience) points, and he provides strict guidelines for achieving 'ease' in the tender point that is being palpated (locating the position of ease usually involves a 'folding' or crowding of the tissues in which the tender point lies). A number of variations exist as to the use of the concepts that Jones developed, and these are fully explained in *Positional Release Techniques* (Chaitow 2002). Additional texts by Deig (2001) and D'Ambrogio & Roth (1997) are also recommended (see Figs 4.5A,B,C). An example is offered of the use of SCS positional release in Figure 8.22A,B,C.

2. **Functional technique** uses palpation of distressed tissues or joints to position them into 'ease', *without using pain sensitivity as a guide* (as in SCS, above). Functional approaches therefore rely on a skilled palpation sense (Johnstone 1997, Schiowitz 1990).

3. A variety of 'facilitating' methods are used to encourage functional and pain-reducing changes, including gentle compression, distraction or respiratory strategies (Goodheart 1984).

4. Physical therapy has evolved methods such as 'mobilization with movement' and 'unloading' taping that incorporate aspects of PRT.

McKenzie exercise methods incorporate concepts of movement towards 'ease' that are also close to PRT concepts (Horton 2002, Morrissey 2002).

5. In chiropractic, aspects of the use of sacro-occipital technique's 'blocking' methods incorporate placing tissues into an exaggeration of existing distortion (i.e. making whatever is short, shorter) and are also in line with PRT methodology (Blum et al 2003).

6. In craniosacral techniques much of the treatment involves indirect pressure, taking distortions into a 'crowded' state, so allowing change to take place spontaneously (Sergueef et al 2002). Upledger & Vredevoogd (1983) give a practical explanation of indirect methods of treatment, especially as related to cranial therapy. The idea of moving a restricted area in the direction of ease is, they say, 'a sort of "unlatching" principle. Often in order to open a latch we must first exaggerate its closure'.

In normal tissues there exists in the mid-range of motion an area of 'ease' or balance, where the tissues are at their least tense. When there is a restriction in the *normal range of motion of a joint or an area*, whether of osseous or soft tissue origin, the now limited range will almost always still have a place, a moment, a point, which is neutral, of maximum comfort or ease, usually lying somewhere between the new restriction barrier in one direction and the physiological barrier in the other. Finding this balance point – also known as 'dynamic neutral' – is a key element in PRT.

Placing the dysfunctional tissues into this 'ease' state, for an appropriate length of time (see below), offers restrictions a chance to 'unlatch', release, normalize. In this way it is suggested that the positioning/fine-tuning element of the process is the preparation for the treatment to commence, and that the 'treatment' itself is self-generated by the tissues (nervous system, circulatory system, etc.) in response to this careful positioning.

Safety

The nature of indirect approaches is essentially safe, since barriers are avoided and tissues are held in comfort. Numerous studies demonstrate that these methods are safe as well as being effective (Cislo et al 1991, Ramirez 1989, Wong et al 2004a,b). Hospital studies involving treatment of recently surgically traumatized tissue validate the essential safety of positional release methods (Dickey 1989).

Proposed mechanisms

Proprioception.   Walther (1988) summarizes a 'strain' situation as follows:

> When proprioceptors send conflicting information there may be simultaneous contraction of the antagonists ... without antagonist muscle inhibition, joint and other strain results [and in this manner] a reflex pattern develops which causes muscle or other tissue to maintain this continuing strain. It [strain dysfunction] often relates to the inappropriate signaling from muscle proprioceptors that have been strained from rapid change that does not allow proper adaptation.

Such patterns exist in acute settings such as torticollis, as well as in acute lumbar spasm. It is also recognizable as a feature of many types of chronic somatic dysfunction in which joints remain restricted due to muscular imbalances of this type, occurring as part of an adaptive process. This is a time of intense neurological and proprioceptive 'confusion', and is the moment of 'strain'. SCS appears to offer a means of quieting the neurological confusion and the excessive, or unbalanced, tone.

D'Ambrogio & Roth (1997) state that:

> Positional release therapy (PRT) appears to have a damping influence on the general level of excitability within the facilitated segment. Weiselfish (1993) has found that this characteristic of PRT is unique in its effectiveness, and has utilized this feature to successfully treat severe neurologic patients, even though the source of the primary dysfunction arose from the supraspinal level.

Nociception.   Bailey & Dick (1992) suggest that strain dysfunction is far more complex than the simple proprioceptive example:

> Probably few dysfunctional states result from a purely proprioceptive or nociceptive response. Additional factors such as autonomic responses, other reflexive activities, joint receptor responses [biochemical features] or emotional states must also be accounted for. Nociceptive responses would occur (which are more powerful than proprioceptive influences) and these multisegmental reflexes would produce a flexor withdrawal, dramatically increasing tone in the flexor group.

Korr's (1976) explanation for the physiological normalization of tissues brought about through positional release is that:

> The shortened spindle nevertheless continues to fire, despite the slackening of the main muscle, and the CNS is gradually able to turn down the gamma discharge and, in turn, enables the muscles to return to 'easy neutral', at its resting length. In effect, the physician has led the patient through a repetition of the dysfunctioning process with, however, two essential differences. First it is done in slow motion, with gentle muscular forces, and second there have been no surprises for the CNS; the spindle has continued to report throughout.

Other hypotheses

Jacobson et al (1989) have suggested a circulatory hypothesis for the benefits of PRT. Another hypothesis relates to the presumed effects of slackening fascial tissues during positional release. D'Ambrogio & Roth (1997) summarize what may happen to the fascia, during PRT, as follows:

> By reducing the tension on the myofascial system, the fascial components of dysfunction may be engaged. The reduction in tension on the collagenous cross-linkages appears to induce a disengagement of the electrochemical bonds and a conversion back [from the gel-like] to the sol [solate] state. Whether proprioceptive, nociceptive, neurological, circulatory or fascial factors are involved in positional release effects remains a matter for further research.

Tensor fascia lata (iliotibial band) techniques

Ober's test. To test for a tight iliotibial band have the patient lie on the unaffected side, with hip and knee flexed to 90°. The patient is asked to hold that leg to the table. The other leg is supported by the practitioner, who is standing behind the patient. The straight leg is extended, to the point where the iliotibial band lies over the greater trochanter. The practitioner's cephalad hand supports the leg at the knee, while the caudad hand supports the ankle. The knee is then flexed to 90° and the hand supporting the leg at the knee is removed, allowing the knee to fall towards the table. If the iliotibial band has shortened, this will not occur and the leg will remain suspended. The band will palpate as tender under such conditions, as a rule.

The iliotibial band (ITB) comprises a thick fascial structure that runs from the iliac crest, down the lateral side of the thigh, to insert on the lateral patellar retinaculum, tubercle of the tibia, and proximal fibular head. The ITB provides attaches to the tensor fascia lata (TFL), gluteal muscles, and vastus lateralis (Orchard et al 1996).

ITB friction syndrome is a common source of overuse injury and knee pain, in athletes (Fairclough et al 2006). When the ITB is shortened it is capable of producing or contributing to a range of pelvic (e.g. SI joint), hip, leg and knee and pelvic symptoms.

Fredericson et al (2002) note that a variety of soft tissue problems (including myofascial trigger points, hip abductor muscle inhibition and fascial adhesions) can contribute to increased tension on the ITB making a comprehensive stretching protocol an important component of rehabilitation.

Because of its massive fascial component, the ITB has attracted a variety of treatment approaches, with an abiding question as to whether this structure can itself be effectively stretched at all.

NMT treatment method 1

Treatment may employ a direct approach, as advocated by Mennell (1969) or by use of MET methods, as described below.

'Twig snap' method. First the patient is placed side-lying, with both legs flexed comfortably. The first contact is with that part of the band distal to the greater trochanter. The anterior fibres are stretched first to create a 'C' bend in the tissues. (Fig. 8.23A). The fingers are laid over the anterior fibres of the band, distal to the trochanter, just above the knee. The thumbs rest, as a fulcrum,

(A)

Figure 8.23A Anterior iliotibial band treatment, using a 'twig snapping' approach to address extreme shortness and fibrosity of these tissues. This is applied sequentially up and down the band using a degree of force that is easily tolerated.

(B)

Figure 8.23B The posterior fibres of the iliotibial band are treated using the heel of one hand alternately to thrust against the band while it is stabilized by the other hand. An alternating sequence of this sort, applied up and down the band, produces marked release of hypertonic and shortened fibres.

and are placed against the posterior aspect of the anterior fibres, and a rapid snapping action is applied. The main force is transmitted through the thumbs, which should stretch the fibres without pressing them against the osseous structures (which would bruise the tissues). A rapidly applied series of 'thrusts' such as this, starting at the knee, and working up and down the band, is carried out.

(b) 'Piston thrust' method.   The posterior fibres are then treated. The heel of each hand is pushed in a piston-like manner against the fibres, alternately. As the heel (thenar or hyperthenar eminence) of one hand thrusts against the fibres, the other stabilizes them by grasping the anterior aspect (Fig. 8.23B). A series of thrusts is made from above the knee to the trochanter and back again. The thrust must be against the fibres and not against osseous structures, or bruising will ensue.

(c) Treatment over the trochanter.   The region overlying the trochanter is treated by rolling it backwards and forwards over the bony prominence. The thumbs are the motive force, being pressed downwards and backward or forward, to achieve this. The roll is attempting to take the band posteriorly, and then anteriorly, over the trochanter. As the trochanter rolls backwards, the heel of the foot on the treated leg should rise from the table (but only if the band is tight).

(d) NMT.   The area above the trochanter is treated by deep, kneading massage or NMT. This is often easily achieved when the patient is prone, and the tissues are contacted by the fingers of the treating hand, with the practitioner standing on the side opposite the area being treated. The fingers may be insinuated into the tissues, and a degree of lifting, drag, as well as pressure medial-wards, is achieved by the practitioner leaning backwards and drawing the treating hand towards him or her (see Figs 6.8A,B) This may be done as part of NMT treatment. These structures require maintenance stretching, via exercise, if improvement is to be held (see below).

Treatment method 2

MET – involving either isometric or isolytic contraction (see Fig. 8.6B). Note: See ITB Study 1 below, for confirmation of stretch occurring in the positions used in this approach.

Isometric contraction.   In the first instance the patient is supine, with the unaffected leg flexed and the affected leg extended (see Fig. 8.24).The practitioner takes the extended leg into maximum adduction, placing a maximum degree of stretch onto the lateral fibres (the abductors and fascia). To achieve this, the leg will be adducted and brought under the other, flexed, leg. Standing on the side of the unaffected leg, against which the practitioner applies stabilizing pressure, the practitioner adducts the treated leg, taking out the slack, and asks the patient to make an attempt to abduct the affected leg using 25% of available strength. This is resisted for 10 seconds as the patient inhales. Release coincides with exhalation, at which time a little more slack is taken out and the affected leg is adducted slightly beyond its resistance barrier. The procedure is repeated two or three more times.

Isolytic contraction.   The position is the same as that given above. Should the above method be only partly effective, then, as the patient attempts to abduct the affected leg (commencing with only a portion – say 25% – of available strength, but with increasing degree of effort, if the procedure is repeated several times) the practitioner overcomes this, and forces it further into adduction. This process may be uncomfortable, and the patient should be forewarned. This will produce

Fig. 8.24   Ultrasonographic measurements on the ITB conducted with modified Ober's test.

microtrauma and reduce fibrous contractions. Progressively more effort on the part of the patient should be introduced on subsequent isotonic eccentric contractions.

ITB studies

1. Wang et al (2008) used a combination of MRI scans and real-time ultrasound imaging (RTU) to establish that when placed in a modified Ober's position, actual stretch occurs in the ITB, and not only in the associated musculature (gluteals, vastus lateralis, TFL). They note that: 'Band width changes indicated that the ITB was subjected to a significant stretching force during hip adduction.' Such as is described above (see Fig. 8.24).

2. Using a variety of high-tech instruments, including four cameras to film the positions of skin markers, Fredericson et al (2002), evaluated both the efficacy of three stretching protocols (see Fig. 8.25ABC), as well as the subsequent degrees of lengthening, in the ITBs of the athletes participating in the study. Between 9 and 11% increase in length was noted, following three static, 30 second stretches. Variations on these stretch positions should be given as home self-care to individuals with ITB shortness.

A caution offered as to what is being stretched:

One of the limitations of this study was that we did not directly measure ITB length; rather we estimated changes in length from angular changes in markers. It is possible that extensibility of other tissues such as the gluteals, tensor fascia lata, and vastus lateralis could have contributed to the changes.

Fig. 8.25 Three stretching positions for ITB. All produced benefits after 3×30 second repetitions, with C the most beneficial. (Adapted from Fredericson M, White J, MacMahon J 2002 Quantitative Analysis of the Relative Effectiveness of 3 Iliotibial Band Stretches Arch. Phys. Med. Rehabil. 83:589–592, Fig. 2.)

References

Abrams A: *New concepts in diagnosis and treatment*, San Francisco, 1922, Physicoclinical Co.

Agarwal N, Pacher P, et al: Cannabinoids mediate analgesia largely via peripheral type 1 cannabinoid receptors in nociceptors, *Nat Neurosci* 10:870–879, 2007.

Ali Z: Intradermal injection of norepinephrine evokes pain in patients with sympathetically maintained pain, *Pain* 88(2):161–168, 2000.

Arbuckle B: 1977, The selected writings of Beryl Arbuckle, National Osteopathic Institute and Cerebral Palsy Foundation.

Bailey M, Dick L: Nociceptive considerations in treating with counterstrain, *J Am Osteopath Assoc* 92(3):334, 337–341, 1992.

Baldry P: *Acupuncture, trigger points and musculoskeletal pain*, Edinburgh, 1993, Churchill Livingstone.

Ballantyne F, Fryer G, McLaughlin P: The effect of muscle energy technique on hamstring extensibility: the mechanism of altered flexibility, *Journal of Osteopathic Medicine* 6(2):59–63, 2003.

Barnes M: The basic science of myofascial release, *Journal of Bodywork and Movement Therapies* 1(4):231–238, 1997a.

Barnes M, Gronlund R, Little M, et al: Efficacy study of the effect of a myofascial release treatment technique on obtaining pelvic symmetry, *Journal of Bodywork and Movement Therapies* 1(5):289–296, 1997b.

Blum CS, Esposito V, Esposito C: Orthopedic block placement and its effect on the lumbosacral spine and discs. Three case studies with pre- and post-MRIs, *Journal of Chiropractic Education* 17:48–49, 2003.

Brodin H: Lumbar treatment using the muscle energy technique, *Osteopathic Annals* 10(12):23–24, 1982.

Cassidy D, Lopes A, Yong-Hing K: The immediate effect of manipulation versus mobilization on pain and range of motion in the cervical spine: a randomized controlled trial, *J Manipulative Physiol Ther* 15:570–575, 1992.

Castlio Y: Effect of direct splenic stimulation in infectious diseases, *American Academy of Osteopathy Yearbook* 1955:121, 1955.

Chaitow L: *Beat fatigue workbook*, London, 1990, Thorsons.

Chaitow L: INIT in treatment of pain and trigger points, *British Journal of Osteopathy* XIII:17–21, 1994.

Chaitow L: *Muscle energy techniques*, ed 3, Edinburgh, 2006, Churchill Livingstone.

Chaitow L: *Positional release techniques*, ed 3, Edinburgh, 2007, Churchill Livingstone.

Chengnan S, editor: *Chinese bodywork*, Berkeley, California, 1990, Pacific View Press.

Cislo S, Ramirez M, Schwartz H: Low back pain: treatment of forward and backward sacral torsion using counterstrain technique, *J Am Osteopath Assoc* 91(3):255–259, 1991.

Clelland J, Savinar E, Shepard K: Role of physical therapist in chronic pain management. In Burrows G, Elton D, Stanley GV, editors: *Handbook of chronic pain management*, London, 1987, Elsevier, pp 243–258.

D'Ambrogio K, Roth G: *Positional release therapy*, Missouri, 1997, Mosby, St Louis.

Deig D: *Positional release technique*, Boston, 2001, Butterworth Heinemann.

Degenhardt B, Darmani N, Johnson J, et al: Role of Osteopathic Manipulative Treatment in Altering Pain Biomarkers: A Pilot Study, *J Am Osteopath Assoc* 107:387–400, 2007.

Dickey J: Postoperative osteopathic manipulative management of median sternotomy patients, *J Am Osteopath Assoc* 89(10):1309–1322, 1989.

Drover J, et al: Influence of Active Release Technique on quadriceps inhibition and strength: A pilot study, *J Manipulative Physiol Ther* 27:408–413, 2004.

Fairclough J, Hayashi J, Tounmi H, et al: The functional anatomy of the iliotibial band during flexion and extension of the knee: implications for understanding iliotibial band syndrome, *J. Anatomy* 208:309–316, 2006.

Feland J, Marin H: Effect of submaximal contraction intensity in contract-relax proprioceptive neuromuscular facilitation stretching, *Br J Sports Med* 38(4):E18, 2004.

Ferber R, Osternig LR, Gravelle DC: Effect of PNF stretch techniques on knee flexor muscle EMG activity in older adults, *J Electromyogr Kinesiol* 12:391–397, 2002.

Fernández-de-las-Peñas C, Sohrbeck-Campo M, Fernández-Carnero J, et al: Manual therapies in the myofascial trigger point treatment: a systematic review, *Journal of Bodywork and Movement Therapies* 9:27–34, 2005.

Fernández-De-Las-Peñas C, et al: The immediate effect of ischemic compression technique and transverse friction massage on tenderness of active and latent myofascial trigger points: A pilot study, *Journal of Bodywork and Movement Therapies* 10(1):3–9, 2006.

Fernández de las Peñas C, Arendt-Nielsen L, Gerwin R, editors: *Physical Therapy for tension type and cervicogenic headache: physical examination, muscle and joint management*, Boston, 2009, Jones & Bartlett.

Field T: *Touch therapy*, Edinburgh, 2000, Churchill Livingstone.

Fielder S, Pyott W: The science and art of Manipulative Surgery, *American Institute of Manipulative Surgery*, Salt Lake City, Utah, 1955.

Fielding S: *J Altern Med*, 1983.

Fredericson M, White J, MacMahon J: Quantitative Analysis of the Relative Effectiveness of 3 Iliotibial Band Stretches, *Arch Phys Med Rehabil* 83:589–592, 2002.

Fryer G: Muscle Energy Concepts – A Need for a Change, *J Osteop Med* 3(2):54–59, 2000.

Fryer G: MET: Efficacy & Research. In Chaitow L, Editor: *Muscle Energy Techniques*, ed 3, Edinburgh, 2006, Elsevier.

Fryer G, Fossum C: 2009, Therapeutic Mechanisms Underlying Muscle Energy Approaches, In: George J: The effects of Active Release Technique on hamstring flexibility: A pilot study, *J Manipulative Physiol Ther* 29:224–227, 2006.

George J: The effects of Active Release Technique on hamstring flexibility: A pilot study, *J Manipulative Physiol Ther* 29:224–227, 2006.

George J: The effects of active release technique on carpal tunnel patients: A pilot study, *Journal of Chiropractic Medicine* 5(4):119–122, 2006.

Goldberg J: Effect of two intensities of massage on H-reflex amplitude, *Phys Ther* 72(6):449–457, 1992.

Goodheart G: *Applied kinesiology workshop procedure manual*, ed 21, Detroit, 1984, Privately published.

Greenman P: *Principles of manual medicine*, ed 2, Baltimore, 1996, Williams and Wilkins.

Hamilton L, et al: The effects of high-velocity, low-amplitude manipulation and muscle energy technique on suboccipital tenderness, *International Journal of Osteopathic Medicine* 10:42e–49e, 2007.

Hoag J: *Osteopathic medicine*, New York, 1969, McGraw Hill.

Horton SJ: Acute locked thoracic spine: treatment with a modified SNAG, *Man Ther* 7(2):103–107, 2002.

Hou C-R, Tsai L-C, Show Cheng K-F: Immediate effects of various physical therapeutic modalities on cervical myofascial pain and trigger-point sensitivity, *Arch Phys Med Rehabil* 83(10):1406–1414, 2002.

Hovind H, Nielson SL: Effects of massage on blood flow in skeletal muscle, *Scand J Rehabil Med* 6:74–77, 1974.

Hruby R, Hoffman K: Avian influenza: an osteopathic component to treatment, *Osteopathic Medicine and Primary Care*, 1(10):2007.

Ikimi F, Hunt J, Hanna G, et al: Interstitial fluid plasma protein, colloid, and leukocyte uptake into initial lymphatics, *J Appl Physiol* 81(5):2060–2067, 1996.

Ironson G, et al: Relaxation through massage associated with decreased distress and increased serotonin levels, *Touch Research Institute*, Miami, 1993, University of Miami School of Medicine.

Jacobson EC, Lockwood MD, Hoefner VC, et al: Shoulder pain and repetition strain injury to the supraspinatus muscle: etiology and manipulative treatment, *J Am Osteopath Assoc* 89(8):1037–1045, 1989.

Janda V: *Muscle function testing*, London, 1990, Butterworths.

Janda V: Muscle and back pain. In *Physical Medicine Research Foundation presentation*, Vancouver, British Columbia, 1992.

Jay G: Sympathetic aspects of myofascial pain, *Pain Digest* (5):192–194, 1995.

Johnson A: *Principles and practice of drugless therapeutics*, Los Angeles, 1939, W Straube.

Johnstone W: Functional technique. In Ward R, editor: *Foundations for osteopathic medicine*, Baltimore, 1997, Williams & Wilkins.

Kamani H, Walters N: Muscle energy technique. The effect on joint mobility and agonist/antagonist muscle activity. *2nd International Conference on Advances in Osteopathic Research (ICAOR)*, London, 2000, The Law Society.

Klinge D, Magnusson S, Simonsen E, et al: The effect of strength and flexibility training on skeletal muscle electromyographic activity, stiffness, and viscoelastic stress relaxation response, *Am J Sports Med* 25(5):710–716, 1997.

Korr I: *Collected papers of I.M Korr*, Newark, OH, 1976, American Academy of Osteopathy.

Kuchera M, Kuchera W: *Considerations in systemic dysfunction*, Columbus, Ohio, 1994, Greyden Press.

Kuchera W, Kuchera M: *Osteopathic Principles in Practice*, Missouri, 1992, Kirksville College of Osteopathic Medicine.

Leahy P: Active release techniques, Hammer W Functional soft tissue examination and treatment in manual methods, ed 2, Aspen, 1999, Gaithersberg Maryland.

Lederman E: *Fundamentals of Manual Therapy*, London, 1997, Churchill.

Lenehan K, et al: The effect of muscle energy technique on gross trunk range of motion, *J Osteopath Med* 6(1):13–18, 2003.

Lewit K: *Manipulative therapy in rehabilitation of the motor system*, London, 1985, Butterworths.

Lewit K: *Manipulative therapy in rehabilitation of the locomotor system*, ed 2, London, 1992, Butterworths.

Lewit K: Role of manipulation in spinal rehabilitation. In Liebenson C, editor: *Rehabilitation of the spine*, Baltimore, 1996, Williams & Wilkins.

Lewit K: *Manipulative therapy in rehabilitation of the locomotor system*, ed 3, London, 1999, Butterworths.

Liebenson C: Manual Resistance Techniques in Rehabilitation. In Chaitow L, editor: *Muscle Energy Techniques*, Edinburgh, 2006, Churchill Livingstone.

Liebenson C: Manual resistance techniques in rehabilitation. In Chaitow L, editor: *Muscle energy technique*, ed 2, Edinburgh, 2001, Churchill Livingstone.

Lupandin L, Kuz'mina K: Interaction of thermoreceptive and vestibular signalling in regulating the activity of flexor and extensor motor nuclei during cold tremor, *Fiziol Zh SSSR Im I M Sechenova* 11(71):1433–1438, 1985.

McHugh M, Kremenic I, Fox M, Gleim G: The role of mechanical and neural restraints to joint range of motion during passive stretch, *Med Sci Sports Exerc* 30(6):928–932, 1998.

McPartland JM, Simons DG: Myofascial trigger points: translating molecular theory into manual therapy, *Journal Manual and Manipulative Therapies* 14:232–239, 2007.

McPartland J: Expression of the endocannabinoid system in fibroblasts and myofascial tissues, *Journal of Bodywork and Movement Therapies* 12:169–182, 2008.

Magnusson M, Simonsen EB, Aagaard P, et al: Contraction specific changes in passive torque in human skeletal muscle, *Acta Physiol Scand* 155(4):377–386, 1995.

Magnusson M, Aagaard P, Simonsen EB, et al: A biomechanical evaluation of cyclic and static stretch in human skeletal muscle, *Int J Sports Med* 19:310–316, 1998.

Magnusson M, Simonsen E, Aagaard P, et al: Mechanical and physiological responses to stretching with and without pre-isometric contraction in human skeletal muscle, *Archives of Physical Medicine & Rehabilitation* 77:373–377, 1996a.

Magnusson M, Simonsen E, Aagaard P, et al: A mechanism for altered flexibility in human skeletal muscle, *Journal of Physiology* 497(Part 1):293–298, 1996b.

Mehta M, Hatton P: The relationship between the duration of sub-maximal isometric contraction (MET) and improvement in the range of passive knee extension, *Journal of Osteopathic Medicine* 5(1):40, 2002.

Mennell J: *Joint pain*, Boston, 1969, Little Brown.

Mennell J: The therapeutic use of cold, *J Am Osteopath Assoc* 74(12):1146–1158, 1975.

Mitchell F Jr : *Tutorial on biomechanical procedures*, Carmel CA, 1976, Yearbook American Academy of Osteopathy.

Mitchell F Jr, Moran P, Pruzzo N: *An evaluation and treatment manual of osteopathic muscle energy procedures*, Valley Park, Illinois, 1979.

Mitchell F Jr, Mitchell PKG: *The Muscle Energy Manual*, vol 1, Michigan, 1995, MET.

Mock L: Myofascial release treatment of specific muscles of the upper extremity (levels 3 and 4), *Clinical Bulletin of Myofascial Therapy* 2(1):5–23, 1997.

Moore M, Kukulka C: Depression of Hoffman reflexes following voluntary contraction and implications for proprioceptive neuromuscular facilitation therapy, *Phys Ther* 71(4):321–329, 1991.

Morrissey D: Unloading and proprioceptive taping. In Chaitow L, editors: *Positional release techniques*, ed 2, Edinburgh, 2002, Churchill Livingstone.

Morrison M: *Lecture notes - Seminar*, London, 1969, Charing Cross Hotel.

Norris C: Functional load abdominal training (part 1), *Journal of Bodywork and Movement Therapies* 3(3):150–158, 1999.

Orchard JW, Fricker PA, Abud AT, Mason BR: Biomechanics of iliotibial band friction syndrome in runners, *Am J Sports Med* 24:375–379, 1996.

Oschman J: What is healing energy? Pt 5: gravity, structure, and emotions, *Journal of Bodywork and Movement Therapies* 1(5):307–308, 1997.

Owen C: An endocrine interpretation of Chapman's reflexes, *Academy of Applied Osteopathy*, Ohio, 1977, Newark.

Pertwee R: The therapeutic potential of drugs that target cannabinoid receptors or modulate the tissue levels or actions of endocannabinoids, *AAPS Journal* 7:E625–E654, 2005.

Polstein B: DiGiovanna E, editor: *Osteopathic approach to diagnosis and treatment*, Philadelphia, 1991, JB Lippincott.

Puustjarvi K, et al: Effects of massage in patients with chronic tension headaches, *Acupuncture and Electrotherapeutics Research* 15:159–162, 1990.

Rathbun J, MacNab I: Microvascular pattern of rotator cuff, *J Bone Joint Surg* 52:540–553, 1970.

Retzlaff EW, Bemy AH, Haight AS, et al: The piriformis muscle syndrome, *Journal of American Osteopathic Association* 73:799–807, 1974.

Rich GJ: *Massage therapy: the evidence for practice*, Edinburgh, 2002, Churchill Livingstone.

Ruddy T: *Osteopathic rhythmic resistive duction therapy*, 1961, Yearbook of Academy of Applied Osteopathy 1961, Indianapolis, p 58.

Sandler S: The physiology of soft tissue massage, *British Osteopathic Journal* 15:1–6, 1983.

Sergueef N, Nelson K, Glonek T: The effect of cranial manipulation on the Traube–Hering–Mayer oscillation as measured by laser-Doppler flowmetry, *Altern Ther Health Med* 8(6):74–76, 2002.

Schiowitz S: Facilitated positional release, *American Osteopathic Association* 90(2):145–156, 1990.

Shoemaker J, Tiidus P, Mader R: Failure of manual massage to alter limb blood flow: measures by Doppler ultrasound, *Med Sci Sports Exerc* 29(5):610–614, 1997.

Simons D, Mense S: Diagnosis and therapy of myofascial trigger points, *Shmerz* 17(6):419–424, 2003.

Simons D, Travell J, Simons L: *Myofascial pain and dysfunction: the trigger point manual*, vol 1, upper half of body. ed 2, Baltimore, 1999, Williams & Wilkins.

Sleszynski SL, Kelso AF: Comparison of thoracic manipulation and incentive spirometry in preventing postoperative atelactesis, *Journal of American Osteopathic Association* 93:834–838, 843–845, 1993.

Schmitt G, Pelham T, Holt L: From the field. A comparison of selected protocols during proprioceptive neuromuscular facilitation stretching, *Clinical Kinesiology* 53(1):16–21, 1999.

Simons D, Travell J, Simons L: ed 2, *Myofascial Pain and dysfunction: The trigger point manual*, vol 1, Baltimore, 1999, Williams & Wilkins.

Smith M, Fryer G: A comparison of two muscle energy techniques for increasing flexibility of the hamstring muscle group, *Journal of Bodywork and Movement Therapies* 12(4):312–317, 2008.

Stoddard A: *Manual of osteopathic practice*, London, 1969, Hutchinson Medical.

Te Poorten B: The piriformis muscle, *Journal of American Osteopathic Association* 69:150–160, 1969.

Taylor P, Tole G, Vernon H: Skin rolling technique as an indicator of spinal joint dysfunction, *J Can Chiropractic Assoc* 34(2):82–86, 1990.

Travell J: Ethyl chloride spray for painful muscle spasm, *Arch Phys Med Rehabil* 33:291–298, 1952.

Travell J, Simons D: *Myofascial pain and dysfunction*, vol 1, Baltimore, 1983, Williams & Wilkins.

Travell J, Simons D: *Myofascial pain and dysfunction*, vol 2, Baltimore, 1992, Williams & Wilkins.

Upledger J, Vredevoogd J: *Craniosacral therapy*, Seattle, 1983, Eastland Press.

Wallace E, McPartland J, Jones J, et al: Lymphatic manipulative techniques. In Ward R, editor: *Foundations for osteopathic medicine*, Baltimore, 1997, Williams & Wilkins.

Walther D: *Applied kinesiology*, SDC Systems, 1988, Pueblo.

Wang H-K, Shih T, Lind K-H, Wang T-G: Real-time morphologic changes of the iliotibial band during therapeutic stretching; an ultrasonographic study, *Man Ther* 13:334–340, 2008.

Washington K, Mosiello R, Venditto M, et al: Presence of Chapman reflex points in hospitalized patients with pneumonia, *Journal American Osteopathic Association* 103:479–483, 2003.

Weiselfish S: *Manual therapy for the orthopedic and neurologic patient*, Hertford, CT, 1993, Regional Physical Therapy.

Wilson E, Payton O, Donegan-Shoaf L, et al: Muscle energy technique in patients with acute low back pain: a pilot clinical trial, *Journal of Orthopaedic & Sports Physical Therapy* 33:502–512, 2003.

Wittlinger H, Wittlinger G: Textbook of Dr Vodder's manual lymph drainage, vol 1, basic course, ed 3, Heidelberg, 1982, Karl F Haug.

Wong C, Schauer-Alvarez C: Effect of strain/counterstrain on pain and strength in hip musculature. Reliability, validity and effectiveness of strain/counterstrain techniques, *Journal of Manual and Manipulative Therapy* 12(2):107–112, 2004a.

Wright P, Drysdale I: Comparison of PIR and RI muscle energy techniques applied to piriformis, *Intl Jnl Ost Med* 11:158–159, 2008.

Xujian S: Effects of massage and temperature on permeability of initial lymphatics, *Lymphology* 23:48–50, 1990.

Zhao-Pu W: *Acupressure therapy*, Edinburgh, 1991, Churchill Livingstone.

Zink G, Lawson W: An osteopathic structural examination and functional interpretation of the soma, *Osteopathic Annals* 12(7):433–440, 1979.

9

NMT in clinical use

CHAPTER CONTENTS

Contextual thinking and synchronicity   203
    Three examples of contextual thinking   204
        Evaluation before treatment   205
        A focus on trigger points   207
            Trigger points and pelvic pain   207
                Local facilitation   208
                Treatment methods   208
        Lief's approach: general vs specific 209
Speransky and Selye: common findings   210
NMT and sports injuries: Moule's methods   211
                When is NMT useful?   213
                The INIT hypothesis   216
                    INIT methods   216
                Summary and comment   217

Wherever possible, statements made in this text up to this point have carried citation references. Those statements not referenced represent the personal opinion of the author, based on 45 years of clinical experience as an osteopathic and naturopathic practitioner, in both private and National Health Service settings, in office practice, residential clinic and academic settings, in Britain, Greece and the USA.

It is therefore suggested that any 'unsubstantiated' (by citations) statements are seen as demanding personal evaluation, by the reader, before being used clinically.

Contextual thinking and synchronicity

Contextual thinking is a valuable approach when confronted by symptoms that are other than obvious (sprained ankle, whiplash injury, etc.). The tendency in clinical practice to consider symptoms in a linear manner, in which cause and effect are plotted almost mathematically, is often flawed. It is possible to learn to see the patient's symptoms in terms of the tip of an iceberg. As is obvious, the bulk of the iceberg is invisible, as are the interacting systemic, constitutional, inherited and acquired, biochemical, biomechanical and psychosocial influences operating within individual patients. And just as the iceberg is influenced by the ocean in which it floats, so the patient functions in a physical and psychological environment in which unseen and uncontrollable forces operate. Unless we take these additional factors into account, we are doomed to see symptoms as arising from simplistic backgrounds, which in the case of chronic problems is seldom the case.

Another way of expressing the idea of *context*, is to speak of synchronicity. There are linear and spatial ways of interpreting what happens in life in general, and to the body in particular. Cause and effect represent the way many people in the West understand the relationships between events (causality). One thing causes, or is caused – or is at least strongly influenced – by another.

A different way of viewing two events is to see them as being part of a complex continuum, each being part of the same (larger) process, but with neither dependent on the other, linked by a synchronistic connective principle. The words synchronicity or 'simultaneity' have been used to describe this way of viewing patterns and events. Such spatial thinking may represent the most effective way of evaluating health problems, avoiding simplistic cause and effect approaches (Jung 1973).

Three examples of contextual thinking

1. Hyperventilation and anxiety: which 'causes' which?

Hyperventilation is commonly associated with anxiety. Therefore, if we think in simple terms of cause and effect, we might assume that hyperventilation 'causes' anxiety. However, anxiety commonly leads to hyperventilation; therefore, again, if thinking simplistically, we might assume that anxiety 'causes' hyperventilation. Or, if thinking more contextually, we might observe (more accurately) that anxiety and hyperventilation not only 'feed' each other, but can be triggered and/or aggravated by – for example: low blood sugar levels (Brostoff 1992), increased progesterone levels in the post-luteal phase of the menstrual cycle (Cimino 2000), sympathetic arousal ('stress') and adrenal stimulation (Nixon & Andrews 1996), metabolic acidosis, for example in pregnancy (Slatkovska et al 2006), climatic conditions, altitude, emotional stimuli, allergic reactions (Brostoff 1992), extreme fatigue, and so on. Therefore, we might conclude that anxiety and hyperventilation are part of a continuum, involving all or any of these (and numerous

other) associated aetiological factors, interacting with the unique genetic and acquired biochemical, biomechanical and psychological individuality of the person affected. And we might reflect that treatment that takes account of the broader context is more likely to succeed than a simple, linear, 'cause and effect' assessment.

2. Possible 'usefulness' of trigger points

Clinical experience suggests that myofascial trigger points may, at times, form part of a functional system for sustaining tension, where this is required by the body – for instance in posturally compromised tissues, as *repositioners* (e.g. for the mandible due to forward head posture), or for sustaining tension across the sacroiliac joint when it is unstable, by strategically increasing hamstring tone (Vleeming et al 1997). In such a situation the body is doing exactly what it was set up to do, as changes occur leading to trigger point development. Simons et al (1999) have shown that, in the absence of adequate levels of adenosine triphosphate (ATP), and in the presence of calcium, the actin and myosin elements of muscles are designed to lock in a shortened position. Trigger points function effectively in the absence of ATP (therefore displaying an economy of resources), and are often strategically located in tissues that are straining to accommodate dysfunctional posture, or habits of use. And trigger points often clear up spontaneously when the immediate causes (and/or other stressors such as dietary imbalance, breathing dysfunction, dehydration, etc.) are corrected (Chaitow & DeLany 2002).

Trigger points also appear to demonstrate a built-in, silent (latent) and non-silent (active) alarm mechanism, when the structures with which they are associated are being abused. Therefore, to release trigger points without regard to correcting the underlying causes (the abuse), to which they are responding, may result in a less than ideal outcome, not least of which could be a rapid, or chronic, return of the trigger point activity. Rather than always being seen as dysfunctional entities, trigger points might be considered as low-energy-consuming contractile devices, established by the absence of available

ATP, to maintain a structural or localized tensional element, for immediate or long-term adaptation/compensation purposes, until no longer required. Additionally they may be seen as alarm signals when tissues are being overloaded and abused. In this way of thinking, it is the individual's posture, patterns of daily use, or lifestyle, that are dysfunctional, not the tissues housing the trigger point, which may be doing exactly what they were designed to do. When this is true – *and when we can recognize that it is* – it is the context from which trigger points emerge that requires attention, not the trigger points.

Of course there are times – arguably in the majority of cases – when trigger points remain active well past their possible usefulness as stabilizing agents, or when they exist as historical remnants of previous overuse or trauma. In such instances they are nuisances, and may be disturbing normal function, and so require appropriate deactivation. Even when trigger points are potentially useful as stabilizers but are nevertheless causing pain, if more appropriate stabilization can be achieved, via (say) improved core stability, then deactivation – manually or by other means – would be seen to be appropriate.

3. Assessment of sacroiliac dysfunction

Lee (2002) reports that Hungerford & Gilleard (1998) have shown that normal individuals, performing a one-legged, standing, hip flexion ('stork') test, vary their motor control strategy *each time they perform the test*, implying that different muscles can be used to perform the same osteokinematic motion. This will vary the amount of compression each time they lift the leg, and thus vary the range of motion. Lee (2002) has written:

> *Unless trials are repeated and motions averaged, reliability is impossible – not because the tester can't feel what's happening, but because the subject keeps changing from moment to moment . . . Unless the specific muscle activation pattern is noted during whatever range of motion test (active or passive) is being evaluated for reliability – there is no way of knowing what amount of compression the SIJ is under (at that moment) and therefore what the available range of motion should be.*

As if this is not enough to create hesitation as to the validity of such tests, a range of other possible influences has been noted. For example, what if:

- the patient's head was slightly turned toward the side being tested, causing increased tension in the hip extensors (i.e. hamstrings) (Murphy 2000)?
- the patient's eyes were turned one way or the other, or were looking slightly up or down, changing markedly the tone in hip flexors, extensors and rotators (Janda 1988, Lewit 1999)?
- the patient's suboccipital muscles had recently been stretched, altering tone in the extensors of the leg (Pollard & Ward 1997)?
- the patient was anxious, hyperventilating (Garland 1994), suffering an allergic reaction (Randolph 1976), or had fallen arches (Myers 2001)?

There are multiple influences, only some of which can be controlled, during tests of this sort, suggesting that clinical reasoning as to what single tests 'mean' is essential. A single test result cannot define dysfunction, offering at best a shadowy indication, and becoming more relevant only when other assessment findings, and the patient's symptom picture and history are added. Assessment is therefore a spatial exercise, not a linear one, seeking synchronous pieces of evidence that, together, lead to a working hypothesis as to what is happening – and what to do.

Conclusion

Hopefully these three examples, hyperventilation, trigger points and sacroiliac joint assessment, offer sufficient evidence to point towards a need to think contextually, to look for synchronicity, and to be cautious regarding linear thinking, especially when dealing with the complexity of the human body.

Evaluation before treatment

If therapeutic intervention is to be structured and organized, and something other than hit-and-miss, there is an absolute requirement for sound evaluation and assessment as to the causes, extent and possible influences on other areas and tissues, of patterns of pain and restriction, such as myofascial trigger points, locally traumatized areas, shortened and/or weakened muscles, joint restrictions and/or general/systemic factors (such as exist in arthritic conditions).

As discussed above, the contexts in which symptoms exist, and out of which they emerge, are of profound importance in arriving at a stage where a programme of intervention and therapeutic modification can be formulated.

NMT provides one such diagnostic/assessment tool and also offers, by switching from its assessment to its actively therapeutic mode, a means whereby precisely focused and modulated degrees of force can be directed towards influencing restricted tissues, directly or reflexively. Myofascial release techniques, as well as ischaemic compression (osteopathic inhibitory technique), can be applied to precise targets via the contacting thumb or finger in NMT.

Perhaps NMT's greatest usefulness in assessment relates to the opportunity it offers for the identification of local soft tissue dysfunction in a gentle, non-invasive manner.

In the USA, as well as in the UK, the focus of many therapists using NMT is primarily on myofascial trigger points (and the often widespread musculoskeletal and other dysfunctional patterns that produce them). To use NMT to its full advantage, it is useful to have a clear understanding of the process of facilitation that can occur paraspinally, or locally, in muscle and fascia (trigger points), as described in detail in Chapter 3.

By learning how to use NMT diagnostically and therapeutically, a good deal of information can be obtained regarding the patterns of dysfunction that are operating.

It is important to stress, once more, that NMT may be used in both a diagnostic mode and a therapeutic mode, and that to some extent these overlap, and may be carried out simultaneously. Having identified the structures and tissues that require greater attention, NMT is available as a tool with which to make contact and give direct localized treatment to areas that are contracted or tightened (Fernandez de las Penas et al 2005).

Specific associated and complementary techniques exist to deal with reflex activity, as is noted in trigger points (Fryer & Hodgson 2005). Muscle energy technique methods, as described by Lewit (1999), and elaborations on these derived from a variety of sources, provide a further array of techniques that can be brought into operation, depending on the particular indications. Many of these associated techniques were described in Chapter 8.

What about joints?

(Chaitow 1983, 1991a,b, Jones 1981, Mitchell et al 1979)

Soft tissue manipulation, which includes positional release methods ('strain/counterstrain'), NMT and MET, is capable of normalizing a great many joint problems, without recourse to active manipulative effort (Schenk 1994, Wilson et al 2003, Speicher et al 2004). MET and NMT are symbiotic, and it is possible to achieve more by combining their repertoire of useful techniques than either can achieve individually. By adding the knowledge of suitable techniques by which to influence reflex activity, demonstrated by the presence of localized areas of soft tissue dysfunction (trigger points, Chapman's points, localized fibrosis, etc.), as well as by using the tender points described by Jones, in gentle functional techniques, the scope of soft tissue manipulation methods should become apparent.

Employment of these approaches does not necessarily preclude the need for active joint mobilization and/or manipulation, in correcting restriction, but can make for a lesser need to use high-velocity thrusts, or long lever techniques, while making such manipulation simpler and far less likely to traumatize the local tissues, or the patient. By combining MET and NMT, some degree of the potential problem of avoiding tissue damage is likely to be solved. NMT, applied to a region containing fibrotic change, will allow for subsequent use of 'normal' MET, or of an isolytic contraction, with less discomfort or likelihood of microtrauma (see Ch. 8).

Are some musculoskeletal problems best left untreated?

The enormous privilege that the patient allows in permitting the practitioner to make physical contact also grants a degree of 'power' to the practitioner. Defences are lowered, and the patient is likely to be amenable to discussing areas of their emotions and thoughts, that they might resist in other situations. This presents opportunities for therapeutic intervention on levels other than the physical. The practitioner should be aware of the opportunity to exploit the potent 'placebo' effect that such situations allow. Suggestions, and positive guidance, can have powerful influences on the patient, and so care should be exercised, and diligent application of therapeutic techniques undertaken, knowing that the recipient is commonly receptive and highly suggestible (Pollo & Benedetti 2008).

When considering treatment of soft tissue changes that relate to an emotional or psychogenic background, it is important to realize the need for an adequate ability on the part of the practitioner/therapist to handle any emotional repercussions resulting from 'releasing' (or attempting to release) the soft tissue manifestations of emotional turmoil, as well as there being a need to have an adequate referral system in place to support the patient in times of crisis (Field et al 2005, Loga 2008).

If the patient is not capable of processing whatever emotional baggage is attached to a particular pattern of soft tissue dysfunction, then it is probably best left intact, until the patient is ready and equipped to process the issues that are submerged in the soma (Mancuso et al 2004).

A scenario is conceivable in which a patient with obvious musculoskeletal dysfunction, but without obvious mento-emotional problems, could be left in a fragile and vulnerable state following apparently appropriate bodywork. The oft-quoted phenomenon of 'emotional release', which may occur during or following treatment, is something therapists could usefully reflect upon and possibly re-evaluate. Just how beneficial – or how dangerous – is such a reaction without further support, such as counselling or psychotherapy?

Additionally, there are times when apparently purely physical symptoms, such as active trigger points in a tight hamstring, as in the example given earlier in this chapter, may best be left untreated until underlying, contextual, causes have been evaluated and dealt with.

A focus on trigger points

Travell & Simons (1983) have demonstrated the clear connection between myofascial trigger point activity and a wide range of pain problems and sympathetic nervous system aberrations. Wall & Melzack confirm that there are few chronic pain problems that do not have myofascial trigger point activity as a component, with these acting, in many instances, as prime maintaining factors of the pain (Melzack & Wall 1988, Wall & Melzack 1989, Fernandez de las Penas et al 2007).

Active trigger points (and other non-referring pain points), commonly lie in muscles that have been stressed in a variety of ways, including postural imbalances (Barlow 1959, Goldthwaite 1949, Simons et al 1999), congenital factors such as warping of fascia via cranial distortions (Upledger 1983), short leg problems, small hemipelvis (Travell & Simons 1992), occupational or leisure overuse patterns (Rolf 1977), emotional states affecting soft tissues (Latey 1986), referred/reflex involvement of the viscera producing facilitated segments paraspinally (Beal 1983, Korr 1977), and trauma.

The repercussions of trigger point activity go far beyond simple musculoskeletal pain, however distressing that may be. Take, for example, the involvement of trigger points in cases of hyperventilation, chronic fatigue and apparent pelvic inflammatory disease. Trigger point activity is particularly prevalent in the muscles of the neck/shoulder region, which also act as accessory breathing muscles (scalenes, upper trapezius, etc.). In situations of increased anxiety the incidence of borderline or frank hyperventilation is frequent (Bass & Gardner 1985) and may be associated with chronic fatigue (Nixon & Andrews 1996). Clinically these muscles palpate as tense, and often fibrotic, with active trigger points being common (Garland 1994, Roll & Theorell 1987). Successful breathing retraining and normalization of diminished energy levels, seem to be accelerated and enhanced, following initial normalization of the functional integrity of the involved muscles (Chaitow et al 2002).

Trigger points and pelvic pain

Slocumb (1984) demonstrated that, in a large proportion of chronic pelvic pain problems in women, destined for surgical intervention, the prime cause of pain involves trigger point activity in muscles of the lower abdomen, perineum, inner thigh and even on the walls of the vagina:

The search for common pathological processes, such as endometriosis, active inflammation, or pelvic adhesions is a major objective in assessing the patient with chronic pelvic pain. However, the frustration of finding normal pelvic structures too often results in the conviction that psychogenic causes might account for the pain. What is probably the most alarming aspect of the inadequacy of gynecologic management of chronic pelvic pain is the frequent recourse, by physicians, to operative exploration and removal of pelvic structures for normal physiologic variations ... As a result of concentrating patients with pelvic pain in a single clinic I have identified a neurological syndrome that can be shown to account for the majority of those patients with chronic abdominal pain ... Several unusual and unexplained phenomena were repeatedly observed. First, the same pain sensation was reproduced by pressure over localized points in several different tissues seemingly anatomically unrelated. These hyperpathic points are consistent with the term trigger points described by Travell and Simons and appear to cause referred pain symptoms as well as sharp pain.

Slocumb describes how the following areas can all produce the *identical* referred pelvic pain:

1. Pinching the skin over the lower abdominal wall
2. Single-finger pressure in one abdominal wall location
3. Single-finger pressure on tissue overlying the pubic bone
4. Lateral pressure with single finger over one or both levator muscles
5. Single-finger or cotton-tip applicator pressure lateral to the cervix
6. Single-finger or cotton-tip applicator pressure over vaginal cuff scar tissue more than 3 months after hysterectomy
7. Single-finger pressure over the dorsal sacrum.

Slocumb demonstrated, in one research study involving 130 patients, that he was able to remove chronic pelvic pain in nearly 90% of cases by deactivating such triggers.

The significance of this and other studies is that trigger points are the cause of serious levels of suffering (see Box 7.1 for evidence relating to trigger point influence on the painful symptoms associated with interstitial cystitis and urgency), and that we need to have an array of tools with which to deal with their activities (Weiss 2001). Further discussion on this topic is to be found in Chapter 7, under the sub-heading 'NMT and chronic pelvic pain dysfunction'.

Local facilitation

According to Korr (1977), a trigger point is a localized area of somatic dysfunction that behaves in a facilitated manner, i.e. it will amplify and be affected by any form of stress imposed on the individual whether this is physical, chemical or emotional. A trigger point is palpable as an indurated, localized, painful entity with a reference (target) area to which pain or other symptoms are referred (Chaitow 1991a).

Muscles housing trigger points can frequently be identified as being unable to achieve their normal resting length, using standard muscle evaluation procedures (Janda 1983). The trigger point itself commonly lies in fibrotic tissue, which has evolved as a result of exposure of the tissues to diverse forms of stress.

Treatment methods

A wide variety of methods have been advocated for treating trigger points, including inhibitory (ischaemic compression) pressure methods (Lief 1989, Nimmo 1966), acupuncture and/or ultrasound (Kleyhans & Aarons 1974), dry needling (Gerwin & Dommerholt 2002), microcurrent (McMakin 2003), chilling and stretching of the muscle in which the trigger lies (Simons et al 1999), procaine or xylocaine injections (Slocumb 1984), active or passive stretching (Lewit 1992) and even surgical excision (Dittrich 1954).

Clinical experience, confirmed by the diligent research of Travell & Simons (1992), has shown that, while all or any of these methods can successfully inhibit trigger point activity in the short term, more is often needed to eliminate the noxious activity of the structure completely.

Common sense, as well as clinical experience, dictates that the next stage of correction of such problems should involve re-education (postural, breathing, relaxation, etc.) or the elimination of factors that contributed to the problem's evolution. This might well involve ergonomic evaluation of home and workplace, as well as the re-education and rehabilitation methods mentioned above.

Travell & Simons (1992) have also shown that, whatever initial treatment is offered to inhibit the neurological overactivity of the trigger point, the muscle in which it lies has to be made capable of reaching its normal resting length, following such treatment, if the trigger point is to be prevented from rapid reactivation.

In treating trigger points, the method of chilling the offending muscle (housing the trigger) while holding it at stretch in order to achieve this end was advocated by Travell & Simons (1992), whereas Lewit (1999) has espoused the muscle energy method of a physiologically induced post-isometric relaxation (or reciprocal inhibition) response, before passive stretching. Both methods are commonly successful, although a sufficient degree of failure occurs (trigger points may rapidly reactivate, or fail to 'switch off' completely) to require investigation of more successful approaches.

One reason for failure may relate to the possibility that the tissues that are being stretched are not the very fibres surrounding the trigger point.

A popular method for achieving tonus release in a muscle, prior to stretching, involves the use of muscle energy techniques, the introduction of an isometric contraction to the affected muscle prior to stretching. See discussion of MET in Chapter 8 (Chaitow 1991b, 2006).

The original use of isometric contractions before stretching was in proprioceptive neuromuscular facilitation (PNF) techniques, which emerged from physical medicine in the early part of the 20th century. In most forms of MET methodology, a partial (not full-strength) isometric contraction is performed before the stretch, in order to preclude tissue damage or stress to the patient and/or therapist, which PNF quite frequently produces (Greenman 1989, Hartman 1985, Fryer & Fossum 2009).

An integrated combination of methods designed to deactivate trigger points effectively, known as integrated neuromuscular inhibition, will be described later in this chapter.

Lief's approach: general vs specific

Stanley Lief, the prime developer of NMT, employed few specific manipulative techniques. His main concern was to attempt to normalize mobility and function (circulation, drainage, nerve function, etc.) and, to this end, his neuromuscular treatment was often accompanied by no more than general mobilization of the cervical and lumbar areas, together with a degree of 'springing' or stretching of the dorsal region. Peter Lief ND DC, son of the primary developer of NMT Stanley Lief, noted: 'NMT is a type of specific soft tissue treatment which is followed [or accompanied] by a general mobilising articular manipulation' (Lief 1963).

Criticism of this approach, by 'specific' manipulators, should be softened by the fact that this general, 'constitutional' treatment approach (some would call it 'engine wiping') achieved phenomenal results in terms of improvements in general well-being, and the alleviation of many specific dysfunctional restrictions.

Brian Youngs ND DO, a colleague of both Stanley and Peter Lief, who is – at the time of writing this in 2009 – still in practice in London in his nineties, has written, regarding Lief's approach, as follows (Youngs 2008):

Usually accompanying this physical approach (NMT) would be recommendations for dietary changes, exercise, breathing re-education, relaxation and short fasting episodes, as appropriate to the individual's needs. In this way long-term benefit, deriving from the NMT procedures, would be supported and modified by responses resulting from the accompanying nutritional and lifestyle changes.

This approach represented a package of nonspecific interventions, designed to impact on total health – a veritable personalized holistic recipe! The physiological effects of the NMT procedures were, in many ways, akin to those resulting from exercise, setting in train improved physiological function (Youngs 1963).

There was an increase of general mobility; head on neck, on shoulders; increased flexion/ extension of spinal movements; increased lung capacity – all of which would continue to improve if accompanying exercise advice was adhered to.

Undoubtedly there exist specific spinal and joint problems that demand individual corrective approaches; however, the improvement of the supporting mechanisms (muscles, fascia, ligaments, tendons) via NMT, on its own, or together with general mobilization techniques, offered by soft tissue manipulation, is able frequently to avoid the need for any more specific technique.

Indeed, it is strongly suggested that the 'adjustment' of joints, that ignores the soft tissue component, is far more likely to fail (in the sense of symptoms speedily returning), than the Lief method.

Speransky and Selye: common findings

(Selye 1984, Speransky 1943)

Early 20th century researcher A.D. Speransky (1887–1961) has offered many pertinent concepts that relate directly to therapeutic approaches including all methods of physical treatment. As a result of decades of research into the functioning of the nervous system in relation to health and disease, he observed that: 'Hence we obtain the rule that only weak degrees of irritation can have a useful significance; strong ones inevitably do damage' (Speransky 1943).

These words should be locked in the minds of all therapists, of whatever school. The term '*irritation*' is used by Speransky, and this is of interest, as a little thought will indicate that whatever is being done to a patient, in terms of therapy, involves to a greater or lesser extent an element of stress (or *irritation*) – stress, in this sense, being defined as any stimulus, pleasant or unpleasant, that calls upon the body to respond, or adapt, in some manner.

Manipulation, acupuncture, pressure techniques, use of heat and cold, hydrotherapy, electrical and mechanical therapies, surgery, and indeed the whole gamut of medications, whether they be drugs or homeopathic dilutions of herbal substances, all call for a response on the part of the body. All are, therefore, to a degree, 'stress' factors. Speransky insists that only mild irritants can have a useful role to play in evoking a positive (i.e. healing) response.

Selye shows stress can be helpful

Hans Selye (1976) has come to precisely the same conclusion in his important research into stress. In experiments carried out in his extensive studies, Selye produced subcutaneous blisters in experimental animals by injecting a given volume of air under the skin. This was followed by the insertion of an irritant of some sort. He first demonstrated that the amount of exudate, and the thickness of the sac wall, varied, as one might anticipate, with the strength and concentration of the irritant substance inserted. He followed this by introducing a form of 'secondary' stress, such as intense cold, or heat or forced immobilization.

The response of the animals varied greatly.

* In those that had been injected initially with a weak irritant, the stress that was then added seemed to aid the recovery, as evidenced by resolution of the irritated area and inhibition of tissue fibrosis.
* Those animals, however, that had had strong irritants injected into the subcutaneous sacs, responded to the subsequent stress factor by showing an increase in inflammation, widespread necrosis, and often death.
* Selye concluded with these words: 'This was the crucial experiment, showing that stress can either cure or aggravate a disease, depending upon whether the inflammatory response to a local irritant is necessary or superfluous.'

We now have Speransky's and Selye's combined evidence, suggesting that what we do to a patient therapeutically can be beneficial or harmful, and that this to a great extent will depend upon the *degree of the irritation* involved in the treatment, whatever form it takes.

Speransky's work further teaches us that Mann's words are true (see Chapter 4): any part of the surface of the body can be an initiator of a process involving neurological changes, which can be pathological or therapeutic.

The classification of certain points as being trigger points, others as being acupuncture alarm points, and yet others as being neurolymphatic or neurovascular – or any other – points, is merely a matter of convenience. It helps us to make a degree of sense out of the enormous amount of information available to us. It should be obvious that, to a large extent, these points may be interchangeable, for many are patently found in precisely the same position, on different 'maps' of points.

Bearing in mind that the distinction between the variously classified points, as discussed in this book, is manmade, we will continue to classify them in these ways as a matter of convenience. It should also be borne in mind that, whenever acupuncture points are mentioned, the availability of these for manual treatment (pressure, chilling, heating, etc.) remains. There is some evidence that needling can achieve particular effects, not available to pressure techniques, but this is equivocal and, for the purposes of soft tissue manipulation, pressure can usually be shown to be as effective as needling, with the one major drawback, that only a limited number of points can be contacted by hand at any one time, compared with the multiple needling that is possible in acupuncture.

Soft tissue adaptation

Selye has described the progression of changes in tissues that are being locally stressed. There is an initial alarm (acute inflammatory) stage, followed by a stage of adaptation or resistance when stress factors are continuous or repetitive, at which time muscular tissue may become progressively fibrotic. If such changes are taking place in muscle that has a postural rather than a phasic function, the muscle will shorten (Janda 1985, Selye 1984).

Such fibrotic tissue, lying in altered (shortened) muscles, cannot simply 'release', in order to allow the muscle to achieve its normal resting length, a prerequisite of normalization of trigger point activity (Simons et al 1999).

Along with various forms of stretching (passive, active, MET, PNF, etc.) inhibitory pressure methods are commonly employed in treatment of trigger points. Such pressure technique methods, together with myofascial release and cross-fibre friction, can focus on normalization of indurated, fibrosed soft tissues, as part of neuromuscular therapy methodology (Chaitow 1991b).

Lewit's 'functional pathology' view

We are in the midst of a change in the concepts of manipulative therapy that have far-reaching implications. One of the major changes is the restoration of the soft tissue component to centre-stage, rather than the peripheral role to which it has been assigned in the past.

Lewit (1985) discusses aspects of this. He describes the 'no man's land' that lies between neurology, orthopaedics and rheumatology, that, he says, is the home of the vast majority of patients with pain derived from the locomotor system, and in whom no definite pathomorphological changes are found.

He makes the suggestion that these be termed cases of 'functional pathology of the locomotor system'. These include most of the patients attending osteopathic, chiropractic and physiotherapy practitioners.

The most frequent symptom of individuals involved in this area of dysfunction is pain, that may be derived from reflex changes involving muscle spasm, myofascial trigger points, hyperalgesic skin zones, periosteal pain points, or a wide variety of other sensitive areas that have no obvious pathological origin. It is a major part of the role of NMT to help in both identifying such areas, and to then offer means for normalizing many of the causative aspects of these myriad and mysterious sources of pain and disability.

NMT and sports injuries: Moule's methods

One practitioner who has achieved outstanding success in applying NMT to athletic injuries of marked severity is osteopath Terry Moule ND DO, son of Tom Moule ND DO, a one-time associate and assistant to Stanley Lief. In the 1970s Terry Moule restored the former captain of England's soccer team, Gerry Francis, to playing fitness. Surgery to the lumbar spine was the only prospect left for Francis after months of agony under orthopaedic investigation. In desperation, Moule was consulted and within a few weeks Francis was playing again. He remained fit for many years before becoming a professional soccer team manager.

A similar return to full function was achieved in the case of the then captain of England's rugby football team, Roger Uttley, whose career appeared to be over following a back injury. Treatment, consisting largely of NMT, resulted in Uttley returning to the England squad in its successful 1980 season.

An even more startling result of the application of NMT to a spinal injury involved then world mile and 1500-metre record-holder, Sebastian Coe (now Lord Coe, leading member of Britain's Olympic Committee). Coe stated in late 1979: 'Last winter I had a back problem. I was having trouble getting a diagnosis, let alone treatment.' Within a few treatments, incorporating NMT, he was running again and setting world record times.

Moule has described NMT as follows (personal communication, 2002):

The principle of NMT is that it is of prime importance to treat connective tissue lesions and abnormalities, prior to any manipulative treatment of the bony structures. If more ortho-dox and less penetrating soft tissue techniques are used, whilst the bony abnormality may be corrected by the application of a specific adjustment, because the soft tissues remain in a similar state to that existing prior to the manip-ulation, there is a strong likelihood of a recur-rence of the lesion. NMT tends to dispense with specific adjustment, for, subsequent to using these specialised soft tissue measures, a general-ised mobilisation adjustment will allow the muscular and connective tissues to encourage the bony structures to return to their normal alignment. This may take a little longer to pro-duce relief from discomfort, but in the long run it means that the correction is more permanent and there is less danger of any damage to the muscular and connective tissues from forceful manipulation.

The great advantage of NMT is that it may be applied to any part of the body. It is particularly effective in dealing with problems related to interference with nerve supply; to any form of muscular or connective tissue lesion; to treat-ment of the abdominal and pelvic organs etc. It is applied mainly by use of the thumb. It may take some years to develop an adequate 'feel' in the hands in general and the thumbs in particu-lar, to effectively diagnose and treat lesions. It is the ability to diagnose through the thumb which is so helpful in the rapid and efficient treatment of all forms of dysfunction. Correctly used it precludes a large number of more conven-tional techniques and saves a considerable amount of time.

NMT has proved invaluable in the treatment of sports injuries, particularly for the diagnostic reasons outlined above and for the fact that it produces a rapid response as compared to ortho-dox soft tissue and physiotherapy techniques. With sports injuries one of the major problems is to get the player back in action as soon as pos-sible, particularly where the injury is to a profes-sional sportsman. NMT has been used very effectively on a large number of sportsmen and women following all types of sports.

One of the most common injuries one encoun-ters is hamstring problems. These are particu-larly prevalent amongst footballers, who in many cases develop the injury through overde-velopment of the quadriceps without adequate attention to the maintenance and mobility (i.e. lengthening and stretching) of the hamstrings at the same time. The normal treatment of ham-string injuries is ultra-sonic and massage. These techniques are not particularly rapid and the resultant loss of overall muscle tone, due to the inability of the leg to be used normally, retards a return to normal function. With NMT a lesion can be accurately and rapidly detected and, by the use of deep thumb manipulation, the soft tis-sue lesion can be dealt with rapidly and effec-tively. Where there is muscular fibre damage this can be felt and literally ironed out. The effect of the technique is to stimulate circulation in the area thus encouraging healing. Where there is inflammation and swelling the technique pro-motes drainage and the restoration of normal tone. With acute lesions the technique is unfortunately painful, but where speed is the prime order in recovery this is a small price to pay.

NMT is also beneficial in the treatment of knee lesions, particularly ligamentous problems and the subsequent inflammation in the joint itself. Correct application of NMT to these lesions will improve drainage from the knee and encourages healing to take place far more rapidly than through orthodox techniques. Where there is knee misalignment or dislocation, reduction of spasm is most important as a prerequisite to satisfactory manipulation of the joint. In many cases injury occurs when the legs become anchored due to studs in the boots. If rotation of the trunk is superimposed onto this static lower limb situation the stress imposed on the knee joint is enormous. The application of NMT prior to attempting correction not only makes the correction less painful but ensures that the result is lasting.

NMT is also beneficial in the treatment of pre-patellar bursitis, and any synovial inflammatory problems.

A problem which plagues many sportsmen, particularly footballers, basketball players and volleyball players, is pain in the groin and down the inside of the leg. This is commonly treated as a sacroiliac or a lumbar problem when, in many cases, it is due to a lesion of the symphysis-pubis. There are a number of techniques for dealing with problems of this joint but none so dramatically successful as the application of NMT.

The technique's effectiveness in producing long-term benefits is perhaps best underlined by the results with sportsmen such as Roger Uttley and Gerry Francis, who had both received short-term benefit from manipulative treatment. The application of NMT, without any change in the manipulative techniques being employed, except to make them less specific, produced long-term improvement which allowed a return to active participation in their respective sports. In both cases the main problem was an imbalance in muscle tone with excessive tension causing persistence of the joint dysfunction. The removal of these soft tissue factors restored balance and encouraged the body to return to normal function, as it always tries to do.

In summary, the benefits of NMT in general are

(1) It is a technique which removes causes rather than dealing with symptoms.
(2) It removes the necessity for the bulk of specific manipulation, instead it encourages the body to normalise itself.
(3) It is applicable to any part of the body.

From the specific sports injury point of view the main advantage of NMT is that it provides (a) a more rapid recovery rate and (b) a more permanent one.

The author's own experience confirms the validity of Terry Moule's comments.

NMT, apart from all the myriad applications discussed in earlier chapters, is the finest soft tissue system for helping to normalize acute and chronic injuries. The successful use of NMT calls for the *applied thought* of the practitioner. The body usually responds rapidly to the help this technique offers. Its limitations are almost always related to the limitations of the practitioner. Its success is in direct proportion to the dedication and intelligence with which it is applied.

When is NMT useful?

NMT may be universally applied to any patient of any age suffering from any condition. This is not to say that it will be curative, or even of marked value, in all conditions, however, it will be of some diagnostic and therapeutic value in every condition, and of enormous value in others, because no one is free from some degree of dysfunction, affecting the overall efficiency and economy of the body.

In general terms, NMT may be applied to all cases of musculoskeletal dysfunction and mento-emotional dysfunction with benefit. The basic spinal and basic abdominal techniques are used as diagnostic and therapeutic tools in the majority of cases. The more specific techniques, such as psoas, piriformis, tensor fascia lata and abdominal release techniques, are used as and when indicated. A general, full-body NMT treatment may be applied as part of a programme of postural reintegration, or breathing rehabilitation.

In specific terms, NMT is applied as follows:

- All conditions of the spine and conditions that involve the arms or legs would receive general spinal technique as well as consideration of local areas, in the limbs affected.
- Such treatments would be repeated once or twice weekly until a degree of normality had been achieved.
- Other complementary modalities and techniques would and should be used if called for. NMT combines with anything of a supportive nature that is aimed at the restoration of normal function, such as (in appropriate conditions) ultrasound therapy, diathermy, manipulation, etc.
- At the outset, the aim of general treatment is to remove the more obvious areas of contraction and stasis.
- All active trigger points should be neutralized by pressure techniques (see INIT in this chapter), if possible and if appropriate.
- If found stubborn, trigger points can also be treated by chill-and-stretch, MET or infiltration methods.
- As therapy progresses, individual patterns of dysfunction will become clearer, and NMT may need to be applied to spinal, abdominal, intercostal and pelvic areas that are slow to improve.
- Manipulative techniques, of a non-specific type (i.e. mobilization/articulation) are often useful in the normalization of spinal integrity, once the initial soft tissue rigidity or dysfunction has been improved.
- NMT can be applied with infinite gentleness or with robust enthusiasm, as it is possible to use the same techniques, with a marked difference in the degree of force employed. This enables its application to areas of acute sensitivity as well as in fragile (e.g. osteoporotic) and tender areas. As long as the practitioner is thinking about the task in hand and not applying the techniques in a mechanical, repetitive manner, there is no danger of injury or harm.
- If treatment is aimed at the removal of symptoms stemming from trigger points, it is essential to normalize all the structures related to the local area of dysfunction. Simply to neutralize the trigger that is causing, say, a headache will produce short-term benefits. If the particular trigger lies in the trapezius muscle, then not only must the trigger be normalized, and the trapezius muscle treated, but the entire cervical and spinal musculature and soft tissues should receive attention, as should the patterns of posture and use that provoked the tissues to the state where headaches became a natural consequence.
- *A general rule should be that no part of the whole should be considered without the whole also being considered.* Thus, even if the spinal areas are receiving the main attention of the therapist on any one visit, the muscles of the lower limb and associated structures should be given some consideration to assess their involvement and possible requirements. The treatment of the back, therefore, calls for the treatment of the front, and this calls for the whole to be considered and treated. The condition in the context of the body, and the body in the context of its (total) environment, are the appropriate areas of investigation and care.
- General abdominal technique is useful in all cases of digestive and intestinal dysfunction of a non-pathological nature. NMT is applicable to all cases of respiratory dysfunction. It is also applicable to all genitourinary conditions of a non-pathological nature. NMT applied to the abdomen will reduce many tension states emerging out of mento-emotional backgrounds.
- General abdominal technique improves circulatory efficiency through the pelvis and abdominal regions, and it enhances respiratory function. The reflex points and zones in the spinal area should always be treated prior to thoracic and abdominal technique, as indicated. In a case of spastic constipation, for example, NMT to the lower spinal areas and the use of neurolymphatic points followed by general abdominal technique would be the pattern recommended. This could be followed by specific abdominal release techniques if areas of marked contractions or 'adhesion' were

elicited during the general treatment. In the author's experience, such an approach, combined with general health measures such as nutritional reform, together with appropriate exercise and relaxation programmes, will promote a return to normal. If the body is being given those factors required for normality, its self-healing tendency (homeostasis), which is constantly acting, will respond positively to the removal of obstacles to recovery (structural, mechanical, dietary).

- In dealing with tension and stress of psychic origin, it is as well to recall that the mind will not be calm or relaxed as long as neuromuscular tensions are present. In applying any form of psychotherapy, the use of NMT, applied to the spine and abdomen, will increasingly improve the patient's ability to relax. NMT is not seen as an end in itself in this regard, but to be a catalyst to the removal or easing of the physical component of a vicious circle. In some cases this physical release of tension, especially when applied to the solar plexus, can produce a sudden emotional release in which the patient may cry and sob. The body becomes a solid mass of tensions and contractions for many individuals, with the tensions of life mirrored by layers of muscular 'armour'. The posture and tensions thus created all carry specific emotional charges and memories and, as the physical components are eased, so the emotional memories and feelings associated with their origins come to the surface. Just how appropriate it is to initiate such 'releases' was discussed earlier in this chapter.

- In restoring total structural and postural integrity to the body, it is necessary to apply NMT to all the supporting structures. This might involve the spinal, thoracic and abdominal soft tissues and the limbs, including the feet. NMT and manipulation, where appropriate, will lay the foundations for a return to normal (or to the patient's individual optimal norm).

- Specific and general exercise, as well as postural re-education, may then follow. It is possible, via such systems as the Alexander technique, to achieve postural and functional normality. With the careful use of NMT and, if necessary, osseous manipulation, such re-education becomes much easier and less arduous. *It must be easier to learn to use a machine correctly if that machine is capable of functioning correctly!*

- The same applies to breathing retraining. Unless the thoracic and diaphragmatic structures are to some extent made pliable by therapeutic interventions, such as those detailed in earlier chapters, such retraining will of necessity involve struggling against great odds.

- In attempting to achieve postural and functional normality, a fairly long-term view is required. Some practitioners suggest that a series of eight to ten treatment sessions will produce this result. It is the author's experience that, while the basic groundwork can be done in eight to ten treatments, some chronic cases require weekly or fortnightly treatment for up to a year if they are to achieve optimal improvement. This should be followed by maintenance visits at intervals of not less than 3 months.

- And just as retraining (posture, breathing) without appropriate bodywork is doomed to partial success at best, so bodywork methods that ignore retraining and re-education will have only short-term benefits, since much of any chronic dysfunctional pattern of use will be firmly locked into habitual neural and behavioural patterns.

- *Structural and functional changes are interdependent: they follow each other causally as well as therapeutically.*

- NMT is universally applicable. It has no side-effects, and combines with all other methods of positive health care. In itself it is capable of improving general function, releasing tension and removing noxious triggers, which may be responsible for myriad symptoms.

NMT has limits, but within the framework of its own area of application its only limits lie in the ability of the practitioner.

The INIT hypothesis

(Chaitow 1994)

When treating myofascial pain, experience suggests that a light isometric contraction, as used in MET procedures, may not activate the particular fibres surrounding the trigger point being treated. Subsequent stretching of the muscle may then not involve critical tissues surrounding and enveloping the myofascial trigger point.

Failure actively to lengthen the muscle fibres in which the trigger is housed may account for the not infrequent recurrence of trigger point activity, in the same site, following treatment. Repetition of the stress factors that produced the active trigger point, in the first place, could undoubtedly also be a factor in such recurrence – which emphasizes the need for re-education (posture, etc.) as a major part of rehabilitation.

A method that achieved precise targeting of these tissues (in terms of tonus release and subsequent stretching) would therefore be advantageous. Clinical experience indicates that, by combining the methods of direct inhibition (pressure mildly applied, continuously or in a 'make and break' pattern), along with the concept of strain/counterstrain and MET, a specific targeting of dysfunctional soft tissues is more likely to be achieved.

INIT methods

Method 1 (Fig. 9.1)

It is reasonable to assume, and palpation confirms, that when a trigger point is being palpated by direct finger or thumb pressure, and when the very tissue in which the trigger point lies is positioned in such a way as to take away the pain (entirely or at least to a great extent), the most (dis)stressed fibres in which the trigger point is housed will be in a position of relative ease. See discussion of strain–counterstrain (SCS) in Chapter 8, and Figs 8.21A, B, C.

Having been digitally compressed, and then placed into 'ease', the trigger point would ideally have already experienced direct inhibitory pressure, and would then have been positioned so

that the tissues housing it are relaxed (relatively or completely).

In the INIT sequence, at that time the patient would be asked to induce an isometric contraction into the tissues surrounding the trigger

Figure 9.1A   First stage of INIT in which a tender/pain/trigger point in supraspinatus is located and compressed ischaemically, either intermittently or persistently.

Figure 9.1B   The pain is removed from the tender/pain/trigger point by finding a position of ease which is held for at least 20 seconds, after which an isometric contraction is achieved involving the tissues that house the tender/pain/trigger point.

Figure 9.1C After holding the isometric contraction for an appropriate period, the muscle housing the point of local soft tissue dysfunction is stretched. This completes the INIT sequence.

point – and to hold this for 5 to 7 seconds. This contraction would involve the very fibres that had been repositioned to obtain the strain/counterstrain release.

Subsequently there would be a reduction in tone in these tissues, allowing them to be gently stretched (locally), as in any muscle energy procedure (see Chapter 8), with the strong likelihood that the most specifically involved fibres would be stretched.

Subsequently the whole muscle would be stretched, as in any other MET procedure, following a further isometric contraction.

Method 2

There is another possibility – a variation in which, instead of an isometric contraction followed by stretch being commenced following the period of ease (strain/counterstrain position), an isolytic (isotonic eccentric) approach could be used.

The muscle receiving attention is actively contracted by the patient at the same time as a stretch is introduced, resulting in mild trauma to the muscle and the breakdown of fibrous adhesions between it and its interface and within its structures (Mitchell et al 1979).

To introduce this method into trigger point treatment, following the application of inhibitory pressure and SCS release, the patient is asked to contract the muscles around the palpating thumb or finger (lying on the now inhibited pain point) with the request that the contraction should not be a full-strength effort, because the practitioner intends to stretch the tissues gently while the contraction is taking place.

This isotonic eccentric effort – designed to reduce contractions and break down fibrotic tissue – should target precisely the tissues in which the trigger point being treated lies buried. Following the isolytic stretch the tissues could benefit from effleurage and/or hot and cold applications to ease local congestion. An instruction should be given to avoid active use of the area for a day or so.

This method mimics aspects of 'pin & stretch'/active release treatment, as discussed in Chapter 8.

Summary and comment

The integrated use of inhibitory pressure, strain/counterstrain and a form of muscle energy technique – applied to a trigger point or other area of soft tissue dysfunction involving pain or restriction of range of motion (of soft tissue origin) – is a logical approach, because it has the advantage of allowing precise targeting of the culprit tissues.

Clearly, the use of an isolytic approach as part of this sequence will be more easily achieved in some regions than in others – upper trapezius posing less of a problem in terms of positioning and application, perhaps, than quadratus lumborum.

After either INIT method, it has been found to be useful to instruct the patient to learn a method of gentle activation of the antagonist muscles to the muscle housing the trigger point that has been treated. The patient is asked to reproduce this activity a number of times daily for the days immediately after treatment. This activation of antagonists produces a reciprocal inhibition of the previously hypertonic muscle, and assists in maintaining the deactivation.

References

Barlow W: Anxiety and muscle tension pain, *B J Clin Pract*, 13(5):1959.

Bass C, Gardner WN: Respiratory and psychiatric abnormalities in chronic symptomatic hyperventilation, *Br Med J* 290:1387–1390, 1985.

Beal MC: Palpatory testing for somatic dysfunction in patients with cardiovascular disease, *J Am Osteopath Assoc* 82:822–831, 1983.

Brostoff J: *Complete Guide to Food Allergy*, London, 1992, Bloomsbury.

Chaitow L: *Neuromuscular technique*, Wellingborough, UK, 1983, Thorsons.

Chaitow L: *Palpatory literacy*, London, 1991a, Thorsons.

Chaitow L: *Soft tissue manipulation*, Vermont, 1991b, Healing Arts Press, Rochester.

Chaitow L: INIT in treatment of pain and trigger points, *British Journal of Osteopathy XIII* 17–21, 1994.

Chaitow L: *Muscle energy technique*, ed 3, Edinburgh, 2006, Churchill Livingstone.

Chaitow L, DeLany J: *Clinical applications of neuromuscular technique*, vol 2, Edinburgh, 2002, Churchill Livingstone.

Chaitow L, Bradley D, Gilbert C: *Multidisciplinary approaches to breathing pattern disorders*, Edinburgh, 2002, Churchill Livingstone.

Cimino R: Does the ovarian cycle influence the pressure-pain threshold of the masticatory muscles in symptom-free women? *J Orofac Pain* 14:105–111, 2000.

Dittrich R: Somatic pain and autonomic concomitants, *Am J Surg*, 1954.

Fernández de las Peñas C, Palomeque del Cerro L, Carnero J: Manual treatment of post-whiplash injury, *Journal of Bodywork and Movement Therapies* 9(2):109–119, 2005.

Fernández-de-las-Peñas C, Simons D, Cuadrado M, et al: The role of myofascial trigger points in musculoskeletal pain syndromes of the head and neck, *Curr Pain Headache Rep* 11(5):365–372, 2007.

Field T, Hernandez-Reif M, Diego M, et al: Cortisol decreases and serotonin and dopamine increase following massage therapy, *Int J Neurosci* 115(10):1397–1413, 2005.

Fryer G, Fossum C: Muscle Energy Techniques. In Fernadez-de-las-Penas C, Arndt-Nielsen L, Gerwin R, Dommerholt J, editors: *Tension-type and Cervicogenic Headache*, Boston, 2009, Jones & Bartlett.

Fryer G, Hodgson L: The effect of manual pressure release on myofascial trigger points in the upper trapezius muscle, *Journal of Bodywork and Movement Therapies* 9(4):248–255, 2005.

Garland W: *Somatic changes in hyperventilating subject*, Paris, 1994, Presentation at Respiratory Function Congress.

Gerwin R, Dommerholt J: Treatment of myofascial pain syndromes. In Weiner R, editor: *Pain management; a practical guide for clinicians*, Boca Raton, 2002, CRC Press, pp 235–249.

Goldthwaite J: *Essentials of body mechanics*, Philadelphia, 1949, JB Lippincott.

Greenman P: *Manual medicine*, Baltimore, 1989, Williams & Wilkins.

Hartman L: *Handbook of osteopathic technique*, London, 1985, Hutchinson.

Hungerford B, Gilleard W: SIJ angular rotation during the stork and hip drop tests in normal subjects: pilot study results, Vienna, 1998, Third Interdisciplinary World Congress on Low Back and Pelvic Pain, pp 332–334.

Janda V: *Muscle function testing*, London, 1983, Butterworths.

Janda V: Glasgow E, editor: *Aspects of manipulative therapy*, Edinburgh, 1985, Churchill Livingstone.

Janda V: Grant R, editor: *Physical therapy in the cervical and thoracic spine*, New York, 1988, Churchill Livingstone.

Jones L: *Strain/counterstrain*, Colorado Springs, 1981, Academy of Applied Osteopathy.

Jung C-G: *Synchronicity: an acausal connecting principle*, Princeton, New Jersey, 1973, Princeton University Press.

Kleyhans & Aarons: 1974, Digest of Chiropractic Economics September.

Korr I: *Spinal cord as organiser of the disease process. 1976 Yearbook of the Academy of Applied Osteopathy*, Colorado Springs.

Latey P: *Muscular manifesto*, London, 1986, Published privately.

Lee D: Palpation issues, *Journal of Bodywork and Movement Therapies* 6(1):26–27, 2002.

Lewit K: *Manipulative therapy in rehabilitation of the motor system*, London, 1985, Butterworths.

Lewit K: *Manipulation in rehabilitation of the locomotor system*, ed 2, London, 1992, Butterworths.

Lewit K: *Manipulation in rehabilitation of the locomotor system*, ed 3, London, 1999, Butterworths.

Lief S: Cited. In Chaitow L, editor: *Neuro-muscular technique/ soft tissue manipulation*, Wellingborough, UK, 1989, Thorsons.

Lief P: Neuromuscular technique, *British Naturopathic Journal and Osteopathic Review Autumn* 304, 1963.

Loga S: Integrative treatment in psychiatry, *Psychiatr Danub* 20(3):349–351, 2008.

McMakin C: Microcurrent Therapy. In Chaitow L, editor: *Fibromyalgia Syndrome – A Practitioner's Guide to Treatment*, Edinburgh, 2003, Churchill Livingstone.

Mancuso C, Tanzi M, Gabay M: Paradoxical reactions to benzodiazepines: Literature review and treatment options, *Pharmacotherapy* 24(9):1177–1185, 2004.

Melzack R, Wall P: *The challenge of pain*, London, 1988, Penguin.

Mitchell F, Moran P, Pruzzo N: *Evaluation of osteopathic muscle energy procedure*, Valley Park, Illinois, 1979, Pruzzo.

Murphy D, editor: In *Conservative management of cervical spine syndromes*, New York, 2000, McGraw Hill.

Myers T: *Anatomy trains*, Edinburgh, 2001, Churchill Livingstone.

Nimmo R: Receptor tonus technique, *Lecture notes*, London, 1966, British College of Naturopathy and Osteopathy.

Nixon P, Andrews J: A study of anaerobic threshold in chronic fatigue syndrome (CFS), *Biol Psychol* 43:264, 1996.

Pollard H, Ward G: A study of two stretching techniques for improving hip flexion range of motion, *J Manipulative Physiol Ther* 20:443–447, 1997.

Pollo A, Benedetti F: Placebo Response: Relevance to the Rheumatic Diseases, *Rheumatic Disease Clinics of North America* 34(2):331–349, 2008.

Randolph T: Stimulatory withdrawal and the alternations of allergic manifestations. In Dickey L, editor: *Clinical ecology*, Springfield, Illinois, 1976, Charles C. Thomas, pp 156–175.

Rolf I: *The integration of human structures*, USA, 1977, Harper & Row.

Roll M, Thorell T: Acute chest pain without obvious cause before age 40 – personality and recent life events, *J Psychosom Res* 31(2):215–221, 1987.

Selye H: *The stress of life*, New York, 1984, McGraw-Hill.

Schenk R, Adelman K: The effects of MET on cervical range of motion, *J Manual Manip Ther* 2:149–155, 1994.

Simons D, Travell J, Simons L: *Myofascial pain and dysfunction: the trigger point manual*, vol 1: *Upper half of body*, ed 2, Baltimore, 1999, Williams & Wilkins.

Slatkovska L, Jensen D, Davies A, et al: Phasic menstrual cycle effects on the control of breathing in healthy women, *Respiratory Physiology & Neurobiology* 154:379–388, 2006.

Slocumb J: Neurological factors in chronic pelvic pain, trigger points and abdominal pelvic pain, *Am J Obstet Gynecol* 49:536, 1984.

Speicher T, et al: Effect of strain counterstrain on pain and strength in hip musculature, *J Manual Manip Ther* 12(4):215–223, 2004.

Speransky A: *A basis for the theory of medicine*, New York, 1943, International Publishers.

Travell J, Simons D: *Myofascial pain and dysfunction: the trigger point manual*, vol 1, Baltimore, 1983, Williams & Wilkins.

Travell J, Simons D: *Myofascial pain and dysfunction: the trigger point manual*, vol 2: *The lower extremities*, Baltimore, 1992, Williams & Wilkins.

Upledger J: *Craniosacral therapy*, USA, 1983, Eastland Press.

Vleeming A, Mooney V, Dorman T, Snijders C, Stoeckart R, editors: *Movement, stability and low back pain*, Edinburgh, 1997, Churchill Livingstone.

Wall PD, Melzack R, editors: *Textbook of pain*, ed 2, Edinburgh, 1989, Churchill Livingstone.

Weiss J: Pelvic floor myofascial trigger points: manual therapy for interstitial cystitis and the urgency–frequency syndrome, *J Urol* 166:2226–2231, 2001.

Wilson E, Payton O, Donegan-Shoaf L, Dec K: Muscle energy technique in patients with acute low back pain: a pilot clinical trial, *Journal of Orthopedic and Sports Physical Therapy* 33:502–512, 2003.

Youngs B: The physiological background of neuromuscular technique, *British Naturopathic Journal and Osteopathic Review* 5:176–178, 1963.

Youngs B: Lief's Neuromuscular Technique: a recollection. In Chaitow L, et al, editor: *Physical Medicine*, Edinburgh, 2008, Churchill Livingstone.

American neuromuscular therapy

10

Judith DeLany

CHAPTER CONTENTS

History **221**
Platform of NMT American version™ **222**
Categories 222
The original six factors of NMT 223
Application of NMT **224**
Order of the routine 225
Clinical application of NMT 225
NMT techniques **226**
Pressure considerations 229
Application of static pressure 229
Use of pressure bars 230
NMT methods **230**
Trapezius 231
Levator scapula 231
Posterior mid-thorax 232
Posterior cranium 234
Cervical lamina supine 234
Splenii tendons 236
Sternocleidomastoid 238
Spinal lamina groove 239
Intercostal muscles 240
Iliolumbar ligament and sacroiliac ligament 241
Erector spinae 242
Quadratus lumborum 244
Overview of differences **244**

History

As detailed in Chapter 2, neuromuscular therapy (NMT) evolved out of the work of a number of clinicians working in both Europe and the USA.[1] The 'evolutionary' development of NMT produced some confusion regarding the name itself. In its earlier stages, American 'NMT' represented neuromuscular 'therapy', whereas, in Europe, the preferred term had been neuromuscular 'technique'. In the past decade, as a number of methods emerged, practitioners began to use these two terms interchangeably. Distinctions between the various NMT methods still exist, although there is less separation with regards to the use of the terms 'therapy' and 'technique', apart from osteopathic training in the UK, where the 'T' element of NMT refers to 'technique'.

The first American protocols of NMT, developed in the late 1970s and early 1980s were based largely on the methods devised and taught by the late Raymond Nimmo (DeLany 1999). Nimmo's research into the pathological influences and relevance, as well as the therapeutic implications of treating 'noxious pain points' mirrors closely that of his contemporary, Janet Travell, in relation to her research into myofascial

---

[1]Variations existing between the European and American versions of NMT are highlighted in this chapter by brief comments, given in footnotes. The European version is commonly known as 'Lief's NMT', which is how it is described in these notes.

trigger points. Nimmo's protocols were subsequently modified and expanded by Paul St John, who studied with Nimmo, and then by St John and Judith (Walker) DeLany, who worked together in the 1980s. Both St John and DeLany have continued expanding their separate NMT programmes over the last decade.

While the American protocols of NMT were initially based on that of Nimmo, the platform of application was strongly influenced by the writings and research of Travell & Simons (1983, 1992), Vannerson & Nimmo (1971), Cailliet (1977), Chaitow (1980) and others. Both St John's and DeLany's variations on Nimmo's protocols resulted in revisions of previous concepts and methodology, leading to significant changes in recommended treatment techniques. St John incorporated structural homeostasis of the body and cranium as the basis of his St John Method™, while DeLany took a broader view in NMT American version™ (Chaitow & DeLany 2000, 2002, 2008), where she utilized a systematic approach with attention paid to biochemical, biomechanical and psychosocial factors.

In 2000, DeLany and co-author Leon Chaitow, published the first of two volumes that present NMT American version™ alongside the European NMT protocols, positional release, muscle energy techniques and other modalities that can be used as adjuncts to its application. *Clinical Application of Neuromuscular Techniques*, volumes 1 (2nd edn 2008) and 2 (2002), distinguish NMT American version™ as a practical, systematic approach for training palpation and assessment skills, as well as for clinical application.

The following introduction to NMT American version™ will concentrate on the basic techniques and examples of application to selected muscles. Although these techniques can easily be practised from the descriptions given, it is important to remember that those given are incomplete protocols, and that 'missing elements', such as treatment of anterior, lateral and deep abdominal muscles, must be included for safe and effective application. There is no substitute for supervised hands-on instruction, which is highly recommended as the safest means of acquiring NMT skills.

Platform of NMT American version™

Homeostasis incorporates the processes through which the various functions of the body, including everything from postural adjustments to the chemical compositions of the body's fluids, are maintained in balance (Stedman 1998). It is through this goal of equilibrium that the body deals with the many stresses and demands placed upon it in daily life, accomplishing this through adaptation and compensation. If stresses are excessive, or if compensation mechanisms have been compromised or overloaded, the adverse effects of decompensation, where frank disease and degeneration occur, are likely to emerge (Chaitow & DeLany 2008).

Categories

The broad foundation of NMT American version™ is based on the assessment of three categories capable of adaptation that, on a constant basis, modify, adjust to and compensate for the stresses of life (Table 10.1). Within the three categories – *biomechanical*, *biochemical* and *psychosocial* – are to be found subdivisions of most of the major influences on health, with a number of these features being commonly involved in causing or intensifying pain (Chaitow 1996, 2003,

Table 10.1 Major influences on health that are commonly involved in causing or intensifying pain can be broadly classified into three categories. The examples given can be readily seen as not only individually problematic, but to profoundly interact with each other and create a cascade of effects.

Biomechanical	Biochemical	Psychosocial
Trauma	Inflammation	Stress
Postural	Dehydration	Guilt
Muscular (including trigger points)	Nutritional	Fear
Congenital	Hormonal	Anxiety
'Wear and tear'	Ischaemia	Emotions
Joint dysfunction	Toxicity	Litigation
Overuse, misuse, disuse, abuse	Immune response	Depression
Neural entrapment and/or compression		Somatization

Chaitow & DeLany 2000, 2008). In addressing these categories, it is acknowledged that there can be local and/or global (systemic) causes of pain and dysfunction, as well as numerous perpetuating factors, that, if left untreated, may cause 'mysterious' recurrence of the condition (Simons et al 1999). Local, global and perpetuating factors should all be considered in a thorough recovery programme. These include Chaitow & DeLany (2000, 2008), amongst others, locally dysfunctional states such as:

• hypertonia
• ischaemia
• prolonged local inflammation
• trigger points
• neural compression or entrapment

as well as the following global factors that affect the whole body systemically:

• genetic predisposition (e.g. connective tissue factors leading to hypermobility) and inborn anomalies (e.g. short leg)
• nutritional deficiencies and imbalances
• toxicity (exogenous and endogenous)
• infections (chronic or acute)
• endocrine (hormonal) imbalances and deficiencies (especially thyroid)
• global (systemic) inflammation
• stress (physical or psychological)
• trauma (abrupt as well as cumulative)
• posture (both static and dynamic and including patterns of misuse and muscle substitution)
• hyperventilation tendencies.

In its early stages, NMT American version™ focused largely on six 'subdivisions' from this list, with practitioners focusing on ischaemia, trigger points, neural entrapments/compressions, postural/structural imbalance, nutritional components/deficiencies and emotional/stress factors. As clinical application has broadened and NMTs are working in exceedingly greater multidiscipline interface, it has become more apparent that, while focusing on the six factors alone may get (sometimes astounding) results, this is insufficient in many cases to achieve a long-lasting resolution. As a result of broadening the NMT perspective, it is often necessary for the astute

practitioner to expand clinical understanding beyond the base education of licence requirements. This poses a challenging problem, since application of that knowledge may not lie within the practitioner's scope of practice. The solution to this situation is to build a strong network of practitioners to whom the patient can be referred when presenting symptoms arouse suspicion that the root cause of the problem may be other than myofascial. Any factors that lie outside the scope of practice and licence of the practitioner should be considered for referral.

It should be kept in mind that the influences of a *biomechanical*, *biochemical* and *psychosocial* nature do not produce single changes. Their interaction with one another is profound, and intervention in one category can affect the others remarkably. The practitioner's role may be to alleviate the stress burden or simply to lighten the load. At times, all that may be accomplished is to work towards more efficient handling of the adaptive load by teaching and encouraging the individual to alter daily habits. While it is important to remove or modify as many aetiological and perpetuating influences as can be identified, this must be done without creating further distress or a requirement for excessive adaptation. For each therapeutic intervention applied, adaptation will probably also be required. It is important that the adaptive mechanisms are not overloaded in the healing process.

The original six factors of NMT

Although the current approach of NMT American version™ encompasses consideration of many additional factors beyond the classic six, the original six still remain the primary focus of the approach. When working with a person in chronic pain, these six subdivisions derived from the local and global lists above should be addressed systematically to assess for and, hopefully, reduce underlying causes of discomfort and/or dysfunction. If assessment of one or more of these factors is omitted, the person may plateau or regress in his or her recovery. These particular six factors should be considered, assessed for, and clinically addressed (if needed) by the practitioner in all patients (Chaitow & DeLany

2000, 2008). If the practitioner is without skill or licence in one or more of these foundational tools, it is suggested that the patient be referred to another practitioner who is suitably trained and licensed in the subject. If progress is not seen within a few treatments, or if pain, fatigue, or other primary symptoms return, other factors (hormonal, organ or bone health, toxicity, etc.) should be considered. The six factors, as noted by DeLany (2002), are:

Ischaemia – a state in which the current oxygen/blood supply is inadequate for the current physiological needs of tissue. Causes of ischaemia can be pathological (narrowed artery or thrombus), biochemical (vasoconstriction by the body to reduce flow to a particular area), anatomical (tendon obstruction of blood flow) or as a result of overuse or facilitation. Ischaemia reduces the level of oxygen, nutrients and waste removal and the tension produced by the resultant muscle shortening can alter joint mechanics and/or entrap neural structures. Ischaemia, and its resultant local energy crisis, can also lead to the production of trigger points (Simons et al 1999).

Trigger points (TrPs) – localized areas within muscle bellies (central TrPs) or at myotendinous or periosteal attachments (attachment TrPs) which, when sufficiently provoked, produce a referral pattern to a target zone. The referral pattern may include pain, tingling, numbness, itching, burning or other sensations. In addition to its location (central or attachment), a TrP can be classified as to its state of activity (active or latent) as well as whether it is primary, key or satellite. (See also trigger point formation theories, described in detail in Ch. 3.)

Neural interferences – compression (by osseous structures) or entrapment (by myofascial tissues) of neural structures may result in muscle contraction disturbances, vasomotion, pain impulses, reflex mechanisms and disturbances in sympathetic activity. Since neurovascular structures course along fascial structures (sheaths, planes, etc.), entrapment by fascial distortions is common. Release of the fascia and mobilization of the neural structures should be components of the manual protocols.

Postural and biomechanical dysfunctions – repeated postural and biomechanical insults over a period of time, combined with the somatic effects of emotional and psychological origin, will often present altered patterns of tense, shortened, bunched, fatigued and, ultimately, fibrotic tissues with resultant alterations from healthy postural positioning. Muscle substitution occurs, with resultant alterations in firing patterns that can escalate to further dysfunctional use. Although structural assessment (postural analysis) has inherent value, it fails to consider patterns of use that may not be displayed in static position. Dynamic pronation, alterations in gait, and other use patterns should be assessed and corrected due to their ability to perpetuate obvious and very subtle dysfunctions.

Nutritional factors – nutritional deficiencies/ imbalances, sensitivities, allergies and stimulants all play roles in myofascial health as well as hormonal, emotional and mental health. The author of this chapter considers the nutritional component to be the most important factor in health. Excess or lack of those that provide energy (protein, carbohydrate, fat) as well as those that support metabolism (vitamins, minerals, water) can have a significant impact on health and chronic pain.

Emotional well-being – the degree and type of the emotional and stress loads the individual is carrying can influence various systems of the body. Hormones and neurotransmitters are chemical messengers of the body that are strongly affected by stress, thought and emotions. Likewise, they can impact mental, physical and emotional response to stress, with resultant cascades of further chemical interfaces. Ultimately, if excessive or prolonged, these factors can result in distress and disease.

Application of NMT

Effective application of NMT techniques may be achieved more easily by applying the following guidelines. As knowledge of anatomy is enhanced and the necessary skills are attained, each practitioner will develop his or her own style by blending NMT knowledge with that acquired from other disciplines studied.

Note: In the USA, laws regarding scope of practice vary from state to state and among the many healthcare professions. Most states require a 'licence to touch' in order to treat patients. It is suggested that each practitioner perform within the scope of his or her own licence regardless of what is presented within this text. NMT is practised in multiple disciplines in many different states and countries, and this text may contain techniques or concepts that lie outside of the scope of a particular licence. It is each practitioner's responsibility to know his or her scope of practice and to work within the boundaries of licensure.

Order of the routine

What should be treated first? Where should treatment begin? Sequencing is an important element in bodywork and, to some extent, is a matter of experience and preference. However, in many instances protocols and prescriptions based on clinical experience – and sometimes research – can be offered.

NMT is written about and usually applied as a sequence of steps. Each step of the 'routine' is performed in the initial examination to assure maximum results, as skipping some steps may cause a significant detail to be missed and result in less than optimal outcomes. In subsequent treatment sessions some of the steps may be omitted if particular tissues are not involved.

The techniques are applied to the muscles in a suggested order that is designed to enter the tissues by layers, to treat the proximal portion of an extremity before the distal portion, and to best manage the therapy time. When the order of the routine needs to be altered, two rules should always be applied:

1. Superficial tissues are treated before deeper layers.
2. The proximal portion of any extremity is addressed before the distal.

Clinical application of NMT

The clinical examination that uses NMT moves almost seamlessly from the gathering of information into application of treatment. The process of discovery leads to therapeutic action as the practitioner searches for evidence of tissue dysfunction, and then applies the technique to turn 'finding into fixing'. This transition from examination to treatment and back to examination is a characteristic of NMT and will become habitual as the methods and objectives of NMT and its associated modalities become more familiar. NMT palpation techniques can be blended with the application of muscle energy techniques and positional or myofascial release methods by moving from one modality to the other and back to examination without delay.

A variety of techniques is used in NMT, the choice of which depends on the practitioner's skills and what is discovered in examination, as well as the desired effect on the tissues. The use of skin lubrication will vary from step to step depending upon the technique being applied. Dry techniques, such as connective tissue work or tissue lifting techniques, should be applied before lubrication, because some techniques become more difficult when the skin is oiled. Generally, gliding procedures require lubrication, while friction and tissue lifting techniques do not. Applying the appropriate amount of lubrication is important, since excessive amounts generally decrease palpatory perception and affect control of the hands during the gliding strokes. An inadequate amount may produce skin drag, friction and moderate discomfort.

Application of dry techniques is generally followed by manipulation or lightly lubricated gliding, which is aimed at increasing blood flow and 'flushing' tissues while simultaneously evaluating for ischaemic bands and/or trigger points. Static digital pressure is subsequently employed in order to release ischaemic bands and for treatment of trigger points, and is usually applied after several repetitions of gliding or other forms of manipulation of the tissues have been completed. Pressure bars may be used instead of (or in addition to) finger or thumb compression (Fig. 10.1B,C) in certain areas; however, precautions apply and proper training is suggested. Manually applied gliding strokes are usually repeated after applications of compression, friction or pressure bar techniques.

Figure 10.1A   The fingers support and steady the hands while the thumbs are the primary tools used in most of the gliding techniques.

Figure 10.1B,C   Pressure bars, held properly, are excellent treatment tools that reduce stress on the practitioner's thumbs and fingers.

NMT techniques

The choice of NMT technique depends upon what is discovered in examination as well as the desired effect on the tissues.

* *Skin rolling and tissue lifting techniques* can be applied to soften the fascia associated with the skin and underlying muscles. The skin can be grasped and lifted, thereby creating mechanical tension on the subcutaneous fascia, which assists in changing the state of the fascia's ground substance from a 'gel' to a 'sol' (Oschman 1997) due to its thixotropic properties (DeLany 2000a). The tissue can also be rolled between the fingers and thumb. Subcutaneous tissue layers and/or muscle bellies may be grasped and lifted, then manipulated between the fingers and thumb, if tolerable, thereby stretching fascia and separating fascial layers. Any of these may result in increased blood and/or lymph flow. Areas where the skin is adherent are often an indication that the underlying muscles need further treatment.
* *Effleurage (gliding stroke)* is an important and powerful component of the NMT American version™. It warms the fascia, flushes blood through the tissues, and therefore increases

oxygenation and perfusion of nutrients while simultaneously eliminating waste products from the tissues (Yates 1989). During the gliding process, the practitioner will discover contracted bands, nodules and tender points unique to that individual. Gliding repeatedly on these bands often reduces their size and tenacity, lessening the time and effort needed to modify or eliminate them. Clinical experience indicates that the best results tend to come from gliding on the tissues several times, then working somewhere else and returning to glide again. The direction of application of glides may be either with or across the direction of the muscle fibres, and usually involves a combination of both. Following the course of lymphatic flow is particularly suggested if tissues are congested. Unless contraindicated (by inflammation, oedema, etc.), a moist hot pack can be placed on the tissues between gliding repetitions to enhance the effects further. A short time of rest of the tissues is usual before additional gliding. This allows circulatory and drainage functions to flush the tissues further. Tenderness and ischaemia are commonly reduced rapidly in this way.

- To glide on the tissues most effectively, the practitioner's fingers, spread slightly, support and stabilize the hands (Fig. 10.1A) while the thumbs are (most often) the treatment tools. The hand and forearm move as a unit, with the wrist being stable. Little or no motion is allowed in the wrist joints or the thumb joints. Excessive movement in the wrist or thumb may lead to joint problems and inflammation of the practitioner's forearms, wrists and hands. A proper and stable hand position helps avoid practitioner injury. When two-handed glides are used, the thumbs are side by side (almost parallel), or one ahead of the other, with the tips of the thumbs leading the glide.[2] When the distal tips of the thumbs are touching during the glide and the medial side of the thumbs lead the stroke, excessive strain is placed on the thumb joints and practitioner injury is a considerable risk.
- When dealing with tissue that is not excessively tender or sensitive, the 'glide' should cover 3–4 inches per second (speed of application is reduced for comfort if tissues are sensitive), which is significantly faster than the thumb stroke used in Lief's NMT. It is important to develop a moderate gliding speed in order to ensure adequate opportunity for simultaneous palpation of muscles. Too rapid a movement may cause unnecessary discomfort and may also skim over congestion in the tissues, missing vital information sources. Movement that is too slow may displace the tissues, making identification of an individual muscle difficult. A moderate speed will allow for repetitions that significantly increase blood flow and, at the same time,

palpation of bands or nodules of ischaemia within the tissues.[3]

- *Compression techniques* can be used to press soft tissues against a bone or underlying muscle (*flat compression*), or the non-lubricated tissues may be lifted and grasped between the finger(s) and thumb (*pincer compression*). Pincer compression can be broadly applied with flattened fingers (like a clothes' peg; see Fig. 10.2A) or precisely applied with curved fingers (resembling a 'C' clamp; see Fig. 10.2D).
- *Static compression* (also called TrP pressure release, ischaemic compression or sustained pressure) applies pressure to tissues without movement of the fingers or thumb. Tissues that are ischaemic or those that contain TrPs usually respond well to static compression (see below regarding use of static pressure). For those that are extremely tender, pressure must be modified so as not to be excessive.
- *Compression with manipulation* can be applied by lifting the tissues and then rolling, bending or twisting them between the fingers and thumb. It is an effective way of mechanically distressing the connective tissue and altering its ground substance from a gel to a sol (DeLany 2000b), and may also help to separate the fibres and increase blood flow. Generally, this technique is used after the tissue tenderness has been decreased by the use of gliding strokes and static compression. It can follow those techniques or be used before TrP pressure release.
- *Friction techniques* can usually be applied to myofascial tissues with variations, depending on the condition of the tissues and the desired results. It is most often used to soften fibrotic tissues and to alter the quality of adhesions. Friction techniques may include those applied transversely (cross-fibre friction, strumming, snapping or transverse friction) or those applied with the fibre direction (longitudinal friction). If tissues are tender, caution should be exercised as tenderness may be indicative of inflammation. If significant tenderness is

---

[2]The American NMT glide is seen in this description to vary from the European hand application in which, while placed ahead of the thumbs, the fingers remain static so that only the thumb moves during the assessment/treatment 'glide'. In the American version the whole hand moves.

[3]As noted in the text, NMT in Europe is usually significantly more deliberate and slow than the American version, especially in the assessment mode.

Figure 10.2A,B   (A) Broad, flat compression can be applied between the thumb and fingers. (B) To uncoil the tissue, the fingers should curl completely around the upper trapezius to touch the anterior surface of the muscle under the forward 'lip'.

Figure 10.2C,D   With appropriate positioning of the arm, portions of the middle and lower portions of trapezius may be effectively lifted and compressed on most people. Elevation of the head of the humerus to shorten the fibres may be needed.

Figure 10.2E   A bevelled-tip pressure bar may be used in grooves and under bony ledges not easily reached with the thumbs, such as here in the spinal lamina groove.

present or if application of friction results in tenderness, ice may be applied for 10–15 minutes. Friction on that particular tissue should then be avoided until no evidence of inflammation is present.

Pressure considerations

After gliding and manipulation of tissues, the muscles may be compressed with static (ischaemic compression) pressure. Pressure should be constant and could even be mildly increased as the tissues relax and release. The length of time for which pressure is maintained will vary, although, as a rule, it is found that tissue tension begins to ease within 8–12 seconds when the ideal pressure is being used. The pressure may be sustained, even increase, for up to 20 seconds. The practitioner should feel the tissues 'melting and softening' under the pressure. Patients frequently reports that they believe the practitioner is reducing the degree of applied pressure.[4]

Pain reduction not always an adequate guide

While a reduction of pain may be achieved via static compression that is sustained for longer than suggested, this is usually of only short-term benefit. Increased pain and a reduction in local mobility may result from the irritation caused by sustained or excessive pressure. A greater, longer-lasting, beneficial effect will usually be gained when the practitioner goes back to an area four or five times for a shorter duration, rather than once for one or two minutes. If release of palpated contractions has not commenced within 8–12 seconds, the pressure may be too heavy or too light and should probably be altered.

Degree of pressure

The appropriate degree of pressure utilized in static compression varies with the individual (and even from one part of the body to another); however, it usually matches the tension palpated in the tissues. Pressure that is too light may not produce a tissue response, whereas heavy pressure may result in reflexive spasms. Age, oxygenation, past trauma, exercise status, previous therapies, hydration, nutritional and hormonal imbalances/deficiencies, tissue toxicity and dysfunctional postures all appear to influence the amount of pressure most appropriately applied.

How does one determine the amount of pressure to use? In addition to matching the tension within the tissues, a 1–10 scale of patient discomfort in the tissues being treated can be established and may be used to help guide the practitioner, where 1 = no discomfort and 10 = extreme pain. Only enough pressure to elicit mild to moderate discomfort is used, with a score of 5, 6 or 7 representing an ideal report. A score of 9 or 10 has no place in therapy! 'Biting the bullet' and 'digging it out' has no advantage – and offers real disadvantages – in NMT. Pressure should be adjusted routinely until the ideal level is found *for that particular tissue*.

Application of static pressure

Static pressure can be applied to soft tissues as an effective means of reducing spasm and contractures as well as for deactivating TrPs. While the blanching effects of applied compression may enhance blood flow when pressure is subsequently released, restriction of blood flow can produce an ischaemic state if held for too long. Additionally, the patient may not tolerate long applications of pressure if the tissue is extremely tender or inflamed. The amount and duration of pressure appropriate for an individual can vary greatly – even from one muscle to the next.

It is important to be specific when applying pressure to dysfunctional soft tissues. To treat TrPs most successfully, the practitioner should be directly on the TrP rather than next to it. When the patient keeps asking for more pressure, moving the point of pressure slightly, in one direction or another along the muscle fibres, may reveal that the practitioner was close to but not right on, the desired spot.

As discussed previously, the length of time for which static pressure should be applied will vary; with practice, the practitioner will develop the skill to feel tension released. This should begin

---

[4]The pressure applied in Lief's NMT has two distinct modes: the assessment mode 'meets and matches' tissue tension, whereas the pressure applied in NMT treatment mode is largely in accord with that described for American NMT.

to occur within 8–12 seconds, although compression may be maintained for up to 20 seconds. A reduction of discomfort may be achieved with pressure that lasts longer than suggested, although clinical experience suggests that increased pain and decreased mobility often result when overly sustained or heavy pressure is used. Pressure should be constant and may be mildly increased as the tissues begin to soften. The patient should be encouraged to report if the pressure is too heavy, if a tissue 'melting' sensation is felt and, if there is a referred sensation, to what region it refers. (See Box 3.6 and further discussion in Ch. 3 for details of algometer usage.)

Use of pressure bars

Pressure bars may be used as valuable treatment tools to protect the practitioner's thumbs from excessive pressure and to access crevices that the thumbs may not be able to reach. These classical tools for NMT are constructed of lightweight wood and comprise a 1-inch dowel horizontal cross-bar and smaller vertical dowel shaft. Each has either a flat rubber tip or a bevelled rubber tip at the end of the vertical shaft (see Fig. 10.1B, C). The large flat tip is used to press into large muscle bellies, such as in the gluteal region, or to glide on flat broad muscles, such as the tibialis anterior. The bevelled tip is useful in the lamina groove, under the spine of the scapula, and to friction certain tendons that are difficult to reach with the thumb. The bevelled end of a flat typewriter eraser can also be used, although it is not as easy to hold as the pressure bar. The pressure bars are never used on extremely tender tissues, at vulnerable nerve areas such as above or below the clavicle, or to 'dig' into tissues. Contracted tissues, fibrosis and bony surfaces may be 'felt' through the bars – just as a grain of sand or a crack in the table under writing paper may be felt through a pencil when writing.

The pressure bar is held securely on the shaft while wrapping the hand around the horizontal dowel, as shown in Fig. 10.1B,C. The practitioner's wrist is kept relatively straight so as to avoid strain. The pressure bar and the practitioner's hand and forearm generally move as a unit. Although flexion of the wrist might occur

with certain uses (such as in scraping the palmar fascia), very little ulnar and radial deviation at the wrist should occur.

Pressure bar tips and handles should be cleaned after each use and can be scrubbed as the hands would be, using an antibacterial soap and scrub-brush. The use of alcohol on the rubber tips is not recommended because it may cause them to become dry and brittle. If the tip contacts oil, the rubber may begin to break down, causing it to split open. Scrubbing oil residue off the rubber tip should help prevent this.

The pressure bars should *not* be used on the face, in the cervical region, under the posterior base of the cranium, in soft, fleshy regions (such as the abdomen or groin) or on arteries or veins. Avoid placing the pressure bar tip on a bony surface where nerves are exposed (such as the head of the fibula), above or under the clavicle, behind the knee, or on any other vulnerable part of the body.

The use of pressure bars to treat myofascial tissues is considered to be an advanced massage technique, the use of which requires experience and training to determine when the technique may be used safely and effectively, and to prevent injury or strain of the practitioner's hands. The author suggests that the practitioner seek training in the proper use and handling of pressure bars before attempting to use them.

NMT methods

The following descriptions and illustrations of NMT American version™ are excerpts of the more complete routines taught as the protocols of NMT and are intended only to introduce the reader to the NMT method. They are not meant to be fully comprehensive; they do, however, provide accurate examples of the way in which NMT would be used if restrictions were being addressed and/or trigger points were being sought and treated in these structures. A thorough discussion of NMT routines, as well as regional anatomy, dysfunctional conditions and precautions, and a variety of associated modalities, is offered by Chaitow & DeLany (2000, 2002, 2008).

The following protocols are described for the right side of the body. All steps should be repeated on the left side. It is particularly important to treat both sides of muscles that attach to the spine, because release of one side only could result in reflexive shortening of the muscles of the untreated side and potentially moderate postural distortions.

Trapezius

The patient lies prone with the arm hanging off the side of the table or with the ipsilateral hand placed near the head.

1. Grasp the upper trapezius between the thumb and first two or three fingers with the thumb on the posterior surface and the fingers wrapping all the way around and up underneath the anterior fibres (Fig. 10.2A,B). This 'flat compression' is suitable for this muscle as well as (with slight variations) the sternocleidomastoid and other muscles.

   'Uncoil' the fibres of the outermost portion of the upper trapezius by dragging three fingers over the anterior surface against posteriorly applied thumb pressure. Do not allow the fingers to flip over the uppermost edge of the trapezius as this area can be very tender and often houses violent trigger points. Keep the wrist low to angle the fingers around the most anterior fibres. Thoroughly examine the toothpick size strands of the outermost edge; these often contain trigger points that induce noxious referrals into the face and eyes.[5]

2. Place the prone patient's arm on the table at his or her side. To define the middle trapezius, draw parallel lines from the two ends of the spine of the scapula to form right angles with the spinous processes. The fibres of middle trapezius lie between these two lines. Elevation of the humeral head 3–6 inches by use of a rolled-up towel, wedge, etc. will usually shorten the middle and lower trapezius, which allows it to be treated more easily.

   Grasp the middle trapezius with both hands and compress and/or manipulate the belly of the middle portion (Fig. 10.2C). Repeat the grasping manipulation to the outer (diagonal) edge of the lower trapezius (Fig. 10.2D). This manipulation is similar to skin rolling techniques (see Ch. 8 for details of skin rolling) but includes more than the skin: lifting, evaluating and stretching the fibres of the muscle itself. If trigger points are found, static pincer-like compression is used to treat them.

3. Place the bevelled tip of the pressure bar against the lateral aspect of the spinous process of C7 (in the lamina groove) and at a 45° angle. Friction cephalad to caudad at tip-width intervals all the way down to L1 to treat the trapezius attachments on the spinous processes as well as deeper attachments (Fig. 10.2E).[6] When tissues are excessively tender, gliding strokes applied with the thumb or finger can be substituted for the pressure bar frictional techniques.

4. The bevelled pressure bar may be used on the scapular and acromial attachments of the trapezius. Gliding strokes with the thumb may be substituted for the pressure bar frictional techniques if tissue tenderness warrants a gentler approach. Thumb glides may be used with caution on the clavicular attachments where the pressure bar is *never* used.

   Caution: It is suggested that the pressure bar not be used on clavicular attachments of the trapezius due to the proximity of the brachial plexus.

5. Gliding strokes can be used to soothe the tissues that have been treated with the pressure bar and with the manipulation techniques. Unless contraindicated, moist hot packs can be placed on the trapezius to increase blood flow. A cold pack or lymphatic drainage should follow the hot pack to enhance fluid drainage.

Levator scapula

The patient is prone.

1. Grasp the lower angle of the scapula and ease it toward the patient's ear to elevate the upper angle of the scapula away from the torso. The

---

[5]Lief's NMT would access these structures from a position in which the practitioner is at the head of the table; see position 3 of spinal NMT application in Chapter 6.

---

[6]Lief's NMT would use thumb pressure to achieve the same effect.

Figure 10.3   Fingers are wrapped around the anterior trapezius and placed directly on the upper angle of the manually elevated scapula to access the bony surface where levator scapula attaches.

practitioner's lower hand is used to increase and secure this elevation at the lower angle of the scapula (Fig. 10.3).

2. The practitioner's fingers of the cephalad hand are passed around the anterior fibres of the trapezius and directly on to the anterior surface of the upper angle of the scapula. It is necessary to ensure that the trapezius fibres are bypassed, because trying to access levator scapula by pressing through the trapezius fibres will fail to achieve optimal results. Friction should be applied gently as these fibres are often extremely tender and referral patterns can produce a dull to moderate ache in the shoulder or trapezius area. The cephalad ends of these fibres attach to the atlas transverse process and are therefore involved in its stability.

3. Careful palpation can be applied at its attachments on the transverse processes of C1–C4 and gliding strokes may be applied to the remainder of the muscle. However, caution should be exercised to avoid intrusion into the suboccipital triangle where the vertebral artery lies and the anterior surfaces of the transverse processes, where the brachial plexus courses near sharp foraminal gutters.

Posterior mid-thorax

The patient is prone.

1. Gliding strokes are applied repeatedly to the interscapular region, which lies between the two vertebral borders of the scapulae. Avoid pressing on the spinous processes. Unless contraindicated, moist hot packs can be placed on the rhomboid region between repetitions of gliding strokes. Taut bands within the muscle can be assessed for the presence of trigger points, which can be treated with trigger point pressure release.

2. Place the patient's hand behind the small of the back, if possible, so distracting the vertebral border of the scapula from the ribs; this will allow additional access and deeper palpation. The following steps may be performed more easily if the practitioner stands on the contralateral side and reaches across to apply treatment.

3. Place the thumbs on the medial anterior surface of the scapula and introduce a glide or use cranial/caudal friction to examine the attachments of the serratus anterior and the subscapularis along the entire anterior vertebral border of the scapula (Fig. 10.4A).

4. With the scapula still elevated, rotate the thumbs so that the thumb pads press onto the thorax. Apply pressure anteriorly, deep to the vertebral border of the scapula, and glide or friction while pressing down onto the rib-cage (Fig. 10.4B). This step may address the 'hidden' tendinous attachments of the serratus posterior superior and its associated trigger point. Trigger points in this area refer significantly into the chest and down the arm, duplicating anginal pain. They may be hidden from palpation unless the scapula is sufficiently elevated.[7] An alternative position to better access this area is shown in Box 10.1.

---

[7]Lief's NMT would access these areas from positions 4 and 5 of the spinal sequence as described in Chapter 6.

Figure 10.4A,B   'Hidden' trigger points in serratus posterior superior may be accessed under the vertebral border of the scapula.

Box 10.1   Alternative positioning of the patient

Alternative positions for applying NMT routines sometimes offer advantages over those given in classic protocols. For instance, when the patient is unable to lie comfortably in a prone or supine position, it is usually possible to adapt the techniques for side-lying or sitting positions.

When using a side-lying position, the patient's head is supported on a pillow or bolster so that the cervical spine is maintained in neutral position. The head should not remain unsupported during the session nor should the patient attempt to support the head with an arm, as cervical and upper extremity musculature might become stressed and uncomfortable. This could lead to activation of trigger points as well as produce exacerbation of the current condition or discomfort in additional areas.

In a side-lying position, the lowermost leg (the one lying on the table) is kept fairly straight while the uppermost leg is flexed at the hip and knee, which brings it forward, where it is laid on a bolster or thick support pillow to maintain the leg

in a neutral sagittal plane. This positioning of the legs stabilizes the pelvis, discourages torsioning of the torso and protects the lumbar area while allowing considerable access to the shoulder region, lateral thorax, lateral hip and medial aspect of the thigh of the lower leg.

An example is offered here for treatment of serratus posterior superior, discussed elsewhere in this chapter in prone position. The tissue that lies deep to the medial edge of the scapula is often more easily and effectively accessed when the patient is placed in a side-lying position with the uppermost arm draped across the patient's chest (horizonal adduction) (Fig. 10.5). This allows the scapula to translate laterally on the torso (protract), thereby exposing considerably more subscapular region than in the prone position. The tendon attachment at the angle of the rib and the 'hidden' trigger point associated with this muscle are often much more accessible. This position is especially convenient to use when the patient is unable to reach behind the back as is necessary in the prone position.

Figure 10.5   Alternative positions for classic NMT routines can be adopted when needed. A side-lying posture horizontal adduction of the arm allows easy access to serratus posterior superior.

5. Apply gliding strokes in all directions between the scapulae while avoiding the spinous processes to treat several layers of muscles, including (from superficial to deep) trapezius, rhomboid major and minor, serratus posterior superior, erector spinae and possibly portions of the intercostal group.

Posterior cranium

The patient is prone.

Palpation and friction techniques can be carefully applied to the base of the occiput to assess the suboccipitals and overlying muscles. However, *caution* must be exercised to avoid deep friction to the rectus capitis posterior minor and to the vertebral artery, which lies relatively exposed in the suboccipital triangle. See Box 10.2.

1. The prone patient's chin is tucked slightly, in order to gently open the suboccipital space between the occiput and C1 (atlas). The fingers provide stability and support for the movements of the thumbs (Fig. 10.7). Transverse (medial/lateral) friction is applied in small increments from the mid-line to the mastoid process to assess the cranial attachments of the posterior cervical muscles. Static pressure may also be applied when trigger points are located in the suboccipital muscles or posterior cervical muscles lying

superficial to them, or when tissues are too tender to be frictioned. This suboccipital region is often involved in forward head posture and chronic headache patterns.

2. Use combination friction to examine the belly of the thin, flat, occipitalis muscle which is located about 1.5–2 inches lateral to the occipital protuberance. Movement of this muscle may be palpated on some individuals when the eyebrows are raised repeatedly, as it merges with the cranial aponeurosis and connects with the frontalis muscle. Trigger points in this muscle may refer strongly into the eye and into the frontal sinus area.[8]

Cervical lamina supine

The patient is supine.

1. Lubricate the lamina groove from the occiput to T1. The left hand lifts and supports the head. The fingers of the right hand lie across the back of the neck at the occipital ridge with the thumb placed next to the lateral surface of the spinous process of C1 (Fig. 10.8A). To achieve the best position, the forearm and hand should be fully supinated. Glide from C1 to T1 while simultaneously pressing toward the ceiling. Repeat the gliding movements five or six times, increasing pressure slightly with each repetition, if appropriate. The practitioner's elbow should remain low and the treating arm should remain in the same plane as the spine. Observe the head and neck extending slightly as the gliding movements of the thumb help to restore flexibility to the posterior cervical muscles.

2. Rotate the patient's head contralaterally (away from the side being treated). Move the right thumb laterally one thumb's width (about 1 inch) and repeat the gliding movements five or six times (Fig. 10.8B). The head and neck will not extend while gliding on the lateral strips. *Caution*: Extreme head rotation is not recommended, particularly for the elderly, as it

---

[8]The position 3 of NMT spinal sequence as described in Chapter 6 would effectively assess and treat these structures working from the head of the table.

Box 10.2   Precautions for vertebral artery

Three of the four suboccipital muscles (all except RCPMin) form the suboccipital triangle. The vertebral artery, which courses through the transverse processes of C1–C6, lies relatively exposed and vulnerable to injury (Fig. 10.6). When pressure or friction is applied to this region, the artery should be avoided especially when the tissues are placed on stretch. Knowing the location of the suboccipital triangle and the optimum angle to orient the treating digits is important to safe treatment in this area. It is suggested that direct contact with the artery be avoided in all manner when working in the upper cervical region and extreme head rotation, particularly with extension, should also be avoided.

In the last decade considerable concern has surfaced regarding safe application of manual techniques and the upper cervical unit. Points in the following discussion have been borrowed from a Powerpoint™ presentation titled *Cervical Spine Adjusting and the Vertebral Artery* produced by the Association of Chiropractic Colleges and posted to www.chirocolleges.org (last viewed online 8/2/09). It is with appreciation to those who prepared the material that the author of this chapter takes the liberty to include some of these as points of concern for all manual practitioners.

Approximately 10% of patients have some form of vertebral artery anomaly and compression of the artery is seen in 5% of patients in neutral position and the same in rotation. Of considerable concern is the development of a serious vertebral artery dissection (VAD). This can arise from minor or major traumas and, particularly in the vulnerable patient with pre-existing concerns, from trivial actions, such as painting, nose blowing, receiving a shampoo, vomiting, sneezing, and the application of certain manual therapy techniques.

Dissections arise from intimal tears, which produce an alteration of normal blood flow

through the artery, the creation of a thrombogenic environment, the formation of a thrombus and the potential generation of emboli. The incidence of VAD is of such significance that the provocative tests for vertebral artery competency (such as George's test or DeKlyne's test) are no longer considered to be safe nor effective screening tests.

In 2004, US chiropractic schools collectively agreed to abandon the teaching of and use of provocation tests for vertebral artery insufficiency. To this author's knowledge there are no reliable, safe tests to rule out a VAD in progress. So what is a practitioner to do? – Stop! Ask questions, listen, act and think.

Five 'Ds'	'And'	Three 'Ns'
Dizziness	Ataxia	Nausea
Drop attacks		Numbness
Diplopia		Nystagmus
Dysarthria		
Dysphagia		

If the patient shows any of the above symptoms pay attention, particularly following a cervical injury. Other symptoms of concern are slurred speech, giddiness, a change in voice pattern, lack of context in speech and inappropriate reactions to situations. Many patients present to manual therapists with these conditions. While it is possible to display these conditions without having a VAD, it is also important to search for them as clues to one in progress. One phrase that should be the strongest flag and should not be ignored is 'I have the worst pain in my head (or neck), unlike anything that I have ever experienced before.'

It is best to be conservative and rule out vertebral artery involvement rather than to ignore these symptoms since the consequences can be devastating.

---

may induce stress to the vertebral artery, which lies within the transverse processes.

3. Continue a series of caudad glides with the thumb, moving laterally in strips until the entire lamina groove has been treated (Fig. 10.8C). The treating thumb should remain posterior to the transverse processes. The muscles being treated include trapezius, semispinalis capitis, semispinalis cervicis, splenius capitis, splenius cervicis, levator scapula, rotatores and multifidus.
Caution: It is necessary to ensure that the gliding strokes remain posterior to the transverse processes (indicated in Fig. 10.8 by a dashed line) because the brachial plexus exits the vertebrae on the anterior aspect of the

Figure 10.6   Caution must be exercised when approaching the suboccipital triangle, where the vertebral artery lies relatively exposed and is vulmerable to injury. Reproduced with permission from Gray's Anatomy for Students (2005).

Figure 10.7   Attachments of several muscles may be treated at the base of the occiput.

transverse processes. The foraminal gutters, which cradle the nerves, are sharp and, if placed anteriorly, pressure from the gliding thumb could press the nerves against the sharp processes.

4. Return to any ischaemic bands or trigger points found and treat with static compression.[9]

Splenii tendons

The patient is supine.
   Caution: Use no pressure until the thumb is securely in place, as described below.
1. To treat the right-side splenius capitis, the patient is supine and the practitioner's right-hand fingers cup across the back of the neck like a shirt collar. Place the right thumb anterior to

---

[9]Lief's NMT would have accessed these areas alongside the cervical spine with the patient prone, in positions 1, 2, 3, 4 and 5 of the spinal sequence as described in Chapter 6. Direct strokes over the tips of the spinous processes are included in this sequence, but caution is suggested so that pressure remains light. The interspinous spaces commonly house trigger points, and the attachments to the spinous processes themselves may manifest as periosteal pain points, indicating a need for attention from the muscles that are producing the stress.

Figure 10.8A,B,C Gliding techniques may be applied to the cervical lamina from the occiput to the thorax as far laterally as the posterior aspect of the transverse processes.

the trapezius and posterior to the transverse processes, while pointing the thumb towards the patient's feet. Use the left hand to rotate the head towards the side being treated (Fig. 10.9A).

2. The right hand should rotate with the neck as if glued to the back of the neck, while the forearm and hand fully supinate. This rotation will open a 'pocket' anterior to the trapezius, allowing room for the thumb to slide into position. The thumb is angled towards the nipple of the opposite breast and is pressed lightly against the lateral surface of the spinous processes (Fig. 10.9B,C). This hand position will rotate the thumb so that the thumb pad faces toward the ceiling. Slide the right thumb into the 'pocket' formed by the trapezius. If the 'pocket' does not allow penetration of the thumb due to excessive tension, or if pressure of the thumb produces more than moderate discomfort, press lightly at the 'mouth' of the pocket until the tissues relax enough to allow the thumb to slide in further.

3. Apply pressure inferiormedially, toward the lateral surface of the spinous processes and simultaneously toward the ceiling for 8–12 seconds. The thumb will press into the tendons of the splenius capitis and splenius cervicis, as well as the deeper muscles (rotatores and multifidus). After the initial application of pressure, allow the tissues to rest for a few seconds and then press the thumb into the pocket a little deeper to repeat the manoeuvre. When the tissues prevent any further caudad movement of the thumb, mild to moderate static pressure that is sustained for a few seconds may produce more opening of the pocket and allow the thumb to slide a little further down the spinal column.

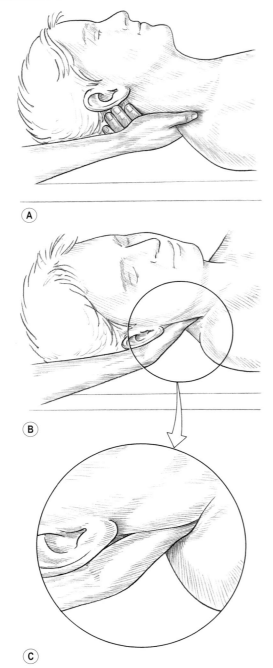

(A)

(B)

(C)

Figure 10.9A,B,C   Originally called the corkscrew technique by Dr Nimmo, treatment of the spleni tendons from C7–T4 is applied 'in the pocket' anterior to the trapezius. The thumb must remain posterior to the transverse processes, with an inferio-medial angle in order to reach the tendons.

4. If tender, repeat the entire process three or four times during a session. This step will usually help restore cervical rotation as well as reduce tilting pull on the transverse processes of C1–3. Trigger points in the splenii tendons can refer strongly into the eye, causing eye (pressure-like) discomfort. Practitioners should rule out glaucoma or other serious eye conditions as a cause of such discomfort, in addition to treating these tissues.

Sternocleidomastoid

The patient is supine.

The release of the SCM muscle is important because of its propensity to distract the head anteriorly. Compensating postural distortions relating to such forward head positions can include anterior rotation of the pelvis and changes in cervical, thoracic and/or lumbar curvature. The effects of compensations can have substantial impact on the body's centre of gravity and thereby, demand a cascade of compensations. Trigger points in SCM can cause severe eye pain, visual changes, temporomandibular joint pain, sore throat, ear pain, hearing loss and tinnitus, and can mimic migraine headaches.

1. Grasp the tendon of the non-lubricated SCM lightly between the thumb and first two fingers as close to the mastoid process as possible. Rotate the head toward the side being treated to rotate the SCM away from the carotid artery. Passively tilt (side-bend) the head toward the side being treated to grasp the SCM more easily and so lift it away from the deeper tissues (Fig. 10.10A). Both heads of the SCM can be grasped in the cephalad half of SCM, although they separate into two distinct bellies in the caudad half. A paper tissue or very thin cloth placed between the treating hand and the patient's skin may help to prevent slippage if the area is oily.
   Caution: If a pulse from the carotid artery is noted while compressing the SCM, release the muscle immediately and reposition the fingers to ensure the artery is not compressed.

(A)

(B)

(C)

Figure 10.10A,B,C Thorough treatment of the sternocleidomastoid often relieves symptoms associated with migraine headaches, temporomandibular joint dysfunction and hearing problems. (C) The medial border of the attachment of longissimus capitis and splenius capitis may be reached under the posterior aspect of the mastoid attachment of the SCM. The suboccipital triangle is avoided due to the location of the vertebral artery.

2. Compress the SCM for 8–12 (up to 20) seconds at 1-inch intervals from the mastoid process to the sternal and clavicular attachments. Each head can be treated separately. Medial to lateral friction may be used on the sternal and clavicular attachments (Fig. 10.10B).
3. Support the head at 45° of flexion and rotate it away from the side being treated. Glide caudally on the upper 1 inch of the mastoid attachment of the SCM, while being careful to avoid the styloid process located anterior to it. Do not glide further down the SCM as gliding pressure across the carotid sinus may stimulate baro-receptors, resulting in a rapid drop in the patient's blood pressure.
4. Place the thumb posterior to the SCM tendon at the mastoid process and displace the tendon anteriorly while simultaneously pressing onto the mastoid attachment of the longissimus capitis (erector spinae) and the splenius capitis. Use static pressure or combination friction to treat them (Fig. 10.10C).[10] Avoid encroaching into the suboccipital triangle where the vertebral artery courses.

Spinal lamina groove

The patient is prone.

Trigger points lying close to the lamina of the spinal column often refer pain across the back, wrapping around the rib-cage and/or anteriorly into the chest or abdomen, and frequently refer 'itching' patterns. Although a more complete protocol would be used, the treatment technique described below is particularly useful if scoliosis is evident as it addresses the many layers of muscular attachment to the posterior aspect of the spine.

1. Angle the bevelled tip of a pressure bar at 45° against the lateral surface of the spinous processes (Fig. 10.11A,B). Use caudad/cephalad friction at tip-width intervals from C7 to the coccyx on each side of the spine. Avoid pressing on the coccyx.
2. When moving the pressure bar, lift it and place it at the next site to avoid gliding it as the

---

[10]Lief's NMT would access and treat dysfunction in these structures with the patient prone, from positions 1, 2, 3 of the sequence described in Chapter 6.

(A)

(B)

(C)

Figure 10.11A,B,C   The bevelled tip of the pressure bar may
be used along the entire length of the spine and sacrum,
both in the lamina (A,B) and between the spinous processes
(C). The cervical region should not be treated with the tool.

bevelled tip may cause tissue irritation. Avoid
treating the cervical lamina with the pressure
bar as the cervical vertebrae are less stable than
those below C7. (See Cervical lamina supine
(above) for procedures used in the cervical
region.)

3. Friction may also be performed between
   spinous processes with the bevelled tip in
   order to treat interspinalis muscles and the
   supraspinous ligament (Fig. 10.11C).[11]

Intercostal muscles

The patient is treated in supine, side-lying and
prone positions in order to access as many of
the intercostal spaces as possible.

Caution: When use of the pressure bar as
described produces excessive discomfort, the tip
of an index finger should be substituted for
the pressure bar tip in the frictional work. Should
this procedure also produce moderate discomfort,
single-digit gliding strokes can be applied
repeatedly with the index finger in each intercostal space and the frictional work delayed until
a subsequent treatment session.

1. Place the bevelled tip of the pressure bar
   inferior to the clavicle of the supine patient,
   just lateral to the sternum, in the first palpable
   intercostal space (Fig. 10.12A). The bevelled
   tip should lie between the ribs and parallel
   with them. Using medial/lateral friction at
   each application site, move the bar laterally at
   tip intervals until just before the pectoralis
   minor is reached. Avoid pressure into
   pectoralis minor because of sensitive neural
   structures in the area.

2. Return to the sternum, move down one rib
   space and repeat the tip-width examination
   while using frictional pressure as described in
   step 1, until just before pectoralis minor is
   reached.

3. Avoid contact with breast tissue. When
   working around the breast, use the patient's
   hand to displace the breast away from the
   treatment site inferiorly, laterally, superiorly
   and medially, as appropriate, in order to

---

[11]Lief's spinal NMT application addresses these tissues with
thumb and/or finger contacts, as described in Chapter 6.

(A)

(B)

(C)

Figure 10.12A,B,C The bevelled tip of the pressure bar may be used at tip-width intervals throughout each intercostal space, especially on people with respiratory ailments. Avoid pressing on the brachial plexus or breast tissue. Friction with a fingertip (or a fingertip gliding stroke) should be substituted when tissue is excessively tender.

allow access for the pressure bar to treat the muscles that lie deep to the margins of the breast.

4. Continue the intercostal work as far caudad and laterally as possible. The patient can also be placed in a side-lying position, which allows access to the more lateral aspects of the intercostal spaces (Fig. 10.12B,C). Treatment is performed on each side of the thorax.

5. With the patient prone, place the pressure bar into the intercostal space lateral to the first thoracic vertebra. With the bevelled tip placed parallel to the ribs and in the rib space, use medial/lateral friction at tip-width intervals in the same manner as that applied on the anterior surface. Continue the treatment in all intercostal spaces as far caudad and laterally as possible.[12] Distinction of the rib spaces may be difficult in the upper posterior thorax where superficial tissue is thicker. The rib spaces will be more distinct in the lower posterior thorax, but caution should be exercised regarding pressure on the last two 'floating' ribs.

Iliolumbar ligament and sacroiliac ligament

1. The iliolumbar ligament attached the transverse process of L5 (and sometimes L4) to the crest and inner surface of the ilium. To contact the iliolumbar ligament most directly, the tip is placed lateral to the erector spinae and under that muscle's lateral edge. A cross-fibre movement is used with the bevelled tip while it is angled in this described manner in order to access the tissues anterior to the lateral edge of the erector spinae muscles (Fig. 10.13), which includes the iliolumbar ligament.

---

[12]Lief's NMT would access the intercostal spaces from the mid-axillary line to the spine, using fingertip pressure while treating the prone patient, as described in Chapter 6 (positions 4, 5, 6 and 7). Anterior intercostal evaluation and treatment would be performed as appropriate, with the patient supine as illustrated in Chapter 7 (lower intercostal only described and illustrated) relating to abdominal application of NMT. The same cautions discussed in the text in this chapter would be issued for manual as for pressure bar applications in the intercostal tissues.

Figure 10.13 The iliolumbar ligament can be treated with the bevelled pressure bar by wedging under the lateral edge of the erector spinae.

2. In order to treat the sacroiliac ligament using NMT, the bevelled tip of the pressure bar is placed at a 45° angle onto the lateral aspect of the sacral tubercles (Fig. 10.14A) with the edge of the bevelled tip being parallel to the tubercles. This position is similar to that previously described for the lamina groove. Commencing at the cephalad aspect of the sacrum, a cephalad/caudad frictional movement is introduced in order to examine the tissues that lie superficial to the sacrum. The pressure bar is then moved one tip-width caudad and the friction is repeated. This continues to the cephalad edge of the coccyx, which should not itself receive any treatment of this sort.

3. Returning to the sacral base, the pressure bar is applied into the soft tissues one tip-width lateral to the initial contact, at 90° to the surface (i.e. to the dorsum of the sacrum) (Fig. 10.14B). The procedure as above is then repeated until the coccyx is reached. In this way the entire sacral dorsal surface should be treated in 'strips'. No pressure should be applied onto the sacroiliac joint (SIJ) or to the tissues lateral to the border of the sacrum. A uniform pattern should be visible with no gaps between the prints left by the tip pressure applications. All the strips of prints should be parallel to the sacral tubercles until the last column, which will angle more diagonally along the medial aspect of the SIJ.

Erector spinae

The patient is prone.
1. The erector spinae muscles are lubricated from the level of C7 to the sacrum. The thumbs or palm are used to glide along this pathway

Figure 10.14A,B If not inflamed, the entire surface of the sacrum can be treated to address sacroiliac ligaments as well as multifidus and erector spinae attachments. Trigger points here will refer sciatica-like pain.

(C7 to sacrum) repeatedly, then alternating from side to side while gradually increasing pressure in order to relax and warm the tissues (Fig. 10.15A).

2. Standing at waist level with the forward foot at shoulder level and the back foot at waist level, face towards the head with knees slightly flexed. The olecranon process of the practitioner's table-side elbow is placed

against, but not onto, the spinous processes at the level of L5 (Fig. 10.15B). With a moderate pressure and speed, the entire length of the paraspinal tissues, including the erector spinae, receives the benefit of a glide from this contact. The pressure should be moderated when the thoracic region is being traversed. Modification of the angle of contact will be necessary when covering the erector spinae

Figure 10.15A,B,C   Long gliding strips, applied with the thumbs, palms, fists or forearm, lengthen thoracic fascia while treating several layers of muscle. When working near the spine, avoid pressing on spinous processes.

medial to the scapulae. Care should be taken not to apply pressure onto the spinous processes themselves (Fig. 10.15C). The stroke ceases at C7, and the thumbs are used in the cervical region.

3. Turn to face the feet. Apply forearm contact in a similar manner as described in step 2 to the erector spinae as a series of glides is performed from C7 to the iliac crest. No pressure should be applied in this way onto the iliac crest itself or the sacrum or spinous processes.

4. The thumbs, knuckles or large pressure bar may be used cautiously to cross-fibre the long tendons of the erectors; however, the spinous processes should not be involved in these contacts.[13]

Quadratus lumborum

The patient is prone.

1. After application of a lubricant, a glide up quadratus lumborum is made using both thumbs, from the crest of the ilium to the 12th rib. The initial contact remains just lateral to the erector spinae as four or five repetitious glides are applied to the medial aspect of the muscle (Fig. 10.16A). The thumbs are then placed approximately 1 inch laterally and the glides are repeated. A series of glides is then performed, in 'strips', moving laterally until the entire muscle has been treated. If necessary, by moving more laterally, the obliques can be treated as well.

2. While standing at chest level and facing the feet of the prone patient, glide caudad from the 12th rib to the crest of the ilium, ensuring that contact is lateral to the erector spinae. A series of glides moving laterally is then performed (Fig. 10.16B) in a manner similar to the upward glides discussed in step 1.

3. Facing the head, and with the fingers of the lateral hand moulded around the curve of the trunk and the thumb angled at 45° to the spine, the thumb is glided medially on the inferior surface of the 12th rib until it reaches the lateral aspect of the erector spinae. Apply static pressure or friction on posterior aspect of the transverse process of L1. In order to avoid trauma, no pressure should be applied onto the lateral aspect of the tip of the transverse process. Follow this with similar applications of friction or pressure onto the lumbar transverse processes at 1–2-inch intervals down to the level of L4 (Fig. 10.16C).[14]

Overview of differences

The key variations existing between the European (Lief's) and NMT American version™ – which emerge from these examples – seem to relate to a far more structured and prescriptive approach in American NMT, with a variety of additional 'tools' being used, including elbows and pressure bars. While Lief's version also has a (different) structured outline, it seems to require fewer 'strokes' or 'glides', while remaining in assessment mode until something is discovered that calls for therapeutic input. In therapeutic mode, the way in which tissues are addressed (ischaemic compression and frictional or cross-fibre methods) seems very similar to the American method, apart from the more restricted variety of contacts (European relies almost solely on finger or thumb contact).

NMT American version™ seems to move directly into a therapeutic 'glide' which has assessment potential, whereas Lief's approach separates assessment from therapeutic input more definitively. Both approaches have proven to be successful training systems for those who are learning NMT techniques as well as reliable clinical protocols, which can be used as primary modalities for treating chronic pain and soft tissue dysfunction.

---

[13]Lief's NMT attention to these same tissues forms a major element of the approach described in Chapter 6, most notably in relation to positions 3, 4, 5, 6, 7, 8 and 9 where thumb and/or finger strokes would be the main means of contact.

[14]Lief's NMT would access these tissues from positions 8 and 9 of the spinal application described in Chapter 6.

Figure 10.16A,B,C   The quadratus lumborum will be treated lateral to the erector spinae by gliding between the crest of the ilium and the last rib. Quadratus lumborum's transverse process attachments may be felt on some people just lateral to the erector spinae. L2 and L3 are palpable on most people. L1 and L4 may be more difficult to locate.

It is suggested that professional training be sought by those practitioners who want to practice NMT American version™ to help assure skill and safety. Although many of the steps can be learned through reading textbook descriptions, supervised training that includes performing and receiving the detailed routines is important. This method will help to develop skills that will be effective while also protecting both the patient and the practitioner.

References

Cailliet R: *Soft tissue pain and disability*, Philadelphia, 1977, FA Davis.

Chaitow L: *Soft tissue manipulation: a practitioner's guide to the diagnosis and treatment of soft tissue dysfunction and reflex activities*, Rochester, 1980, Healing Arts Press.

Chaitow L: *Modern neuromuscular techniques*, ed 1, Edinburgh, 1996, Churchill Livingstone.

Chaitow L: *Modern neuromuscular techniques*, ed 2, Edinburgh, 2003, Churchill Livingstone.

Chaitow L, DeLany J: *Clinical application of neuromuscular techniques*, vol. 1: *The upper body*, Edinburgh, 2000, Churchill Livingstone.

Chaitow L, DeLany J: *Clinical application of neuromuscular techniques*, vol. 1: *The upper body*, ed 2, Edinburgh, 2008, Churchill Livingstone.

Chaitow L, DeLany J: *Clinical application of neuromuscular techniques*, vol. 2: *The lower body*, Edinburgh, 2002, Churchill Livingstone.

DeLany J: *The roots and branches of neuromuscular therapy*, no. 11. Florida, 1999, American Massage Therapy Association, pp 16–17.

DeLany J: Connective tissue perspectives: introduction, *Journal of Bodywork and Movement Therapies* 4(4):273–275, 2000a.

DeLany J: Connective tissue perspectives: neuromuscular therapy, *Journal of Bodywork and Movement Therapies* 4(4):276–277, 2000b.

DeLany J: *Neuromuscular therapy: care of soft tissue pain and dysfunction. Applications pack*, St Petersburg, Florida, 2002, NMT Center.

Oschman JL: What is healing energy? Pt 5: gravity, structure, and emotions, *Journal of Bodywork and Movement Therapies* 1(5):307–308, 1997.

Simons D, Travell J, Simons L: *Myofascial pain and dysfunction: the trigger point manual*, vol. 1: *The upper body*, ed 2, Baltimore, 1999, Williams & Wilkins.

Stedman's electronic medical dictionary, 1998, Version 4.0. Online Available: http://www.stedmans.com.

Travell J, Simons D: *Myofascial pain and dysfunction: the trigger point manual*, vol. 1: *The upper body*, Baltimore, 1983, Williams & Wilkins.

Travell J, Simons D: *Myofascial pain and dysfunction: the trigger point manual*, vol. 2: *The lower body*, Baltimore, 1992, Williams & Wilkins.

Vannerson J, Nimmo R: Specificity and the law of facilitation in the nervous system. Reprinted in Schneider M, Cohen J, Laws S, 2001: *The collected writings of Nimmo & Vannerson, pioneers of chiropractic trigger point therapy*, Pittsburgh, Pennsylvania, 1971, Self-published.

www.chirocolleges.org: 2006, *Cervical spine adjusting and the vertebral artery*, Powerpoint™ presentation available online; last viewed 8/2/09.

Yates J: *Physiological effects of therapeutic massage and their application to treatment*, Vancouver, 1989, Massage Therapy Association of British Columbia.

Progressive inhibition of neuro-musculoskeletal structures (PINS) technique

11

Dennis J. Dowling

CHAPTER CONTENTS

Neuromuscular techniques   **247**
Background   **248**
Inhibition   **249**
Osteopathic point and/or pressure techniques   **251**
Strain/counterstrain   251
Facilitated positional release   252
Still technique   253
Functional technique   253
Additional osteopathic methods using palpated points   253
Non-osteopathic point and/or pressure systems   **254**
Progressive inhibition of neuromusculoskeletal structures (PINS) method   **254**
Procedure   255
Application   261
Possible mechanism of action   **268**
Contraindications and side-effects   **271**
Conclusion   **271**

Progressive inhibition of neuromusculoskeletal structures (PINS) is a manipulative medicine technique that, when properly utilized, can be included in the treatment regimen of patients with neuromusculoskeletal dysfunction. Knowledge of anatomy and neuromuscular physiology, as well as reliance on standard forms of palpatory diagnosis and treatment, are necessary.

As a variant of a technique known as 'inhibition', PINS bears some resemblance to other manual medicine techniques. The practitioner must determine any alteration of the related soft tissues due to dysfunction. Then he or she must gauge the direction and amount of treatment based on palpatory evaluation and patient feedback.

Initially, two related sensitive points are located. One is most commonly in the immediate region of the patient's symptoms, and the other is sometimes at the other end of a structure, such as a muscle, nerve, fascial link or ligament that is anatomically related. The practitioner exerts a mild amount of pressure progressively from one to the other.

Other similar techniques are also discussed. Some theoretical as well as selected practical applications are presented.

Neuromuscular techniques

Manipulative treatments have been used throughout history, although the aetiology of musculoskeletal dysfunction, as well as the processes by

Parts of this chapter that appear in the case study component were used in preparation for application to Fellowship of the American Academy of Osteopathy (FAAO).

which dysfunctions are maintained, have been poorly understood until recently. What is obvious to anyone who practises palpation is that the soft tissues, including the skin, muscles, fascia and ligaments, may be involved. Dysfunction of each of these result in, result from, or both in relation to other structures such as the joints, nerves and viscera. With knowledge of anatomy, separate hypertonic individual muscles, as well as groups of muscles, can usually be discerned in association with somatic dysfunction. While many skeletal muscles are capable of being activated by conscious initiation, many muscular actions operate via reflexive mechanisms.

Clinical experience shows that injured muscles may remain in a state of hyperresponsiveness, as evidenced by their hypertonicity, due to unconscious mechanisms that maintain them in a dysfunctional state. Looking past the usual concepts associated with intent and activity, attention most logically turns towards reflex activity as a maintaining factor. With the capability of being enhanced or inhibited by higher neurological functions, the stimuli that maintain undesirable hypertonicity operate at a spinal cord level. Often, a reflex that seems to be programmed for the purpose of protection is inappropriately maintained afterwards. Muscles innervated by segmental nerves may become activated consciously or reflexively. When the latter occurs, possibly following injury, there can be maintenance of a dysfunctional hypertonic state. The potential for the central nervous system to inhibit or eliminate such activity may have been overridden reflexively.

Understanding these patterns suggests that the process of manipulative treatment should involve more than the 'prodding', 'kneading' or 'folding-and-holding' of dysfunctional tissues. Through a combination of observation, assessment and diagnosis, the manipulative specialist may postulate the causes as well as the most appropriate treatment choices. Appreciation of the connection between the musculoskeletal and the neurological influences involved in somatic dysfunction allows for the therapeutic manual interventions that follow to be designated as neuromuscular techniques.

Many neuromuscular modalities have been developed. Some practitioners and physicians apply these in a narrow regional manner involving localized dysfunction. Others learn to apply the concepts and principles behind any particular technique more widely, involving global appreciation of the interactions between body regions and systems. Jones' strain/counterstrain system, for example, started as a form of treatment for low back pain in an individual patient (Jones et al 1995). It is almost certain that in treating low back pain, others had practised locating a local tender point and then holding the region until it dissipated. The crucial leap beyond these limitations occurred when Jones postulated the underlying principles involved, and then developed the practical methods that flowed from this hypothesis, to locate tender points throughout the body in a similar way. Similarly, as later discussion in this chapter will elaborate, understanding the basic principles involved in manual methods, such as applied pressure, allows for a variety of different methods of application, all of which are neuromusculoskeletal, by definition.

Background

Osteopathy has been practised since the late 1800s. Many osteopathic treatment modalities have been delineated and refined in the 100 or more years of the profession. Several are adaptations of other methods. There are many other modalities developed before or since in other related fields of manual medicine as well. Sometimes, the similarities are greater than the differences. Appropriate clinical selection of any one depends upon experience, skill, suitability, efficacy, ease of use and expected outcome. As a new technique, PINS is a variation of the technique known as inhibition.

Having suffered from headaches over 30 years ago, the author was frustrated with the treatments that were offered. Having little knowledge of anatomy, early attempts involved the application of pressure on various portions of his scalp. The related symptoms involved pain at and near the right eye, increased lacrimation (tearing), facial pain, nasal stuffiness and scalp pain. There were also suboccipital symptoms, which appeared to be distantly related to the periorbital pain. As the symptoms appeared to progress following a great deal of reading, eye strain was a typical initiating condition. Exposure to bright sunlight without the benefit of sunglasses could also precipitate the cephalgia. Each of the symptoms could occur independently and was worsened by stress.

By trial and error, manual pressure was exerted at several sensitive points. There appeared to be a temporary beneficial effect when any point was pressed singly, but sometimes, within seconds, secondary adjacent regions of the scalp developed pain. When these secondary points were likewise pressured, patterns seemed to appear.

Treatment of these patterns as a succession of points was the most successful approach – more so than addressing any individual point or pair of points. When similar symptoms of headache that developed in others were likewise treated, the results were equivalently successful.

Later, after beginning osteopathic medical education at the New York College of Osteopathic Medicine, the author began to integrate knowledge of osteopathic manipulative medicine theory along with clinical observations. As it was utilized more and more, and taught to others, the rationale as well as further expansion of use of this inhibitory technique beyond just headache was determined. During this exploration, similarities and differences were noted in relationship to other methods of 'point therapy'.

Inhibition

PINS is most closely related to the osteopathic modality of inhibition. According to the *Glossary of Osteopathic Terminology* (American Osteopathic Association 1998), inhibition is 'a term that describes steady pressure to soft tissues to effect relaxation and normalize reflex activity.' Inhibition, or this use of 'steady pressure to soft tissues', is perhaps one of the oldest methods of manual treatment, regardless of the name applied. Typically, inhibition is performed by pressing the fingers or other body parts at a constant mild-to-moderate amount of force on regions of persistent hypertonic muscle. Even though the patient may complain of pain or decreased function, the objective of the treatment is to decrease the tonicity of the muscles. The symptoms that the patient has are directly related to this increased dysfunctional muscular tone (Dowling & Scariati 2005).

Large superficial muscles are most easily identified in both the normal relaxed and hypertonic states. A series of regional muscles can be identified and treated in pairs or individually. The supine or prone positions may facilitate the process as the patient will not need to use some of these muscles for postural support of the trunk and neck. With the patient in the supine position, a muscle, such as the trapezius, can easily be located in the cervical, shoulder and upper thoracic regions. The body of the muscle can be grasped, pressed or pinched. A hypertonic muscle is usually found to be firmer, but not necessarily larger, than its counterpart on the other side. An initial response of the tissue to pressure may be an increase in tonus and perhaps sensitivity. Gradually, with sustained pressure, the structures relax.

Another consideration is the relationship between musculoskeletal structures and the underlying organs. The viscera receive innervation from the spinal cord via nerves that originate from the same segments as the nerves that service the more superficial structures. As the sympathetic chain lies just anterior to the rib heads, dysfunction of the vertebra may result in increased sympathetic activity, or stimulation, to the innervated visceral target organs and the segmental musculoskeletal region (Ehrenfeuchter 1997).

The sympathetic system is often referred to as the 'flight or fight' response mechanism. It allows for rapid response to perceived danger or injury. The organism's reactions are channelled towards self-preservation. The heart rate increases, pupils dilate, blood is shunted to the skeletal muscles and away from the internal organs, and the respiratory rate increases. Gastrointestinal activity, among other visceral concerns, effectively shuts down. This normal reaction to stresses becomes abnormal when it does not abate. Inhibition also has a specialized purpose in the thoracic region. In theory, constant pressure to an area, which is the source of increased sympathetic activity, will result in reduction of the autonomic activity.

Raised blood pressure, ischaemic changes, arrhythmias, tachycardias or myocardial infarction secondary to vasospasm of a congested coronary artery may result from the effect of the stimulation on a visceral organ such as the heart. Musculoskeletal response includes spasm, decreased circulation due to vasoconstriction, impaired drainage of waste products, sensitivity changes and trophic alterations. Acute responses to this activity are the same as those to any new injury: redness (rubor), pain (dolor), swelling (tumor), heat (calor) and decreased function (functio laesa) (Robbins et al 1984).

- The skin and subcutaneous tissue may have a 'doughy' consistency and the pain sharp and throbbing.
- As the state persists without relief, the alterations reflect the chronicity of the dysfunction. Muscles and the surrounding fascia become more fibrotic ('ropy').
- The skin responds to the chronicity of the dysfunction by becoming thinner, paler and cooler.
- Pain responses may be more variable from insensitivity ('anaesthetic') to altered sensitivity ('paraesthesia') to hypersensitivity.

External pressure, such as is provided by inhibition, may initially result in a transitory increase in spasm or sensitivity. However, subsequent reduction of some or all of these components can be readily appreciated. Research regarding the visceral responses has indicated reduction of the undesirable autonomic responses (Hermann 1965). However, the persistence may be more dependent on the aetiology. If the visceral organ's structure or function were somehow altered, either primarily or secondarily, then the benefits of surface inhibition might be short lived. The more observable musculoskeletal signs and symptoms might represent a viscerosomatic reflex. When a musculoskeletal injury is the origin, a somatovisceral reflex may occur. Manipulative treatment of the musculoskeletal structures may result in a more persistent reduction of all elements.

In the suboccipital and sacral regions, the intention switches from the sympathetic half of the autonomic system towards resetting parasympathetic activity, the other half of the autonomic nervous system. Rather than being reactive to external danger such as the sympathetic system, the parasympathetics comprise nerves affecting the modifying reconstructive processes. Upgrading of parasympathetic activity coordinates increased gastrointestinal motility, decreased sphincter closure, reduction of heart rate, constriction of pupils, and sleepiness, to name just a few of the reactions.

Parasympathetic fibres travel only to the head and trunk, not to the extremities. Any region that has a visceral organ will have parasympathetic innervation. Although there are other cranial nerves (III, V, VII and IX) with some parasympathetic fibres, the vagus nerve (cranial nerve X) is the major influence to the head, neck, and thoracic and abdominal cavities. The origin of the vagus nerve is in the upper spinal cord and lower brainstem. The pelvic organs and the terminal portions of the gastrointestinal system are influenced by branches of nerves originating from the terminus of the spinal cord and exiting from foramen in the sacrum (S2, S3 and S4). The parasympathetic centres also receive sensory information from the target organs.

Persistent conditions such as nausea, vomiting, diarrhoea, dysmenorrhoea and dyspepsia are parasympathetic in nature. Dysfunction of the upper cervical, occipital and sacral regions may reflect or result in inappropriate parasympathetic activity. Inhibitory treatment results in reduction of the more superficial representation (increased musculoskeletal tone and congestion) and theoretically downregulates the more internal mechanisms. A thorough understanding of the structure and function of all of the factors related to dysfunction should guide accurate treatment.

Andrew Taylor Still first developed the concepts of osteopathy in 1874. An American medical practitioner primarily trained through apprenticeship with his father, a Methodist missionary and itinerant practitioner, Dr. Still practised what could be called conventional medicine until he suffered personal loss as a result of its inadequacy. Despite calling in other practitioners to assist, he watched as members of his family succumbed to meningitis. Realizing that the approaches utilized in the 'heroic' era of medicine, which were the primary tools of the allopathic profession at that time, were often more dangerous than the diseases they were meant to combat, and seeking other means, Still began using manipulative treatments. He found these were quite effective in managing or facilitating his patients' health.

Theorizing that the body was a unit, structure and function were interrelated, and the body had the ability to heal and defend itself, he set about reorganizing medical theory. In 1892, he established the first school of osteopathy in Kirksville, Missouri. As a rural institution, osteopathy spread slowly and experienced much prejudice. In the United States, there are currently 26 medical schools of osteopathy and approximately 66 000 osteopathic practitioners with full medical practice rights. Brought to England at the turn of the century by J. Martin Littlejohn, osteopathy spread to the rest of Europe, and the Empire (now Commonwealth).

The origins of some of Still's treatments apparently predate his professional separation from his allopathic colleagues. When he was a young man suffering from chronic headaches, Still treated himself with a rope-swing. He lowered the rope to a few inches above the ground and slung a blanket across it. Lying on the ground, he positioned himself with the contraption supporting his neck at the base of the skull, and subsequently fell asleep. He awakened refreshed and pain-free. This method may represent inhibition as well as a positional intervention (Still 1908). Some descriptions of both inhibition and stimulation methods were included in Still's early writings (Still 1902).

Some of Still's early students likewise described inhibitory techniques as well as their rationale. Eduard Goetz, one of Still's earliest students, described and illustrated inhibition for various conditions, both somatic and visceral, in his book *A Manual of Osteopathy* (Goetz 1905). Selected photographs in this small handbook clearly demonstrate and detail inhibitory treatment of several regions. Two such areas are the orbital and suboccipital regions of the head. In one such approach, pressure is applied individually to each of these areas for a few minutes.

Dain L. Tasker delivers a more extensive description in *Principles of Osteopathy* (Tasker 1916). Tasker describes a rationale as to the effectiveness of inhibition and that it is a natural phenomenon. Activities such as defecation and urination could not come under conscious and unconscious control without the ability of the individual to perform inhibition. In discussing the ability of externally applied inhibitory pressure, applied by a practitioner of manual medicine, to lessen hyperactivity, Tasker states that it is not the palpation itself but the initiation or alteration of the reflex arc that occurs. Observation reveals that placing a pressure should be a form of stimulation because it is impacting on the soft tissue. The effect of inhibitory pressure is to produce neural resetting of tone, modification of the dysfunction, and a beneficial modulation of distant or deeper reflexively linked structures. In citing Hilton's law 'that the skin, muscles and synovial membrane of a joint, or the skin, muscles of the abdomen and contents covered by peritoneum, are innervated from the same segment of the cord', Tasker states that the 'over-stimulation' caused by inhibition brings about a diminution or elimination of the overreactivity.

Osteopathic point and/or pressure techniques

Strain/counterstrain (see also p. 196)

Several passive direct and indirect systems of osteopathic treatment of somatic dysfunction exist. Standard points and diagnoses are used as fulcrums, or monitoring locations, in practically all. Monitoring by constant palpation at the points allows both practitioner and patient to experience feedback as to the success of the treatment when performing Jones' strain/counterstrain treatment (Glover & Yates 1997, Jones 1981, Jones et al 1995).

The practitioner determines a tender point, such as those that have been identified and mapped by Laurence Jones and his followers. The pressure on the point is designed to create a mild degree of discomfort, which the patient reports on as the tissues are positioned to remove the discomfort. The positioning of the region or the whole patient into a direction of ease is the actual therapeutic intervention. Although the diagnostic points are named for spinal segments, bony landmarks, ligaments or muscles, it appears that the treatment positions bring about shortening, and therefore relaxation of the muscles and ligaments.

In theory, during the period spent in a position of ease, muscle spindle resetting occurs. The muscle spindle apparatus is a sensory organ embedded into the larger muscle. Small, almost primitive, fibres exist in parallel within the larger extrafusal muscle. Two distinct shapes of the muscular fibres, as well as two of the sensory ends of the nerve fibres, exist. The nuclear bag muscle spindle fibre has all the nuclei collected in the centre. Nuclear chain fibres have the nuclei set almost in line. The primary type of sensory fibres to the nuclear bag appear almost like a coiled spring, and are termed annulospiral. The descriptive name 'flower spray' is applied to the endings of the fibres that primarily service the nuclear bag fibres. The muscle spindle fibres, unlike the other large extrafusal muscle fibres, do not have a great deal of contractile ability.

The sensory nerves to these intrafusal spindle fibres are stimulated by stretch of any kind. The annulospiral is more responsive to rate of stretch, and the other to constant stretch. This assists in the regulation of muscle tonicity as stretch brings about reflexive muscular contraction. Ordinarily, this is short in duration and recovery is quick. Sometimes, the reflex persists longer than is appropriate. The signals from the spindle continue as if the tissue were being stretched too rapidly, or overstretched, even though the length may be normal.

Increased neural activity is evidenced by increased sensitivity of a 'tender point'. Applied pressure elicits a report of tenderness. The positioning process during application of strain/counterstrain technique shortens the whole muscle, allowing the spindle reflex mechanism to be reset. The position that relieves the tenderness in the palpated point is typically held for 90 seconds and is then slowly returned to neutral. When successful, the previously hypertonic muscles relax and the sensitivity disappears.

Facilitated positional release

Facilitated positional release (FPR) (Schiowitz 1997) is similar in many respects to strain/counterstrain. It differs in its use of an activating force, usually compression or torsion, after initially positioning the region in neutral (ease). By comparison, strain/counterstrain is a form of positional release, whereas FPR utilizes an additional facilitating force. As with most manipulative techniques, the efficacy is directly proportional to the accuracy of diagnosis. The diagnosis includes relative motion freedom in the sagittal plane (flexion/extension), coronal plane (lateral flexion/abduction/adduction) and horizontal plane (rotation). Any increase in tissue tension in the surrounding tissue is also noted by means of palpation.

Initially, at least with spinal dysfunctions, the region is brought into a neutral position relative to the sagittal (anterior–posterior) plane. The lordosis of the cervical spine and the kyphosis of the thoracic spine are flattened. The practitioner then further brings the somatic dysfunction into the directions of relative ease. A facilitating force, usually compression and/or torsion, follows this. Release of the dysfunction and localized tension is noted almost immediately, as shown by the practitioner's monitoring finger.

Both strain/counterstrain and FPR theoretically utilize the same neurophysiological mechanism. However, because of an inverse myotactic reflex caused by the facilitating force, a release occurs within seconds instead of in 1.5 minutes. The muscle spindle has a specialized motor nerve known as the *gamma* motor neuron. Even though the nuclear chain and bag fibres are weakly contractile, increased *gamma* activity causes the ends to contract and the central regions become stretched. Regardless of whether the whole muscle is stretched or not, the spindle will react as if it were. The reaction results in overall protective contraction. The *gamma* gain, as it is known, tends to persist longer than is necessary and is modified by many factors including stress, pain, anxiety, endocrine alterations, medications and food substances. FPR, with its initial manoeuvres to flatten curves and adding a facilitating force, addresses the *gamma* activity component as well as the spindle stretch response. Diagnosis for FPR is less reliant on the localization of a tender point, but when such a point is found it is used solely for the purpose of monitoring.

Still technique

The recently described Still technique (van Buskirk 1996) shares many similar applications with these two previously described techniques. Richard van Buskirk attributes the writings of Charles Hazzard (Hazzard 1905), as well as those of Still himself, as the sources for the method. The descriptions revolve around the palpatory diagnosis of dysfunctions followed by motion into the directions of freedom/ease, and finally by movement past the neutral point into the barrier directions. A low-velocity, relatively low-amplitude articulatory movement towards the barriers follows positional treatment and the utilization of forces into the directions of ease (freedoms).

Functional technique

Functional technique (Johnston 1997) utilizes the diagnostic tender points to define the somatic dysfunction that exists at that level relative to the two adjoining vertebrae, the one above and the one below. Detection is typically made by percussion testing to scan and screen the regions. Once an anomaly is determined, the practitioner tests the dysfunction more specifically. The practitioner guides the region into a compound position of freedom ('ease', comfort) along various axes. Fine tuning to achieve release of the dysfunction includes side-bending and lateral translation, flexion/extension together with anterior or posterior translation, as well as rotation combined with compression or distraction. Breathing is then held in either exhalation or inhalation, dependent upon which phase is associated with greatest sense of tissue freedom.

Additional osteopathic methods using palpated points

Monitoring points as sites where some form of pressure is exerted to relieve dysfunction is used in other osteopathic techniques. The intent goes beyond monitoring.

Elaine Wallace developed Torque unwinding (Dowling 2005) and has taught this on a limited basis. She advises that the body can be imagined as a collection of adjacent or overlapping cubes. Injuries place forces into a whole 'cube'. Even though the vector force may be straight initially, after entry into the complex body it rarely remains so fixed. The pathway, because of bodily composition, motion or twists, becomes arced or more twisted. The tissues, especially the fascia, maintain memory for these injurious forces. The practitioner's fingers direct rhythmic, balancing, pressures centrally from two opposing cube faces. Placed on the contralateral sides of the head, trunk or extremity, the therapeutic forces negate the residual traumatic ones. A light percussive test on one side that is monitored on the other yields a sense of resonance that confirms the correct selection of the connected points.

Osteopathic literature is filled with many other variations of myofascial or fascial release techniques (Chila 1997, Ward 1997) that utilize point contacts as references, contact points and/or diagnostic reflections. Steven Typaldos (1994) has written about trigger band technique – a method intended to change the pathological cross-linkages of fascial bands. Using an instrument or fingers, the practitioner exerts significant pressure along certain connective pathways. This occurs along involved tissue in a basically linear fashion from an area of relative dysfunction towards the more involved region. Leon Chaitow (Chaitow 1980, 1996) describes the development of neuromuscular technique by two of his relatives, Stanley Lief and Boris Chaitow. Consisting mostly of point localization, reflected dysfunctions are treated by pressure followed by deep stroking and/or rolling of the tissue.

Standardized patterns of Chapman's point treatment (Owens 1937) reflect a neurological/endocrine/lymphatic internal alteration to the surface. The palpatory finding has been described as a lenticular (bean-shaped) subcutaneous structure. Although they may not be tender or sensitive to pressure, clinical correlation should raise suspicion either to locate Chapman's points or possibly to search for a latent visceral correlate. Apparently developed independently, some of the specific points are similar to those of acupuncture. Circular pressures are applied rhythmically by the pad of the manipulator's finger(s) to the nodular findings that are related to visceral conditions.

Non-osteopathic point and/or pressure systems

There are some similarities between typical inhibition technique and some other manual medicine systems of treatment. These include the Cyriax method (Cyriax 1959), trigger point therapy (Chaitow 1990, Travell & Simons 1983), acupressure (Kenyon 1988, Cerney 1974), reflexology, rolfing and shiatsu (Schultz 1976, Weil 1995). Some of the common elements include the practitioner providing the treatment by pressing the patient's soft tissue with the intent of bringing about a persistent alteration. Another similarity is the reliance upon a system of diagnosis and/or treatment points.

James Cyriax was most noted as a medical orthopaedist who practised joint mobilization and massage. He discussed the use of a 'pinching' technique on several locations (Cyriax 1959). The end goal was relaxation and stretching of tissue, as well as a relative hyperaemia. Triggerpoint therapy, developed by Janet Travell, recognizes the relationship between a remote referral point and a damaged myofascial nexus. Manual pressure can be used, but more commonly dry needling, vapocoolant spray, or a combination of anaesthetic and/or steroid agents are injected into the trigger point. By these means the practitioner locates and interrupts the aberrant patterns. Regardless of the method, theoretically restricted soft tissue is released by means of deep pressure applied to the selected points. Another manual version of the triggerpoint concept, Bonnie Prudden myotherapy, consists of primary points, as well as satellite points. Both are treated for short intervals several times a day over several sessions (Burton Goldberg Group 1994, Prudden 1980). After the treatment, stretching is also incorporated.

Like the better-known acupuncture, acupressure utilizes similar surface points that represent reflections of visceral changes. Traditional Oriental concept meridians align the specific point locations. Generally, one or two points are treated at any given time and the technique generally involves the application of pressure as well as circular motions.

Injured in a horse-riding accident as a young girl and treated by an osteopathic practitioner, Ida Rolf developed the eponymous system, Rolfing (Burton Goldberg Group 1994). She proposed utilizing deeply applied pressure on regions of the body as the tool to re-establish symmetry and more normal function. The actual force of deeply applied pressure used in this modality exceeds that which is commonly applied in inhibition. Some initial discomfort to the patient usually results. There is a great deal of emphasis placed on approximating ideal symmetry and alignment. Modifications to this basic theme were made by followers of Rolf, and integrated into other modalities involving movement patterns (Hellerwork, Aston-patterning).

One of the oldest forms of manual therapy, shiatsu, usually involves relatively heavier pressures applied for short intervals. Increases in 'the circulation of vital energy' (Schultz 1976) are reflected by a reduction of the tissue tension. The amount of force, especially in the hands of a traditional practitioner, is intense and brief (10 lb for 10 seconds), as opposed to the lower, steady and unrelenting force used in inhibition. Specific conditions dictate the sequencing of points based on energy flows throughout the body. Some points are adjacent, and others are quite distant to the primary location.

Reflexology correlates treatment points with certain visceral organs that are hypothesized as reflecting onto resonant areas located on the hands, feet and ears. In theory, the name has more to do with the functional contribution to the integrity or energy component of the organ than to the actual physical structure.

Progressive inhibition of neuromusculoskeletal structures (PINS) method

There is no doubt that practically all modalities of manual pressure treatment have merit, given the appropriate circumstances. PINS shares some commonality with several of these, including the localization of points and the application of pressure. The PINS system allows for versatility that is based on the practitioner's ability to utilize anatomical and clinical knowledge to determine treatment. A thorough knowledge of the typical and variant courses of nerves, fascial bands and muscles must be augmented by clinical decision-making skills for efficacy and accuracy. Treatment of contiguous muscles, which is modified by an understanding of 'watershed' areas of innervation (the overlapping zones where more than one nerve can be contributing to sensory and motor innervation), leads to the sequencing of PINS treatment.

Anyone can locate a sensitive point in the region of a patient's chief complaint. The practitioner must also be fully aware of anatomically normal, as well as variable, connections. For example, shoulder pain invites attention to the glenohumeral joint, and when treatment is successful, as evidenced by increasing mobility and decreasing discomfort, investigation can end. However, when localized attention is unsuccessful, more of the same treatment is not the answer. This will prove frustrating to both the patient and the practitioner. Restriction of motion of the shoulder into flexion, abduction and external rotation, as well as reduction of scapulothoracic motion, should instigate further investigation. For example, latissimus dorsi muscle, originating from the mid to lower back and attaching at the bicipital groove of the humerus, would merit assessment. Expanding the focus, in this example, might also incorporate treatment of the upper ribs, pectoralis muscles, lower cervical spine, clavicle, thoracic spine, lumbar spine, pelvis and lower extremity. Fascial planes – and therefore fascial stresses – overlap and influence one another.

In PINS, patients participate in the treatment by describing the amount of pain or other sensitivity. As the treatment proceeds, changes that occur, as well as the comparison of symptom intensity, are evaluated. Frequently, PINS is not the only treatment modality employed. It can be used before or after other methods of treatment, manipulative or otherwise.

Procedure

The development of an appropriate and specific diagnostic and treatment protocol using PINS requires:

1. In examining the patient, any relationship between the presenting symptoms, somatic dysfunctions and soft tissue findings should be determined.
2. The components comprising a somatic dysfunction must be determined. The mnemonic 'S-T-A-R' (Dowling 1998) can be used to track the different aspects:

    S – *Sensitivity* changes are the patient's subjective experiences in response to the palpation performed by the practitioner at the sites of dysfunction. These sensations include tenderness, numbness, radiation, warmth, irritation, throbbing, etc.

    T – *Tissue texture changes* are the soft tissue conditions as found by palpation by the practitioner. They can be *chronic* (prolonged blanching of the skin, ropy or fibrous texture of the muscles and fascia, coolness, dryness, vascular changes) or *acute* (increased redness, swelling and oedema, moist and/or increased temperature). The findings may worsen with palpation, to a slight degree.

    A – *Asymmetry* is the utilization of the non-dysfunctional side of the patient in comparison with the dysfunctional side. An area of dysfunction should be compared to the analogous structure on the other side of the body. An imaginary line down the middle of the body should reveal an almost mirrored ideal functional symmetry of one side to the other in a non-dysfunctional person.

    R – *Restriction of motion* is the most important determinant of dysfunction, especially when motion testing demonstrates asymmetry. The restriction can be by quantity (number of degrees of motion) and quality (stiffness, tremors, cogwheel rigidity, extraneous movement, etc.). Although one or more elements may be present, and the patient may or may not complain of a decrease in available motion, abnormal movement is perhaps the most sensitive and specific determinant of somatic dysfunction (see also p. 196).

3. Complaints of pain can be deceptive and may actually not help in the localization of the patient's true problem. They are, however, a very good indication that there is a problem. Often, spasmed muscles on one side may be relatively pain free while the contralateral muscles that are being stretched are more 'attention seeking'. Exclusive attention to the symptoms may distract treatment from the more needy locations. Pain, or any other symptom, suggests that there is a problem, although the site of pain may or may not correlate with the site of dysfunction.

4. A 'primary sensitive' point is determined by examination of the tissue in the region of the patient's complaint. If a significant one is not found, the practitioner utilizes knowledge of anatomical relationships and widens the search to contiguous areas.

5. Using knowledge of anatomical structures, another point, designated as the 'end point', is located distal or proximal to the primary point. Knowledge and understanding of muscle and ligamentous origins and insertions is a good beginning concept in determining this pair of points. If the primary point is at the origin, the end point may be at the insertion. The reverse can also be true.

   Sometimes the primary point is located in the belly of the muscle. In that case, exploration of both ends of the attachments to bone may reveal the location of an end point. Ligaments, which are generally shorter and more fibrous, have points that are probably also fairly close to one another. Fascia encompasses all structures, and the path between one point and another may seem to traverse other structures. Generally, the more specialized the fascia, the more palpable and tendinous it is.

   Tracing superficial and deep pathways of nerves is useful when determining paths that do not correlate with the other structures. Primary and end points may be found where a nerve passes out of a foramen, between or through muscles, or over and around bony protrusions. Sometimes, if more than one nerve innervates a region, the primary point can be found at the beginning of one nerve and the end point at the beginning of the other. In the case of nerve distribution of an extremity, one point will be found closer to the body while the other will be closer to the end of the extremity.

   There is no substitution for an excellent working knowledge of functional anatomy. Regardless of the aetiology, the chosen primary point will most probably be near to the patient's symptoms. The end point may also elicit symptoms, but to a lesser extent. As the two ends of the same problem, both (and all intervening) points must be addressed. In any case, the practitioner makes the determination of the two ends of the pattern. Sometimes the clue for the practitioner is that the patient relates what appears to them as unrelated complaints. Assuming patient knowledge of anatomy is small, it is left to the practitioner to draw the conclusions necessary to begin treatment. For the purpose of proceeding in a logical fashion, the point that is more sensitive is designated as the initial 'primary'. The other point, which is found distant from it but on a related structure that links the points, is considered as the 'end point'.

   A few examples of primary and end points are shown in Table 11.1.

6. Conceptually, a muscular, fascial and/or neurological pathway is drawn between the primary sensitive point and the end point. The line may be curved rather than straight. The direction of treatment may be from distal to proximal, or vice versa.

7. The physical connection between the two points may involve:

   (a) Nerve innervation:
      (i) Direct connections (The connection of a point near the medial epicondyle at the elbow to a point along the medial arm near the wrist – ulnar nerve.)
      (ii) Overlap or 'watershed regions' of innervation – The ophthalmic division of the trigeminal nerve travels from

Table 11.1 Examples of primary and end points

Primary point	End point	Connection
Supraorbital notch	Suboccipital region	Frontalis–occipitalis muscles
		Trigeminal–greater occipital nerves
Medial elbow epicondyle	Scaphoid wrist region	Flexor carpi radialis muscle
	Pisiform at wrist	Ulnar nerve
Greater trochanter of femur	Fibular head	Iliotibial band
Sternum at 2nd rib	Upper humerus	Pectoralis major
Temporomandibular joint	Side of head	Temporalis muscle
Gluteal region	Greater trochanter	Piriformis muscle
	Popliteal region	Sciatic nerve
Xiphoid process	Public ramus	Rectus abdominis
Maxillary	Angle of mouth	Trigeminal nerve
Temporomandibular joint	Maxillary region	Facial nerve

the supraorbital notch over the frontal region and to the top of the head. The greater occipital nerve exits the suboccipal region in the occipital sulcus and travels over the occiput to the top of the head. Rather than have a region of nerve-free scalp, there is an area at the top of the head that is innervated by both the trigeminal and greater occipital nerves.

(b) Muscle origins and insertions
   (i) Typical – A sensitive point may be found at the medial aspect of the clavicle and another at the mastoid process representing involvement of the sternocleidomastoid muscle.
   (ii) Overlap – The location of a sensitive point medial to the scapula and another in the upper cervical spine might represent splenii, levator scapula and/or trapezius muscles.
   (iii) Contiguity – The tensor fascia lata and iliotibial band actually form a continuity for two possible tender points located, respectively, at the greater trochanter and the fibular head. If a terminal point were actually found near the lateral malleolus instead of the fibular head, there might be a tensor fascia lata, iliotibial band, peroneal muscle connection.

(c) *Fascia* (see Ch. 1; Figs 1.3, 1.4)
   (i) The interosseous ligaments are actually specialized fascia connecting the radius and ulna in the arm, in the same way that the fibula and tibia are connected. These ligaments should be suspected when the pattern appears to overlie their locations. When analysing the line of connection between the two points, there may be no obvious neural, muscular or other ligamentous analogues. For the lower extremity, the symptoms may be of 'shin splints' where forearm symptoms may appear radicular without involving the hand.
   (ii) Septa – Although it contains muscular components to a greater extent, the central tendon and crus of the thoracoabdominal diaphragm are fascial in nature. The diaphragm supports the thoracic viscera, and separates the thoracic and abdominal cavities. Points found around the lower costal cartilage, the 12th rib and T10–T12 may represent a diaphragmatic involvement.
   (iii) Overlaps – The common fascia in the lumbar region acts as an attachment for muscles such as the latissimus dorsi and overlaps muscles such as

the quadratus lumborum, iliocostalis and other erector spinae muscles. Points may be found anywhere within the region and may extend to the lateral edge of the 12th rib (quadratus lumborum) or even to the bicipital groove of the humerus (latissimus dorsi).

(d) Ligamentous attachments

(i) Typical – Points can be found at the attachments of either end of the collateral ligaments in the elbow and knee.

(ii) Relationships to muscles – Surface of the points found on the superior C7 spinous process and the base of the occiput may represent spinalis muscles or the nuchal ligament.

(iii) Relationships to nerves – The flexor retinaculum and palmar aponeurosis are key components to treat when the median nerve in the forearm is involved. There may actually be a need to treat the articular relationships of the four carpal attachments (pisiform, hamate, scaphoid and trapezium) of the retinaculum as well.

(e) *Bones* – Although the bones are the deepest of the musculoskeletal structures, they and their components should be considered as connective tissue as well.

(i) Construction of joints – The joint capsules represent encompassing connections of two or more bones. At joints such as the elbow and the knee, the capsules are stronger and reinforced on their medial and lateral surfaces by collateral ligaments. The anterior and posterior surfaces tend to be more flaccid in one direction of motion or the other. Points may occur in the middle of the capsule and at the bony attachments.

(ii) Lever action – The mechanical activity of the bones is more of a concern for the analysis of the

aetiology of strains and somatic dysfunctions. The bony prominences are relatively strong extensions of the bones. Muscle tendons and ligaments attach to bone and, as a result of frequent usage, lead to the development of enlargements including tubercles, trochanters and other processes. Points theoretically located at tendinous insertions may also represent a contribution from the periosteal anchors.

8. Both the primary point and the end point are pressed simultaneously using the pad region of a finger on each hand (for the sake of simplicity the practitioner can identify the primary point as the 'first point' for the patient). The pressure exerted is a few ounces, enough to elicit the patient's symptoms, and should be of equal degree on both points. The patient may experience a mild to moderate increase in sensitivity. The practitioner should also determine the soft tissue response to pressure by sensing changes in the tissues:

(a) Dysfunctions that are acute may be more sensitive than chronic ones. A muscle that has been hypertonic will usually be more sensitive to pressure than the same muscle on the contralateral side.

(b) Muscles that are used excessively will hypertrophy and be bulkier than their contralateral pairs.

Larger muscles do not necessarily indicate dysfunction. When muscles have been subjected to increased usage or there is preference to one side being used more, such as in sports activities that preferentially utilize muscles in an asymmetrical manner (e.g. bowling, archery), the dominant side will typically be larger, but not necessarily dysfunctional.

Whether dysfunctional or not, hypertonic muscles that have been so for some time may not be quite so sensitive to pressure. This may be due to the chronicity of usage. A more sensitive, but less hypertonic, muscle indicates a problem. This does not necessarily indicate the laterality of the problem. Both sides can be dysfunctional. One may be more symptomatic than the other, but to varying degrees. Given a choice of examined findings versus symptoms, the findings take precedence. The practitioner should initially treat the more dysfunctional tissue, re-examine, and treat the less involved side as well.

(c) Whenever possible, the patient should be in a comfortable position, which generally means one where the muscle is not actively being utilized. Because postural muscles do not fully relax while the patient is seated or standing, a supine or prone position is preferred.

(d) The pressure exerted on both the primary point and the end point should be equal:

(i) Patients may assume that the more sensitive location is receiving more pressure. They should be reassured that the reason for the asymmetrical degree of sensitivity is because of the dysfunctional state of the involved tissue.

(ii) Occasionally, patients will direct the practitioner to apply greater pressure. Increased pressure does not accelerate the treatment. It is not necessary to increase the pressure, and doing so may be counterproductive.

(iii) Pain or tenderness may not be the only sensations experienced as a result of the applied pressure. The chronic nature of some dysfunctions may result in the patient reporting other sensations such as paraesthesia, which may occur alone or in combination with pain.

(e) Maintain constant pressure on the end point throughout the treatment (this can be identified as the 'end point' or 'final point' for the patient).

9. Initiate pressure on the point that produces the greatest sensitivity (primary point). A series of points will be located for application of inhibitory pressure between this 'primary' (i.e. the more sensitive) point and the end point during the course of the treatment.

10. Request that the patient report the initial amount and type of sensitivity. Feedback should be given if the sensation at any sensitive point decreases or increases. When inhibition is utilized properly, the sensitivity will usually have a transient initial increase followed by a typical subsequent decrease in sensitivity as the tissue accommodates to the irritation of the inhibition. Ultimately sensitivity may disappear totally. The duration can vary from several seconds to minutes.

11. The practitioner maintains simultaneous contact with the two points for 20–30 seconds and then seeks another point:

(a) A finger of the same hand that has a finger applying pressure to the primary point is used to locate a 'secondary point'. If the index finger is on the primary point, then the middle finger can be used to palpate for the secondary point.

(b) Usually the secondary point will be approximately 2–3 cm (approximately 1 inch) away from the primary point in the direction of the end point. (The practitioner can identify the secondary point as the 'second point' for the patient.) This will typically follow the predicted course of an anatomical structure (innervating nerve, along the direction of the muscle fibres, or following fascial planes).

12. Equal pressure is exerted onto both the primary and secondary points while maintaining pressure on the end point.

13. The patient is requested to determine which of the two points (primary versus secondary or 'first versus second') is more sensitive. The practitioner can state: 'I am pressing on two points that are close together. Please tell me which of the two, the "first" (practitioner

may move the finger slightly) or the "second" is more sensitive.'

(a) If the second point is more or equally sensitive than the first:

  (i) pressure is relieved and removed from the first point (primary);

  (ii) and then constant pressure is maintained on the second (secondary) sensitive point for 20–30 seconds. It becomes the new 'first' point.

  (iii) The sensitivity at any point does not have to abate completely before moving on to the next point. It is only important that the next point is more sensitive.

  (iv) The initial pressure on a new 'secondary' point will usually cause a response of both increased tension and sensitivity. This typically returns to a baseline after a few seconds, as noted above; the amount of time depends on the soft tissue response.

(b) There are a few considerations if the primary point persists as the more sensitive of the two contiguous points:

  (i) Maintain pressure at the location of the primary point.

  (ii) The practitioner moves the finger pressing on the secondary point more laterally or medially in an arc 2–3 centimetres from the primary point and into the direction of the end point. A point may be found that has more or the same sensitivity as the primary point by searching slightly out of line with the targeted end point. (The anatomical structure, which is being inhibited, may have slight variations in the specific course in this individual.)

  (iii) Once a secondary point that is equally or more sensitive (compared with the primary point) is located, pressure is released from the primary point and maintained on the new secondary point, as described above.

  (iv) The secondary point then becomes the new 'first' point in the continuing sequence of treatment towards the end point.

14. Before searching or inhibiting any subsequent points, the practitioner should wait approximately 20–30 seconds.

15. If no secondary point can be located despite searching in a 2-cm radius from the primary point, the clinician maintains pressure on the primary point (or the new 'primary' point) for an additional 30 seconds. Sometimes certain points require further inhibition before progress can be made. After doing so, a new secondary point may be located where previously there was less sensitivity.

16. The end point will have received inhibitory pressure throughout. Often the patient will forget that this point is being inhibited and it may lose all sensitivity.

17. The process is continued successively until the ultimate 'second' point is 2 cm from the end point.

18. Once there are the two final points being inhibited, the practitioner determines the amount of dysfunction that persists at the end and secondary point locations. The dysfunction may have reduced or disappeared totally.

19. If the dysfunction, including the end point, remains persistent, the practitioner can choose to treat the dysfunction with whatever additional modality is deemed necessary and appropriate. The end point and dysfunction, having been recalcitrant to treatment previously, may now be more amenable. Strain/counterstrain, facilitated positional release, Still technique, muscle energy technique, balanced tension techniques or some other modality may be used. Single-segment somatic dysfunctions that were difficult to position or resistant to thrust technique may now be more responsive to articulatory techniques such as high-velocity, low-amplitude thrust.

20. PINS technique can be the sole approach to the somatic dysfunctions that were found, or may be used in conjunction with any other

modality of manual treatment. Determining this is:

(a) The persistence of the dysfunction or related components after treatment.

(b) The ability of the practitioner to perform other modalities of treatment.

(c) The need or capability of the patient to accept additional treatment.

  (i) After any treatment, some soreness or other symptom may persist despite sufficient treatment. The practitioner should determine extent of treatment based on the findings for the individual; it should not be based on the patient's subjective complaints. Overtreatment can cause as many problems as undertreatment.

  (ii) Based on previous experience or misconceptions, patients may limit types of treatment. This may be due to fears or reactions that they have had to previous types of treatment.

21. The somatic dysfunction is always reassessed.

22. The patient should be advised that, despite the relative comfort of the treatment, there may be a post-treatment reaction. These reactions can include transient soreness, aches and fatigue. In patients who are prone to bruising, or when there are certain other predisposing factors (e.g. medication), ecchymoses can occur. These may also be found if excessive pressure has been used. Generally, all of these side-effects will resolve in 24–48 hours.

Application

The following two case studies are illustrative of the use of PINS to common myofascial conditions.

Case study 1

The patient was a 25-year-old married female osteopathic medical student who presented with a chief complaint of 'migraine headache'. She had been followed for her musculoskeletal complaints by another osteopathic practitioner who was unavailable on the day of presentation to the clinic. The headache was sharp and focused near the right orbit with radiation to the right frontal and temporal region. The patient had some nausea, blurring of vision, increased lacrimation and neck stiffness. The pain had started a few days beforehand and was unrelieved by the use of non-steroidal anti-inflammatory drugs, sleep or frequent doses of sumatriptan succinate, which she took orally. The patient stated that she takes between 21 and 30 pills of this drug per month (recommended usage is 2–3 per month). Loud sounds, light and certain food smells appear to worsen the chief complaint. There were no other visual, auditory or olfactory complaints or other associated symptoms with the presence of headache. The current episode appeared to be unrelated to the patient's menses, since her last menstrual period had been 2 weeks previously.

Past medical history relevant to the chief complaint was significant for paraesthesias to the upper extremities secondary to a motor vehicle accident 2 months earlier. She was the driver of a vehicle that was stopped at a traffic light, when it was struck from behind. She saw the other vehicle in the rear-view mirror and had braced herself for impact. She had had a fall at age 12 years, in which she struck the top of her head, and had migraines since that time. Family history was significant in that other members of the family have had migraines, a brother has allergies, and her mother has 'colon problems'. The patient drank two glasses of wine once per week, during religious observations, and denied use of recreational drugs or tobacco. She had a tonsillectomy, rhinoplasty and sinus cauterization. Other medical history was non-contributory.

Other medications included fexofenadine hydrochloride, oral contraceptives, Excedrin® PM (paracetamol (acetaminophen), aspirin and caffeine) and ibuprofen, as well as the sumatriptan. The last three drugs were taken episodically for headaches. At times in the past, she had gone to the emergency room for treatment of unrelieved migraine headaches.

Cranial nerve, sensorimotor and reflex testing as well as other neurological and orthopaedic evaluation findings for the patient were essentially normal. Although she had several tender points, there was not a pattern that would suggest fibromyalgia as a component of the patient's condition.

Examination of the head, neck, chest and abdomen were essentially normal, with the exception of photophobia. Vital signs were stable and the patient was alert and oriented for all modalities. Examination resulted in findings of somatic dysfunctions, as described below.

Cranial. Cranial examination revealed restrictive patterns on the right side with relative freedom of left cranial motion.

Cervical. Several single somatic dysfunctions were found in the cervical spine including ones at OA (C0–C1), AA (C1–C2), C2, C3, C6 and C7. There was also hypertonicity of the right trapezius and right sternocleidomastoid muscles.

Thoracic and rib. Hypertonicity of the right levator scapula and of the left scalene muscles; right first rib elevation; myofascial restriction of the hyoid and anterior strap muscles; multiple thoracic type II somatic dysfunctions.

Lumbar. A somatic dysfunction was found at L5 on the right accompanied by thoracolumbar paravertebral muscle spasms.

Sacrum and pelvis. Restrictions of the right sacroiliac joint and the related myofascial structures were noted.

The primary diagnosis for the office visit in question included cephalgia (migraine). Other diagnoses included cervical, thoracic, head, lumbar, sacral and pelvic somatic dysfunctions and strain. Although they were present, the areas other than those related to the patient's head were more chronic in nature and not as crucial to the patient's chief complaint. The patient was clearly anxious regarding her condition.

Much of the treatment that was performed on this single visit was similar to that which had been performed previously for the patient. Many modalities of treatment were utilized to address all related and apparently unrelated strains and dysfunctions. All of these interventions were successful, to some extent, in relieving most of the somatic dysfunctions and complaints, with the exception of the chief one – the cephalgia. The complaints of the 'migraine headache' persisted unabated.

PINS, as a modality, was added to the other customary treatment. Sensitive points at the right supraorbital ridge at the trochlear notch and in the suboccipital region were identified. Placing his left hand beneath the patient's head and neck, the author inhibited the suboccipital point with his left index finger ('end point'). Simultaneously, the author's right index finger (Fig. 11.1A,B,C) exerted pressure on the right orbital sensitive point ('primary point').

The patient indicated that the orbital point was the more sensitive of the two. The pressure also seemed to increase her ophthalmic symptoms (nausea, blurring of vision, increased lacrimation). Pressure was maintained for approximately 30 seconds on the anterior, primary point. After this interval, a second point superior to this was simultaneously pressed, with the same amount of pressure as the first, utilizing the author's right middle finger (Fig. 11.2A,B). The patient was asked to identify which of the two anterior points was more sensitive. She stated that the second was more so. Pressure was then maintained on this second point and released on the first.

This was then maintained for 30 seconds before a third point was identified approximately 2 cm above the second point. This now was reported as more sensitive than the second point. Pressure was then relieved from the second point and maintained on the third. The same pattern was followed progressively along a parasagittal line over the frontal, parietal and occipital bones until a final point was identified. This was 1 cm above the end-point location that was being constantly inhibited in the suboccipital region throughout the whole process. The somatic dysfunctions were treated with a combination of other modalities such as cervical strain/counterstrain, facilitated positional release, low-velocity and then high-velocity, low-amplitude techniques to the suboccipital region. These techniques had previously, during this session, either been unsuccessful or could not be performed, because of the patient's symptoms. All the patient's symptoms resolved completely.

Note: Placement and movement of the fingers often requires that the practitioner move the whole hand when selecting subsequent points. This 'finger walking' may mean that the second, third and fourth fingers are primarily used in sequence. Sometimes, the first finger (thumb)

Figure 11.1A   Frontal view.

Figure 11.1B   Lateral view.

Figure 11.1C   Crown view.

Figure 11.1   Pressure is exerted on the end point at the right suboccipital region and the right supraorbital ridge by using a finger of each hand. Redrawn from Dowling (2000), with permission from The American Osteopathic Association.

can be utilized temporarily to locate a new secondary point. Once it has been selected, one of the other fingers can be substituted.

Because she understood the process and her own particular patterns, the patient also tried the technique on herself, with positive results. When used early in the onset of subsequent headaches, it could be quite effective in aborting a migraine headache. When the results were less than optimal, she reported that she could then take a single sumatriptan pill and the symptoms would usually improve to a greater extent. Instead of the 21–30 pills per month, her use of this medication reduced to a more acceptable 2–3 monthly. This remained constant for several months and ultimately she was able to not require the prescription medications.

Cephalgia or headache is complex and complicated by overlapping symptoms and findings. The same symptoms can represent multiple aetiologies. A consideration is that all headaches have elements of muscle contraction, regardless of the cause. When initiated during the prodromal phase or during relatively symptom-free intervals, manipulative treatment of migraine headaches appears to be most successful. Migraine headaches, in particular, are vascular with arterial constriction, dilatation and inflammatory phases nearly paralleling the aural, pain and refractory phases. When considering

(A)   (B)

Figure 11.2A,B   Pressure is typically exerted for 20–30 seconds before searching for a secondary point. The secondary point is usually 2–3 cm from the anterior primary point in the direction of the end point. Pressure is then placed simultaneously on all three locations. If the secondary point is greater or equal in sensitivity to that now experienced at the original primary point, pressure is released from the primary point. The secondary point becomes the new – and temporary – 'primary' point. Each subsequent point between this and the end point is treated similarly. If other 'secondary points' are not found easily in a direct line towards the end point, the practitioner should attempt to press at another location medially or laterally until a point of equal or greater intensity is found. If this is also unsuccessful, a longer period of inhibition on the primary point is performed. Generally, after 1–2 minutes, new secondary points are located more easily. Redrawn from Dowling (2000), with permission from The American Osteopathic Association.

irritation and inflammation of the cranial dura, one must keep in mind that the first branch of the trigeminal nerve innervates the frontal region. The posterior fossa receives a good portion of innervation from the upper cervical region. Generally, treatment during the full-blown sickening headache component of migraine may be more effective in reduction rather than complete elimination of the symptoms.

Other types of headaches, such as muscle tension/contraction and cervicogenic headaches, can mimic some of the more typical migraine symptoms. Because all headaches have muscle contraction as a component, there is no reason why migraine and muscle contraction headaches cannot occur in the same person. Patients with chronic headaches of any sort may seek many means of intervention.

It is well documented that pharmacological interventions, such as non-steroidal anti-inflammatory drugs and vasoconstrictive medications, are frequently the initial and/or most frequently attempted interventions. Caffeine is an ingredient in many other self-treatments, including beverages, foods and pills. Because of their vasoconstrictive effects, they are successful in limiting or eliminating headaches. However, paradoxically, they have also been implicated in recurrences. It is possible to experience a rebound effect once the medication level goes below a critical point. Rather than eliminate headaches as intended, frequent use of anti-inflammatory and/or vasoconstrictive substances may encourage recurrences.

Cephalgia of this type can be approached from a neuromusculoskeletal model by inhibiting discovered sensitive points by using the PINS technique. The location of the initial point, in this particular case, was at the exit of the ophthalmic division of the trigeminal nerve, above the orbit. The same nerve innervates both the dural lining of the brain and the pain-sensitive structures of the forehead. The dura, one of the layers of the meninges, is also a pain-sensitive structure. The attachment of the superior oblique muscle at the trochlear notch of the orbit, as well as sympathetic influences from the upper cervical spine postganglionic fibres, must also be considered.

There are several branchings of the ophthalmic division of the trigeminal nerve (Fig. 11.3), and all project more superiorly along the frontal region. Basically, they track upwards unilaterally into the parietal region and are responsible for sensory appreciation from this region. Near their terminations on the top of the head there is a 'watershed' region at the galea aponeurotica (Fig. 11.4). The greater occipital nerve (Fig. 11.5) begins to also innervate the skin and musculature in this region (Moore 1980). This nerve is derived from C2 and C3 nerve roots and perforates the fascia and suboccipital muscles. These nerve roots control the majority of sensory and motor innervation to most of the occipital region. Fibres also travel anteriorly upwards through the foremen magnum to the dura of the posterior fossa. Without inhibition and other treatment of the suboccipital region, resolution of the headache may not occur. With limited treatment, some of the symptoms may abate but the presence of multiple untreated regions may result in fairly rapid recurrence.

The typical direction of treatment of frontal headache utilizing PINS (Fig. 11.6) proceeds in a pattern that progresses from orbit to occiput along a typical parasagittal line. The direction may vary in some cases and include other

Figure 11.4 Overlapping innervation of the trigeminal nerve and the greater occipital nerves in the watershed region of the scalp (superior view). Redrawn from Dowling (2000), with permission from The American Osteopathic Association.

Figure 11.3 Trigeminal innervation of the face and head (frontal view). Redrawn from Dowling (2000), with permission from The American Osteopathic Association.

Figure 11.5 Greater occipital nerve innervation of the head (posterior view). Redrawn from Dowling (2000), with permission from The American Osteopathic Association.

Figure 11.6   Pattern of inhibition points in this case of cephalgia. Redrawn from Dowling (2000), with permission from The American Osteopathic Association.

divisions or subdivisions of the trigeminal nerve (Fig. 11.7). The approach may be more antero-grade, beginning in the suboccipital region and proceeding to the frontal–orbital region depend-ing on the findings. This depends on the clinical complaints of the patient as well as the experience

Figure 11.7   Some typical inhibition patterns for the face and head. Redrawn from Dowling (2000), with permission from The American Osteopathic Association.

of the practitioner. Generally, the more sensitive of the points is selected as the beginning location. Sometimes, pressure placed onto the suboccipital region reproduces the symptoms and pain in the region of the eye. Although it is infrequently a terminal point, it is also not unusual to find that one of the intermediate points near the vertex of the head also refers pain towards the initial pri-mary point, either to the eye or to the base of the head. Finding this symptom-referring point should be taken as a positive sign in that the pro-cedure is locating and treating the component fac-tors of the dysfunction. In any case, sometimes a 'search and test' approach determines the location of several involved points. Two or more found points may give an indication of the involved structures by tracing a line and identifying the structures that link them.

Case study 2

The patient was a 72-year-old man with chief complaints of pain in the left lower extremity, specifically in the hip area. He also had a history of Parkinson's disease and osteoarthritis. He described the primary symptom as sharp, almost constant, and with radiation of the pain from the left hip towards the knee and ankle. His Parkin-son's disease had progressed slowly and was expressed primarily by stiffness. When added to his arthritis, some activities had become difficult to perform. His posture and gait were stooped, with head forward and moderate bradykinesia. The recent onset of the hip pain added a limp to his already shuffling gait. Shortly after the exami-nation, radiography revealed apparently symmet-rical moderate degenerative joint disease of both hips. The patient denied any changes in bowel or bladder habits.

Range of motion examination revealed equal restriction of motion of both hips. Fabere (Patrick test) and Fadir (Flexion, Adduction and Internal Rotation) ranges of motion, as well as pure flex-ion, were equally limited and equivalent for both hips. Sacroiliac motion was likewise limited with asymmetry. The left side demonstrated slightly less motion than the right. A left unilateral sacral shear was noted. Equal mobility, or relative lack thereof, of ilia motion was demonstrated. The legs appeared to be of equal length. Moderate somatic dysfunctions were noted throughout the lumbar, thoracic and cervical regions as well. Neurological examination revealed that sensorimotor and deep tendon reflex testing of the lower extremities were equal and normal. Strain/counterstrain tender points were noted in the left gluteal, piriformis, midpole sacral and iliotibial band. Left posterior fibular head somatic dysfunction was also noted.

Manipulative treatment based on these findings was performed on one occasion using techniques such as strain/counterstrain, muscle energy, balanced ligamentous tension, and other means of fascial release. Attempted mobilization utilizing high-velocity, low-amplitude (HVLA) thrust of the posterior fibular head was unsuccessful. Ultrasound modality was utilized along the iliotibial band, both during that office visit and

during the twice-a-week physiotherapy sessions, along with other physical medicine modalities. Despite all this, the patient's chief complaint symptoms persisted.

One week later, the same clinical and palpatory findings were noted. PINS technique was then utilized. A sensitive primary point was located at the greater trochanter. The end point was found overlying the fibula head. Location of this point took some trial and error. End points could have been located at the ankle, medial knee, popliteal space, buttock, or even more centrally above the iliac crest. In this case, successive points were also found along the tensor fascia lata/iliotibial band (Figs 11.8–11.10). Following a process of sequential inhibition of these points utilizing PINS, the final 'primary' point that was located close to the end point was approximately 2 cm proximal to the end point. Pressure was

Figure 11.8   Iliotibial band and musculature of the lateral leg. Redrawn from Dowling (2000).

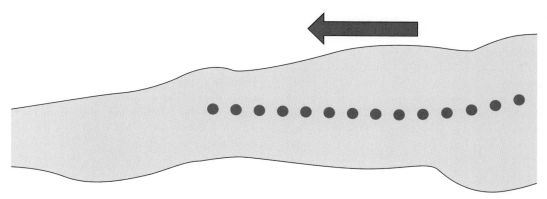

Figure 11.9   Points and direction of treatment of iliotibial band in case study 2. Redrawn from Dowling (2000).

Figure 11.10   Locations of end point (index finger, left hand) and primary point (middle finger, right hand). The index finger of the right hand has located the 'secondary point'. Redrawn from Dowling (2000).

maintained for half a minute simultaneously on the two points. Inhibition alone resulted in a reported reduction of at least 50% of the lower extremity pain and radiation. The fibula head was then mobilized successfully with HVLA mobilization. The patient stated he had only a small amount of residual discomfort after this was performed. Previous attempts at performing HVLA thrust to the fibula head had been unsuccessful.

At the next visit, the patient reported that the improvement had persisted for at least 1 week. Some of the findings were again present, but to a much lesser degree, and were limited to a single tender point near the left greater trochanter. This was easily treated with only strain/counterstrain technique. PINS was not necessary to the treatment protocol on this visit.

Possible mechanism of action

The mechanism of action by which the technique of inhibition works can only be postulated. Unfortunately, this is the status with many other modalities of osteopathic manipulative technique: insufficient research has been performed for many manipulative modalities. However, the clinical outcomes have been reported anecdotally many times. Understanding the processes of injury as well as treatment is typically based on the most likely combination of relevant physiological and anatomical components.

One of the important components of inhibition is the use of a low-level (but using a constant amount of force) pressure applied to a dysfunctional tissue.

Accommodation or habituation is a process wherein a stimulus of a constant level, even if initially irritating, becomes less noticeable over time. At first, the subject may be acutely aware of the intrusion or pressure. The patient may state that there is pain, sensitivity, increased pressure or some other sensation. The practitioner may also note that the local tissue reacts by initially increasing in tension. Firm, spasmed muscle may become more so. When the pressure is maintained constantly, these reactions decrease and may disappear altogether as the system adapts (Bailey 1976). The reticular formation as a screen is but one component involved in the process. There are many other occasions where the body accommodates to stimuli. These are evidenced by the relative non-awareness of body contact with eyeglasses, tight belts, stiff clothing, uncomfortable shoes, as well as constant extraneous auditory and visual stimuli. It is only when attention is called to them by a new, probably irritating, event that awareness resurfaces. A refrigerator in the kitchen or the sounds from a nearby railway often fail to attract the attention of someone accustomed to them – unless the sounds deviate from the usual. Persons who have worn eyeglasses since infancy may be oblivious to their presence and may even casually adjust the positioning with almost unconscious effort.

However, someone who has recently developed the need for visual aids, such as a middle-aged presbyopic adult, may be all too aware of every aspect from the points of contact to the change in appearance of objects. Gradually, this diminishes. This filtering process may also involve lower components, such as the spinal cord, to act as a mediator. Its contribution in this habituation process is to act as a 'brake' when sensory overload occurs (Patterson 1976).

Direct pressure placed upon areas of greatest sensitivity or symptoms may act as a counter-irritant. Rapid, conducting, large nerve afferents gate transmission in the dorsal horn of the spinal cord. Collateral fibres in the substantia gelatinosa or adjacent interneurons then inhibit the transmission of pain to the central nervous system via the spinothalamic tract (Ganong 1995). Pressure acts as a stimulant to the neighbouring tissue, reducing the sensitivity of the original tender point. Scratching in the region of an itch would be an example of this phenomenon. An ischaemia theory concerning the use of a sustained pressure, such as that used in inhibition, describes an effect in the immediate tissue. When a muscle is maintained in prolonged contraction, metabolites are released that were produced from the local tissue damage (Stoddard 1969). Damaged tissue ordinarily demonstrates a decrease in circulation in a progressive fashion. Immediate or acute injury results in hyperaemia and congestion. This is followed by infiltration of vasoactive substances. These appear primarily for the theoretical purpose of dealing with tissue injury. If the injury persists or there is a prolonged reduced function, trophic tissue changes occur. The muscles, ligaments and fascia may develop fibrotic changes. The chronic nature of the dysfunction demonstrates decreased circulation by blanching following any pressure. Normally, the skin shows a brief blanching followed by redness, which also fades. When muscle is maintained in a chronically tightened state, circulation is impaired. The use of further pressure in a therapeutic fashion to cause a relatively increased ischaemia does not initially make sense from the standpoint of nutrient deprivation. One way of appreciating an effect is to postulate that, following pressure, the increased ischaemia reduces the capacity of

the nociceptive receptors to process. Once this pressure is removed, the resultant hyperaemia produced after release results in flushing of the waste products from the region. The local vessels are dammed temporarily, there is a build-up of pressure, and then sudden washing away as the compression is released.

Although there may be no visible abnormality, a dysfunctional muscle may appear to be in its neutral position but still be hypertonic. Any further stretch from the shortened attitude increases activity of the muscle spindle mechanisms. Slight increases in length, even if the muscle is halfway between fully shortened and extended, may result in a reflexive and prolonged contraction. Within skeletal muscle, sensory muscle fibres 'monitor' length changes. These specialized muscular fibres lie deep within the larger extrafusal fibres. Set in parallel, the sensory nerve fibres to these small muscles track back to the spinal cord. Specific motor nerves (*gamma* motor neurons) modulate muscle spindle contractions. The sensory fibres, the annulospiral and flower-spray afferents, react to either contraction of the nuclear bag and chain fibres or the stretching of these. This is an intrinsic means of protection. A rationale for this is the prevention of tearings of the muscle. Factors that increase the sensitivity and gain of these fibres include stress, anxiety, pain, cold and other general components. Sudden, unexpected stretching, as well as overstretching of the intrafusal fibres, also increases activity of the special sensory flower-spray and annulospiral fibres. Mediated by the spinal cord segment, this results in a reflex action by activation of the *alpha* motor neuron. This causes contraction of the larger extrafusal muscle fibres. When the *gamma* motor neuron gain is set too high, the muscle spindles react earlier in the stretch, to a greater degree than is usually necessary, or are inappropriately maintained for longer than is necessary (Becker 1976, Buzzell 1967, Ganong 1995, Korr 1976).

Slow stretching is encouraged, especially before and after exercise, to prevent contractions as a means of 'training' the extrafusal muscles, but also to lower the reactivity of the muscle spindles. Pressure applied during inhibition introduces a gentle stretch while allowing re-setting of the stretch receptors (Korr 1979b). This localized pressure may add a stretch in a region of only a few centimetres without challenging the whole muscle. The component that is initially irritating is at a subcritical level. Once the small, localized component is overwhelmed, any affected adjacent area can subsequently be inhibited, with similar results. The use of digitally applied pressure along the muscle, such as is used in PINS, may be a very effective method as it deals with a series of irritated parts. In this way, the practitioner completes the treatment by progressively treating all of the involved elements.

Myotendinotic changes, which are usually characterized by increased tone, thickening, resistance and decreased plasticity, have been described by some authors (Dvorak & Dvorak 1990). These occur within the muscle. They are particularly tender when the muscle is palpated perpendicular to the direction of the fibres. The tenderness may be elicited when using pressure that should not ordinarily be irritating. Along with the increase in sensitivity, changes in these fibres can be palpated from the origin to the insertion. Other non-pathological fibres that are located in the same or nearby muscles do not evidence the same pattern of irritation. The pathological and physiological fibres can be parallel to one another. However, the pathological aspects of the fibres may occur in relatively isolated bundles from the neighbouring unaffected ones. These tender bands can be found in patterns that are similar to trigger points. The appearance may be related to relatively non-traumatic events. After a variable latency period in which only one site is irritable, the rest of the muscle and attachments become irritable. This phenomenon may explain some of the correlation between locations of Jones' strain/counterstrain tender points and Travell's trigger points (Travell & Simons 1983). Jones' points tend to be related to muscle bands, are sensitive to light pressure, but elicit only tenderness at the site of pressure. The Travell points themselves may be sensitive or not, but the hallmark of their existence is the pain patterns that radiate when they are compressed. The differences in quality between the two types of point may represent a matter of duration and degree of the dysfunction.

A complementary muscular reflex system to the muscle spindle is that of the Golgi tendon system. The Golgi tendon organs are set in series and located in a net-like fashion in the tendon, unlike the muscle spindles, which are set in parallel with the extrafusal muscles. Tendons are the least contractile element of a muscle. The Golgi unit has sensory fibres that become relatively stretched during muscular contraction. This is unlike the activation of the muscle spindles, which occurs during muscular stretch. The Golgi tendon organs can also become activated by passive stretch of the whole unit. Unlike the muscle spindle, increased Golgi tendon organ activity brings about reflex relaxation of the muscle as a whole. The sensory neuron from the Golgi apparatus influences the *alpha* motor neuron indirectly through the mediation of an inhibitory interneuron. The reflex is also known as the clasp-knife reflex, and the results can be quite dramatic and sudden. The progressive tightening of muscles recruits more and more Golgi tendon activity. Therefore, the signals bring about greater inhibition of the muscular contraction. When muscles are hypertonic, an intervention whereby initial stretch results in further contraction is then followed by resultant relaxation (Ganong 1995). This reflex system is the one most probably involved in direct active techniques (i.e. muscle energy technique) and in passive stretch interventions where the region is held at a pathological barrier for a significant amount of time.

A narrow view of compression is that only blood flow is impeded. Impaired flow can be of vascular, lymphatic or neuronal origin. Pressure on the axons can impair the transport of necessary neuropeptides and other substances when considering nerves (Korr 1979c). According to Korr & Appeltauer (1979), the speed with which this flow naturally occurs is quite slow at 40 to several hundred millimetres per day. These rates would therefore not easily explain any immediate effect of inhibitory pressure. The reduction in the soft tissue hypertonicity and the persistence of this effect in response to soft tissue treatments such as PINS may be due in some part to alleviation of the pressure upon nerves (Korr 1979a).

The persistence of somatic dysfunction, as has been expressed previously, can occur despite adequate treatment. Sometimes the breakthrough in successful treatment comes with the recognition of the connection of various apparently unrelated elements. Beginning with the postulate that some dysfunctions support others, failure to recognize and initiate improvement of some aspects allows for continuation or recurrence. The more symptomatic elements may receive the attention, while the supportive ones remain relatively silent in the background: the 'noisy' ones are treated while the 'quiet' ones are not. After treatment, the whole problem may resolve, the secondary components may assert themselves, or they may instigate a recurrence of the original problem. Using the analogy of a reverberating circuit, all elements should be 'shut down' to eliminate the process entirely. It is tempting, on first presentation, to focus solely on the region of the patient's chief complaint. If there is good resolution, there may be no need to search further. However, when limited results are obtained, there is a need to search further. As a treatment modality, the PINS approach offers an additional means of analysing and treating persistent or difficult dysfunctions.

Contraindications and side-effects

Over the years, repeated use of PINS has demonstrated few contraindications and side-effects. Any condition in which pressure placed on or through the skin might be expected to cause a worsening of the symptoms or signs should preclude the use of PINS. Localized inflammation, abscesses or infection should not be pressed; surgical or other medical interventions may be more appropriate. The aetiology in these instances would preclude the use of PINS or any other technique that may cause more damage. Other manipulative interventions could then possibly include lymphatic or other fluid techniques instead. PINS could be applied to treat any residual sensitive points if sensitive points persist after the resolution of the inflammatory or infectious process. As the pressure applied is just enough to ensure a response of sensitivity, the likelihood of real injury should be minimal. There is always a possibility that the patient may develop some temporary symptoms such as aches or fatigue.

These generally begin within 24 hours, are usually vague, and almost always resolve by 48 hours. Preparing the patient for the possibility goes a long way in reassuring and meeting their expectations from treatment. As with all manipulative interventions, the intensity is generally less than the symptoms and disability experienced by the patient before treatment, the localization varies, and the duration is relatively brief.

Conclusion

Inhibition or the use of pressure on dysfunctional areas is one of the oldest forms of treatment. PINS represents a variant of the more traditional approach to using inhibition. Standard methods of palpatory and other techniques of palpatory diagnosis are utilized. PINS offers a theoretical model for searching out the primary and related locations that maintain somatic dysfunction. As a technique, it follows a theoretical framework while allowing for adaptations based on the palpatory findings. As a modality, it can be used solely or in combination with other methods of manipulation. Even though it bears some similarities to previously described methods, PINS is distinctive enough to warrant inclusion as an individual method of osteopathic manipulation. Knowledge of physiology and anatomy is necessary for the determination of primary and end points, as well as of the intervening points. Further adaptations may be necessary for analysis of alterations from the norm, the patient's subjective responses, and the use of appropriate low-level force to inhibit specific connected locations leads to reduction of the underlying aetiology. Rather than being used exclusively, if there are still remnants of the dysfunction, other manipulative techniques should be employed. Previously ineffective treatment modalities may be attempted after PINS, and may then be found to be more effective.

PINS does require an investment of time. The amount of time can be anywhere from 2 to 10 minutes, depending on the process of locating and treating the number of points. Compared with other methods, this may seem excessive: some other point techniques, such as facilitated positional release, take only a few seconds, and strain/counterstrain typically takes 90 seconds. However, when typical interventions are of limited success with recalcitrant dysfunctions, alternative means are required. PINS, by eliminating inappropriately maintained reflexes, restrictions and abnormal function, can be a tool utilized to facilitate the person's intrinsic function. By freeing the restricted elements, this maximizes the individual's self-healing and repair functions.

References

American Osteopathic Association 1998 Glossary of Osteopathic Terminology: *American Osteopathic Association Yearbook and Directory of Osteopathic Practitioners*, Chicago, Illinois, 1998, AOA.

Bailey HW: Some problems in making osteopathic spinal manipulative therapy appropriate and specific, *J Am Osteopath Assoc* 75:486–499, 1976.

Becker RF: The gamma system and its relation to the development and maintenance of muscle tone. In *1976 year book of the American Academy of Osteopathy*, Colorado Springs, 1976, American Academy of Osteopathy, pp 26–40.

Burton Goldberg Group: *Alternative medicine: the definitive guide*, Puyallup, Washington, 1994, Future Medicine Publishing.

Buzzell KA: The potential disruptive influence of somatic input. In *The physiological basis of osteopathic medicine*, Postgraduate Institute of Osteopathic Medicine and Surgery, New York, 1967, Insight Publishing, pp 39–51.

Cerney JV: *Acupuncture without needles*, West Nyack, New York, 1974, Parker Publishing.

Chaitow L: *Neuro-muscular technique*, Wellingborough, UK, 1980, Thorsons.

Chaitow L: *Osteopathic self-treatment*, Wellingborough, UK, 1990, Thorsons.

Chaitow L: *Modern neuromuscular techniques*, New York, 1996, Churchill Livingstone.

Chila AG: Fascial – ligamentous release: an indirect approach. In Ward RC, editor: *Foundations for osteopathic medicine*, Baltimore, 1997, Williams & Wilkins, pp 819–830.

Cyriax J: *Text-book of orthopaedic medicine*, vol. II, Treatment by manipulation and message, ed 6, New York, 1959, Harper & Row.

Dowling DJ: Myofascial release concepts. In DiGiovanna EL, Schiowitz S, Dowling DJ, editors: *An osteopathic approach to diagnosis and treatment*, ed 3, Philadelphia, 2005, Lippincott Williams & Wilkins, pp 95–102.

Dowling DJ: S.T.A.R.: a more viable alternative descriptor system of somatic dysfunction, *American Academy of Osteopathy Journal* 8(2):34–37, 1998.

Dowling DJ: Progressive inhibition of neuromuscular structures (PINS) technique, *J Am Osteopath Assoc* 100(5):285–297, 2000.

Dowling DJ, Scariati PD: General physiologic considerations. In DiGiovanna EL, Schiowitz S, Dowling DJ, editors: *An osteopathic approach to diagnosis and treatment*, ed 3, Philadelphia, 2005, Lippincott Williams & Wilkins, pp 38–52.

Dvorak J, Dvorak V: *Manual medicine: diagnostics*, ed 2, New York, 1990, Thieme.

Ehrenfeuchter WC: Soft tissue techniques. In Ward RC, editor: *Foundations for osteopathic medicine*, Baltimore, 1997, Williams & Wilkins, pp 781–794.

Ganong WF: *Review of medical physiology*, 1995, Lange.

Glover JC, Yates HA: Strain and counterstrain techniques. In Ward RC, editor: *Foundations for osteopathic medicine*, Baltimore, 1997, Williams & Wilkins, pp 809–818.

Goetz EW: *Manual of osteopathy*, ed 5, Ohio, 1905, Cincinnati.

Hazzard C: 1905, *The practice and applied therapeutics of osteopathy*.

Hermann E: 1965, *The D.O. October*, pp 163–164.

Johnston WL: Functional technique: an indirect method. In Ward RC, editor: *Foundations for osteopathic medicine*, Baltimore, 1997, Williams & Wilkins, pp 795–808.

Jones LH: *Strain and counterstrain*, Newark, Ohio, 1981, American Academy of Osteopathy.

Jones LH, Kusenose R, Goering E: *Jones strain–counterstrain*, Jones Strain–Counterstrain Company, Idaho, 1995, Boise.

Kenyon J: *Acupressure techniques: a self help guide*, Rochester, Vermont, 1988, Healing Arts Press.

Korr IM: Proprioceptors and somatic dysfunction. In *1976 year book of the American Academy of Osteopathy*, Colorado Springs, Colorado, 1976, American Academy of Osteopathy, pp 41–50.

Korr IM: Neurochemical and neurotrophic consequences of nerve deformation: clinical implications in relation to spinal manipulation, *J Am Osteopath Assoc* 75:409–414, (reprinted in: The collected papers of Irvin M Korr) American Academy of Osteopathy, 1979a, Colorado Springs, pp 196–199.

Korr IM: Proprioceptors and somatic dysfunction, *J Am Osteopath Assoc* 74:638–650, (reprinted in: The collected papers of Irvin M Korr), American Academy of Osteopathy, Colorado Springs, 1979b. pp 200–207.

Korr IM: The nature and basis of the trophic function of nerves: outline of a research program, *J Am Osteopath Assoc* 66:74–78, (reprinted in: The collected papers of Irvin M Korr), American Academy of Osteopathy, 1979c, Colorado Springs, pp 96–99.

Korr IM, Appeltauer GS: Continued studies on the axonal transport of nerve proteins to muscle, *J Am Osteopath Assoc* 69:76–78, (reprinted in: The collected papers of Irvin

M Korr), American Academy of Osteopathy, 1979, Colorado Springs, pp 100–101.

Moore KL: *Clinically oriented anatomy*, London, 1980, Williams & Wilkins.

Owens C: *An endocrine interpretation of Chapman's reflexes*, ed 2, Chattanooga, Tennessee, 1937, Chattanooga Printing and Engraving Company.

Patterson MM: A model mechanism for spinal segmental facilitation, *J Am Osteopath Assoc* 76:62–72, 1976.

Prudden B: *Pain erasure: the Bonnie Prudden way*, New York, 1980, Ballantine Books.

Robbins SL, Cotran RS, Kumar V: *Pathologic basis of disease*, ed 3, Philadelphia, 1984, WB Saunders.

Schiowitz S: In DiGiovanna , Schiowitz S, editors: *An osteopathic approach to diagnosis and treatment*, ed 2, Philadelphia, 1997, Lippincott-Raven, p 91.

Schultz W: *Shiatsu: Japanese finger pressure therapy*, New York, 1976, Bell Publishing.

Still AT: *The philosophy and mechanical principles of osteopathy*, Kansas City, Missouri, 1902, Hudson-Kimberly.

Still AT: *Autobiography of AT Still*, Revised ed, Kirksville, Missouri, 1908, Self-published.

Stoddard A: *Manual of osteopathic practice*, London, 1969, Hutchinson Medical.

Tasker DD: *Principles of osteopathy*, ed 4, Los Angeles, 1916, Bireley & Elson.

Travell JG, Simmons DG: *Myofascial pain and dysfunction: the trigger point manual*, vol. I: The upper extremities, Baltimore, 1983, Williams & Wilkins.

Typaldos S: Introducing the fascial distortion model, *American Academy of Osteopathy Journal* 4(2):1994.

Van Buskirk VL: A manipulative technique of Andrew Taylor Still as reported by Charles Hazzard, DO, in 1905, *J Am Osteopath Assoc* 96(10):597–602, 1996.

Ward RC: Integrated neuromusculoskeletal release and myofascial release: an introduction to diagnosis and treatment. In Ward RC, ed. *Foundations for osteopathic medicine*, Baltimore, 1997, Williams & Wilkins, pp 846–849.

Weil A: *Spontaneous healing*, New York, 1995, Ballantine Books.

Thai massage and neuromuscular technique

12

Howard Evans

CHAPTER CONTENTS

Thai massage – past and present   276
Sen, nadi, meridian, myofascial pathway?   277
Sen and Chinese meridians   278
Sen and Ayur-vedic nadis   278
Sen and myofascial pathways   279
Myofascial sen   282
Myofascial leg lines   283
Myofascial arm lines   284
Myofascial back lines   285
Thai massage as myofascial massage   286
Thai massage and neuromuscular technique   287
Conclusion   288

In his book *The Human Machine and Its Forces* published in 1937, Dr. Dewanchand Varma says:

We have discovered that the circulation of the nervous currents, slows down occasionally because of the obstruction caused by adhesions; the muscular fibres harden and the nervous currents can no longer pass through them. We have demonstrated effective and positive methods designed to restore nervous equilibrium which promotes the healthy circulation of blood, so that new tissues begin to be built up again

(Chaitow 2003, pp. 32–33)

Based in Paris, Dr. Varma practised a form of soft tissue manipulation which he called 'Pranatherapy'. This was derived from Ayur-veda, the traditional medical system of India, Dr. Varma's homeland. His system was to become one of the sources of what we now know as neuromuscular technique (NMT).

Stanley Lief, who had trained in America as a chiropractor and naturopath, heard of Dr. Varma's work and travelled to Paris to receive a series of treatments from him. Lief was so impressed by the results that he persuaded Varma to teach him his system. With the help of his cousin and assistant, Boris Chaitow, Lief further developed and refined the techniques and coined the name 'neuromuscular technique' (Chaitow 2003, pp. 32–33).

When I studied NMT in 1995 with Leon Chaitow, Boris Chaitow's nephew, I was intrigued by the way in which aspects of neuromuscular technique resonated with Thai massage, a system I had already been practising for three years. Around the same period I also discovered the work of Ida Rolf and experienced its practical application in the form of ten sessions of 'Rolfing'. These two influences began to inform my understanding of Thai massage which, back in the nineties, was taught as a practical work with very little theory.

Thai massage – past and present

In common with Dr. Varma's 'Pranatherapy', Thai massage is said to derive from Indian Ayur-vedic medicine; Jivaka Kumar Bhaccha, a North Indian physician, is generally regarded as the father of Thai medicine. The Foundation of Dr. Shivaga Komarpaj in Chiang Mai preserves his name in its Thai version. The foundation runs the Old Medical Hospital where it has offered short courses in Thai massage since 1962.

Jivaka Kumar Bhaccha was a member of the community (sangha) that gathered around the Buddha 2500 years ago. According to an account in the Vinaya Pitaka, a Theravadin document that records the life of that original sangha, Jivaka's father was King Bimbisara, a contemporary of the Buddha, and the ruler of the Magadha Empire in North India. Jivaka's mother was the wife of a merchant who fell for the charms of the king while her unfortunate husband was away on business. Soon after his birth Jivaka was taken by his mother to the king and was raised in the royal household.

As a young man Jivaka realized that medicine was to be his vocation. With his father's permission he went to study under Atreya, the renowned Rishi physician. Atreya was the personal physician to King Bimbisara's father, Padma dPal. The years of study bore fruit and Jivaka stood out as the most brilliant student in his class. He quickly developed a reputation as a great physician and his pride grew to match his fame. He is said to have boasted that nobody could cure a somatic disorder, as could he; just as nobody could cure a psychological disorder, as could the Buddha. In time, like many of his contemporaries, Jivaka went to the Buddha to learn the path by which he could free himself from his suffering (Rapgay 1981).

It is generally believed that Jivaka's name and the medical system he practised came to Thailand with the teachings of the Buddha, although it is not known exactly when that was. Some accounts suggest that Asoka, India's first Emperor, sent missionaries in the second century BC. Asoka embraced Buddhism in response to the terrible cruelty he saw during the conquest of Kalinga and came to be known as 'The Prince of Peace' (Kinder & Hilgemann 1978).

A stone inscription from 1292 AD records the declaration of Rama Khamheng, King of Siam, that Buddhism be recognized as the country's official religion (Gold 2007, p. 65). Beyond that little more is known. When the Burmese invaded Thailand in 1767 they destroyed the old royal capital of Ayutthia and with it most historical and medical texts.

In 1832 King Rama III gathered what fragments of the medical texts survived and had them carved on stone and set into the walls of Wat Pho, the main Buddhist monastery in Bangkok. These carvings comprise 60 figures and are said to indicate treatment lines and points on the human body along with explanatory notes (Brust 1990, p. 5).

Until the late 1980s Thai massage was little known outside of Thailand. Even within the country the traditional medical system to which the massage belonged was losing favour. In common with many of its Asian neighbours, Thailand was embracing a Western model of industrial and economic development and the modern medical system it brought with it.

Thai massage is now enjoying a new lease of life in Thailand as well as finding its way into massage centres and hotel spas around the world. This revival owes much to the interest shown by Western travellers, some of whom found their way to the traditional massage schools or studied directly with village massage practitioners. Lacking the necessary language skills they learned Thai massage as a practical study with little theory to explain the techniques. Despite, and possibly because of this lack of theory some of these early Western students discovered an affinity with the practice and went on to become teachers themselves.

Between the late 1980s and the present day much has changed in the world of Thai massage. There are now many more schools offering courses in Thailand as well as around the world. There is now an abundance of books on the subject. 'Thai Reflexology' and 'Thai Head Massage' have emerged as standalone therapies. Even aspects of Thai herbal medicine have entered the mainstream and it is now quite common to see the use of 'Thai herbal compresses' in hotel spas. Despite the global reach of Thai massage there has been little development in understanding the medical system to which the massage belongs.

We do know that Thai massage is one of the three branches of traditional Thai medicine; the others being naturopathic medicine and spiritual practices. Traditional Thai medicine is intimately entwined with Theravada Buddhism, the esoteric and monastic branch of Buddhism practised in Southeast Asia and Sri Lanka. In Thailand this traditional medicine is still typically offered under the auspices of the Buddhist monastic community.

Given that Thai massage is but a small part of a Buddhist approach to medicine it is, perhaps, not so surprising that our knowledge is so limited. Buddha taught Jivaka Kumar that the cause of all suffering, whether physical or mental, is the greed, anger and ignorance generated by the unenlightened mind. Although traditional Buddhist medicine includes naturopathic remedies and physical therapy, of far greater importance is the spiritual teaching and practical guidance offered by the lama physicians of the monastic community. Buddhist medicine is taught within the broader context of Buddhist philosophy and medical intervention is similarly prescribed.

Although some Westerners have made the effort to learn the Thai language and explore more deeply Thailand's culture and religion I am not one of them. For this reason, in this discussion of Thai massage, I will disengage it from its spiritual context and look at it exclusively as a form of bodywork. We will see that in the West, although Thai massage carries with it no more than a fragment of the medical system to which it belongs, in this may lie its strength. Freed from the weight of a substantial theoretical foundation and from the rigour to be expected of a medical system it nevertheless stands its ground as an excellent massage technique. We will seek here to understand why.

Sen, nadi, meridian, myofascial pathway?

There are three main activities involved in the practice of Thai massage:

- the manipulation of treatment lines known as 'sen'
- the application of passive stretches and postures derived from Hatha Yoga
- the induction of a deep 'meditation-like' relaxation in the patient.

The balance of these three activities is quite individual and the massage will vary considerably depending on the massage practitioner's preferences. Some massage practitioners are more attracted to the yoga aspects of the work and offer quite dynamic massage sessions. Some are drawn more to the stretches, and practise Thai massage with a 'no pain, no gain' style similar to that found in sports massage. My own approach to Thai massage focuses mainly on the manipulation of the sen and inducing relaxation. This is the style encouraged by my teachers, both of whom studied at the Old Medical Hospital in Chiang Mai.

The 'sen' are the lines documented in the stone carvings of Wat Pho. It is said that these carvings refer to a network of 72 000 lines or channels permeating the body. Ten of these are used for massage. These are known as the 'ten sen'. In addition to the sen, the stone carvings of Wat Pho also record descriptions of treatment points.

When I first studied Thai massage in 1992, as well as diagrams of the sen, we were given others indicating treatment points on the hands, feet and face. These looked to me like Chinese acupressure and Western reflexology charts. There was little information to explain their use so I disregarded them and concentrated my efforts on the manipulation of the sen.

Asokananda (AKA Harald Brust), with whom I studied advanced Thai massage in 1995, says of treatment points: 'Thai massage never developed a standardised set of points but therapy always was and is centred around intensive and complete line work' (Brust 1996, p. 18). If we accept, therefore, to leave aside the idea of treatment points we are left with a simple massage based around the manipulation of treatment lines.

Even though it is said that there are ten main sen used in Thai massage this is actually open to debate. The ten sen are known as: sen sumana, sen ittha, sen pingkhala, sen kalathari, sen sahatsarangsi, sen thawari, sen lawusang, sen ulangka, sen nanthakrawat and sen khitchanna. However, sen lawusang and sen ulangka follow the same path but on the left side and right side of the body. The same goes for sen thawari and sen sahatsarangsi and for sen ittha and sen pingkhala. In all we really only find seven unique pathways.

The story is further confused by the fact that Thai massage only uses aspects of the sen mentioned above and there are many differences of opinion as to where these aspects run. This lack of clarity leads many Western Thai massage practitioners to other systems for the theory to support their practice. These include traditional Chinese medicine, Ayur-vedic medicine and Hatha Yoga, each of which incorporates a system of lines or channels with some similarities to the sen.

Sen and Chinese meridians

Of these traditional systems the best known in the West is traditional Chinese medicine (TCM). TCM is based on a Western anatomical model but with the addition of acupuncture channels and acupuncture points. The channels are used to describe the interconnection of the various functional systems of the body. In TCM however, there are not 7, nor 10 but 14 main channels. There are, in addition, numerous secondary channels. These include connecting channels, muscle channels and cutaneous regions. The connecting channels branch further into minute connecting channels, blood connecting channels and superficial connecting channels (Maciocia 1991). These form an intricate web involved in the distribution of fluids and energies throughout the body. Although there is no specific reference to 72 000 channels in TCM it is quite likely that this web of channels does have something in common with the system of sen referred to in traditional Thai medicine especially when we consider that both systems are thought to originate from around 2500 years ago.

Often, Western writers who liken the sen to acupuncture channels also generalize Thai massage as a form of 'energy work' similar to Japanese shiatsu or Chinese acupressure (Mercati 1998, Brust 1990, p. 6, Gold 2007, p. 12). From my own studies in traditional Chinese acupuncture with JR Worsley in the early 1980s I could recognize some similarities between the sen used in Thai massage and the channels used in acupuncture. However this is a perilous comparison. What it reveals are major shortcomings in our knowledge of the sen. In Thai massage there is no sense of a complete system of sen comparable with acupuncture channels and there is no system of diagnosis with which to justify the term 'energy work'.

Sen and Ayur-vedic nadis

Another common source of information used to explain Thai massage is to be found in India. Here in the homeland of Jivaka Kumar, patron of traditional Thai medicine, a vast historical record exists in the form of the Upanishads and the Vedas. These document the development of the medical and spiritual system that forms the basis of the Hindu and Buddhist religions. The oldest Upanishads, the Brhadaranyaka and the Chandogya, have been dated to the eighth century BC while the Vedas date from 1000 BC (Milne 1995).

Ayur-veda, a naturopathic approach to medicine still practised in India today, dates from the Vedic Period (1800–1000 BC) and is thought to be the source of traditional Thai medicine. The oldest existing encyclopaedic medical work is the Sushruta-Samhita. Although much of this work was completed in the early Christian era, parts of this collection are pre-Buddhist (Feuerstein 1990, p. 88).

Hatha Yoga, the style of yoga practice most familiar in the West, is documented in a series of Upanishads written between the sixth and fourteenth centuries AD. This period saw the birth and development in India of the philosophy of Tantrism, the aim of which was 'to overcome the dualism between the ultimate Reality (Self) and the conditional reality (ego) by insisting on the continuity between the process of the world and the process of liberation or enlightenment' (Feuerstein 1990, p. 251).

Although for many Westerners Hatha Yoga represents little more than a system of exercise, for its founders it was the distillation of centuries of research. The result is a psycho spiritual system designed to integrate the spiritual life with the physical reality of the body. Hatha Yoga means 'yoga of the force' and its aim is nothing less than 'the blissful state of ecstatic merging with the Divine' (Feuerstein 1990, p. 246).

In the Yoga-Upanishads we find reference to 'nadis', the Ayur-vedic equivalent of the sen. The renowned, contemporary Hatha Yoga teacher, BKS Iyengar, refers to the nadis as channels 'through which nervous energy passes' (Iyengar 1984, p. 117). In common with the Thai system, some of the Yoga-Upanishads refer to 72 000 nadis. Others, however, refer to 350 000. Similarly, some refer to ten important nadis but others refer to fourteen or fifteen (Motoyama 2003, p. 135).

There are other similarities between the Thai sen and the Ayur-vedic nadis. In both systems three channels are considered to be particularly important. In Thai massage they are sen sumana, sen ittha and sen pingkhala. In Ayur-veda they are sushumna-nadi, ida-nadi and pingala-nadi. As well as the similarity of name, sen ittha and ida-nadi are in both systems symbolized by the moon and associated with the feminine quality while sen pingkhala and pingala-nadi are symbolized by the sun and associated with the masculine quality.

Hereafter we discover more differences than similarities. For instance, in the Thai description, sen sumana starts at the navel and ascends inside the throat, terminating at the base of the tongue. Sen ittha and sen pingkhala are described as lines that run either side of sen sumana and then continue down into the legs. In the Yogic tradition these lines are usually depicted as a caduceus; sushumna-nadi forms a central core while ida-nadi and pingala-nadi weave a double helix, intersecting sushumna-nadi at a series of seven centres along the vertical axis of the body. In Sanskrit these centres are called 'chakras', meaning wheel or vortex. They are thought to relate to nerve plexuses (Motoyama 2003, pp. 197–198).

According to the Yogic tradition, sushumna-nadi means 'the current that is most gracious' (Feuerstein 1990, p. 260). BKS Iyengar calls it the nadi of fire and locates it inside the spinal column. He says it is the main channel for the flow of nervous energy (Iyengar 1984, p. 439). Although there are some variations, most traditional Yogic sources agree that sushumna-nadi begins at the perineum and continues up to a point called 'Brahman Gate' at the top of the head (Motoyama 2003, p. 141).

The Yogic tradition goes still deeper, identifying within sushumna-nadi another channel called vajra-nadi and within that yet another called citrini-nadi (Feuerstein 1990, p. 260). According to the Shat-Chakra-Nirupana, written in 1577 by a Bengali guru known as Purananda there is within citrini-nadi yet another called the Brahma-nadi (Motoyama 2003, p. 164).

It soon becomes clear when reviewing Yogic literature that the nadis are part of a complete and complex system involved not only in medicine but also in the development of consciousness. What we know of this system in the West is generally limited to the practice of yoga asanas. According to the Yoga Sutras, compiled some time between the second century BC and the second century AD by Patanjali, the asanas are but one of the eight disciplines of Yogic practice. Hiroshi Motoyama, a Japanese Shinto priest, veteran yoga practitioner and scientist says of this practice:

> There are those who may claim that it is too grandiose a wish for us humans to become more than human. But it must be stated that this wish is neither impossible nor too dangerous, as long as the correct practices are performed without error. It should also be added that the guidance of a qualified teacher is essential in case difficulties are encountered along the way
> (Motoyama 2003, p. 29).

Sen and myofascial pathways

In 1990 Dick Larson, an acupuncturist and Rolfer, wrote a paper discussing the link between the fascial planes used in Rolfing and the channels used in acupuncture. According to Larson, the ancient Chinese were well aware of the significance of connective tissue and its relationship to acupuncture meridians. During the Han Dynasty (206 BC–220 AD) 'Prince Mang ordered physicians and butchers to perform surgery on live political prisoners to measure their organs and to establish the source and route of blood vessels' (Larson 1990, p. 25). Larson suggests that the writers of the Qing Dynasty (1644–1912) further clarified this relationship and described a system whereby, 'the meridians themselves are recognised as flowing through the superficial fascia of the body', and:

> *The system of branches which come out from the meridians run through the entire body, just as the superficial fascia does. Thus, when the branches 'spirally wrap' the paired organs, they permeate the fascial envelopes that encircle the organs*
>
> *(Larson 1990, p. 27).*

Larson refers to the earlier work of another Rolfer, Stanley Rosenberg, who in 1986 suggested that:

> *. . . the acupuncture meridians are a map of the planes of fascia. By putting my hands on the meridians in certain ways (other than traditional acupressure), I can produce some predictable improvements in structure, easily and with little effort*
>
> *(Larson 1990, p. 29).*

Ida Rolf had already sensed this connection herself, although she related it to reflexology rather than to acupuncture. In her book 'Rolfing', originally published in 1977, she says:

> *Many people are aware that reflex points can be found on the sole of the foot. When individual visceral organs become congested, pressure on a specific point on the sole elicits pain, sometimes intense in quality . . . In such reflex situations, fascial planes may be the route of mechanical transmission*
>
> *(Rolf 1989, p. 39).*

Kiiko Matsumoto and Stephen Birch, who were studying the relationship between acupuncture channels and connective tissue in the 1980s,

suggest that: 'Perhaps the fascia, the tissues that cover and line the body and organs, have some special qualities, properties or functions that were recognised by the medical authors of the Han Dynasty' (Larson 1990, p. 26).

Fascia (and, more generally, connective tissue) does indeed have some special qualities. The first is that it provides a physical means of communication from the outside of the body to the heart of every cell and from the heart of every cell to the heart of every other cell. Each individual cell contains a connective tissue cytoskeleton that provides a framework of support, structure and communication for the various cellular and nuclear elements within. Proteins called integrins reach out from the cytoskeleton, across the cell surface to the surrounding connective tissue matrix. At the outermost layer of the skin, tonofilaments reach in from the epidermis and are attached via hemidesmosomes to the dermal connective tissue. From here, anchoring fibrils link in to the connective tissue matrix (Oschman 2000, pp. 45–47). Thus do we find a route from the massage practitioner's hands to every cell of the patient's body.

Another of the special qualities of connective tissue is the presence of collagen fibres within the matrix of ground substance, fibres and cells. Collagen is the 'longest molecule that has ever been isolated' and is 'stronger in tensile strength than steel wire' (Juhan 2003, p. 72), qualities ideal in its role of providing support and connectivity in the body. Collagen is also hollow, which suits its role in circulation and communication. James Oschman, a researcher into 'energy medicine' talks of life energy as 'bioelectric, biomagnetic, biomechanical, and bioacoustic signals moving through collagen fibres, ground substance, and associated layers of water molecules' (Larson 1990, p. 25).

Curiously, it has been shown that within the collagen tubule is not only, as we might expect, lymph or ground substance but also cerebrospinal fluid (Juhan 2003, p. 73). This phenomenon provides evidence of an extraordinary communication from the sources of cerebrospinal fluid in the ventricles in the middle of the brain to, potentially, every cell in the body; a point not lost on craniosacral therapists who consider cerebrospinal fluid to be the carrier of the 'breath of life'.

Fascia is the general name for the dense irregular connective tissue layer surrounding muscles, bones, and joints. It consists mainly of randomly arranged collagen fibres within the ground substance. It provides support and protection and gives structure to the body. Ida Rolf says of it, 'fascia forms an intricate web coextensive with the body, central to the body, central to its well-being, central to its performance. Clearly fascial tone, fascial span, is a basic contributing factor to bodily well-being' (Rolf 1989, p. 39).

Fascia consists of three layers: the superficial, the deep and the subserous. The superficial fascia is located directly under the subcutis of the skin. Its functions include the storage of fat and water and it provides passageways for nerves and blood vessels. In some areas of the body, it also houses a layer of skeletal muscle, allowing for movement of the skin.

The deep fascia lies beneath the superficial fascia. It aids muscle movement and, like the superficial fascia, provides passageways for nerves and blood vessels. In some areas of the body, it also provides an attachment site for muscles and acts as a cushioning layer between them.

The subserous fascia lies between the deep fascia and the membranes lining the cavities of the body. There is a potential space between it and the deep fascia that allows for flexibility and movement of the internal organs.

Myofascia extends from the deep fascia as a thin, elastic and dynamic membrane that covers, supports and separates the skeletal muscles. As endomysium it wraps and separates each muscle fibre. As perimysium it wraps each bundle of muscle fibres into a fascicle. As epimysium it wraps each muscle itself. These three varieties of myofascia each contribute collagen fibres to the connective tissue that attaches the muscle either to bone or to other muscles. These attachments may also extend beyond the muscle as tendon or aponeurosis (Tortora & Grabowski 1996, pp. 240–241).

Between adjacent muscles the epimysium provides a protective route for blood vessels, nerves and lymph ducts. The muscles, ideally, act as cushions for these vessels. However, the quality of cushioning depends on the tone of the muscle as well as the dynamism of the myofascial pathways. If the surrounding muscles are hypertonic they will limit the flow of blood and lymphatic fluid through the epimysium and reduce the flow to the surrounding tissue.

This may be exactly the condition Dr Varma describes in the quote at the beginning of this chapter. It is echoed in the words of Andrew Taylor Still (1828–1917) the founder of osteopathy. Still always reminded his students that the physician's task 'was to remove with gentleness all perceived mechanical obstructions to the free-flowing rivers of life (blood, lymph, and cerebrospinal fluid). Nature would then do the rest' (McPartland & Skinner 2005). Perhaps an ancient appreciation of the significance of myofascia in relation to those rivers of life was what inspired the development of some of the traditional medical systems still available to us today.

Yoshio Manaka, who died in 1989, contributed much to our modern understanding of acupuncture through scientific research. Although he did not specifically refer to the connective tissue he said: 'While we can offer no clear description of the body's hardware, we propose that it is better to examine and define the software first' (Manaka 1995, p. 55). Manaka referred to the 'X-signal system', so called because it could not yet be fully explained, even if he considered it to be *the biological system that lies at the very heart of acupuncture and moxibustion theory and practice.*' He considered it to be a primitive signalling system, as yet unknown to biologists and impossible to explain with neurophysiology because, 'it manifests and is manipulated clinically with minute stimuli or influences that cannot be clearly said to affect the nervous system' (Manaka 1995, p 18). It seems highly likely from what we now know that the connective tissue provides a significant part of the hardware in this signalling system.

Recent research would seem to confirm this. Helene Langevin and colleagues at the University of Vermont College of Medicine used high frequency ultrasound scanning acoustic microscopy to study acupuncture channels and the effects of acupuncture needling. Langevin observes that 'Acupuncture points and meridians typically are located between muscles or between a muscle and a tendon or bone' (Langevin 2001, p. 2279).

In other words, acupuncture meridians may be myofascial pathways.

In one experiment, Langevin explored a phenomenon discussed for more than 2000 years in acupuncture texts and of great clinical significance to acupuncturists. This phenomenon, known as 'de qi' or 'needle grasp', is described as a tug on the needle 'like a fish biting on a fishing line' (Langevin 2001, p. 2275). Microscopic observation shows that as the acupuncture needle is turned collagen fibres wind around its shaft. Not only does this explain the tug on the needle but it also suggests that acupuncture achieves some of its effects through mechanical influence on the connective tissue matrix. Langevin says that:

> *The ancient maps of acupuncture points and meridians may essentially be a guide to insert the needle into connective tissue. Spreading of matrix deformation and cell activation along connective tissue planes thus may mediate acupuncture effects remote from the acupuncture needle site*
> *(Langevin 2001, pp. 2279–2280).*

This would certainly fit Manaka's theory of a signalling system requiring no more than minute stimuli and free from the need for mediation through the nervous system. Hiroshi Motoyama draws similar conclusions in his study of yoga practice and the Ayur-vedic nadis. He says, 'I consider the nadis to be essentially equivalent to the meridians of Chinese acupuncture; from my research, it appears that these channels are formed of connective tissue and filled with body fluid' (Motoyama 2003, p. 43).

Perhaps one day we will construct an anatomical model with which to explain exactly how traditional Chinese acupuncture works. Researchers like Matsumoto, Motoyama and Langevin call our attention to the connective tissue matrix as an important part of that model. That matrix might have 72 000 pathways; it might have 350 000 pathways; it might have as many pathways as cells. In the practice of Thai Massage we have only ten sen but if these are myofascial pathways perhaps they are the more significant routes through the connective tissue matrix or, at least, those into which we can most easily press our thumbs. Perhaps we have the beginnings of a way in which to explain the physical benefits of manipulating these lines.

Myofascial sen

> *In Thai Massage all the schools seem to agree that there are ten main lines, but nobody seems to agree on where they run*
> *(Brust 1996, p. 15).*

If we consider the sen not as lines but as myofascial planes or pathways we can be very clear in our description of where they run because they always relate to muscles and bone and the myofascial channels between them.

As mentioned before, when it comes to the practice of Thai massage we concern ourselves only with fragments of the ten sen. Here they are referred to as treatment lines (Fig. 12.1).

There are only a couple of rules when it comes to manipulating these treatment lines:

Figure 12.1   General view of the treatment lines used in Thai Massage.

- only work where the tissue is soft
- never apply pressure towards the bone.

This means we are always working to soften and deepen myofascial channels between muscle and muscle and muscle and bone.

Myofascial leg lines

When I first studied Thai massage we were taught five treatment lines on the legs. Nowadays some people teach six, more in keeping with the traditional Chinese meridian model. On the lateral surface of the leg there are two treatment lines, usually referred to as the 1st outside leg line and the 2nd outside leg line (Fig. 12.2).

The 1st outside leg line begins just above the ankle and follows the lateral edge of the tibia between the bone and the tibialis anterior muscle towards the knee. The technique when working

Figure 12.2   Lateral view of the leg showing the path of the 1st outside leg line and the 2nd outside leg line.

this line is to rest the thumbs on the lateral edge of the tibia and then allow them to drop off the bone into the myofascial channel between the bone and the muscle. Each pass along the line aims to gain a little more softness and depth.

On the upper leg the 1st outside leg line follows the lateral border of the rectus femoris muscle. The line begins at the little dip on the superior, lateral corner of the kneecap and continues up to the anterior superior iliac spine (ASIS).

The 2nd outside leg line begins on the lower leg, just superior to the lateral malleolus and follows the anterior border of the peroneus longus muscle. The aim in working this line is to soften and open the myofascial channel between the peroneus longus muscle and the tibialis anterior muscle. This is achieved by pushing the muscle downwards under the bone. It is tempting to medially rotate the leg to see where the line runs but this is best avoided as the rotation will tighten the fascial web, contrary to the aim of softening it.

Above the knee the 2nd outside leg line follows the anterior border of the iliotibial tract from just above the knee towards the head of the femur. The method of working this line involves pressing the fascial band of the iliotibial tract down and under the femur.

The 3rd outside leg line actually starts at the back of the leg in the centre of the achilles tendon and passes between the two heads of the gastrocnemius muscle into the soft tissue at the back of the knee. Above the knee the 3rd outside leg line follows the lateral border of the biceps femoris muscle from the knee to the hip (Fig. 12.3).

On the medial surface of the leg there are two treatment lines, usually referred to as the 1st inside leg line and the 2nd inside leg line (Fig. 12.4).

The 1st inside leg line follows the medial edge of the tibia between the bone and the soleus muscle. The fascial binding associated with this line is often quite tight and extra care is needed to avoid causing pain. Above the knee the line begins at the little dip on the superior, medial corner of the kneecap. From there the 1st inside leg line follows the medial border of the rectus femoris muscle up towards the groin.

The 2nd inside leg line begins at the ankle on the medial border of the achilles tendon and

Figure 12.3   Posterior view of the leg showing the path of the 3rd outside leg line.

Figure 12.4   Medial view of the leg showing the path of the 1st inside leg line and the 2nd inside leg line.

follows the medial border of the gastrocnemius muscle up to the knee. Above the knee the line begins at the posterior border of the sartorius muscle, just above its attachment to the head of the tibia. Moving up towards the groin, the line follows the posterior border of the gracilis muscle.

Myofascial arm lines

Using a myofascial approach to Thai massage we find four treatment lines on the forearms. These prove very useful in working an area that is often poorly attended in other massage systems (Fig. 12.5)

The middle arm line begins at the wrist, between the tendons of palmaris longus and flexor carpi radialis. The line travels superior to the wrist between the palmaris longus muscle and the flexor carpi radialis muscle to the elbow crease.

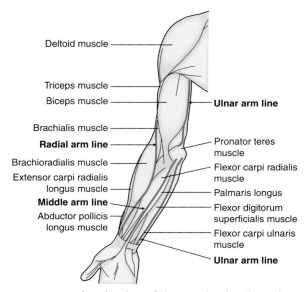

Figure 12.5   Anterior view of the arm showing the path of the radial arm line, the middle arm line and the ulnar arm line.

The ulnar arm line starts medial to the flexor carpi ulnaris tendon at the crease of the wrist. It follows the myofascial pathway between the flexor carpi ulnaris muscle and the flexor digitorum superficialis muscle. In order to find depth in this myofascial channel it is necessary to bend the flexor digitorum superficialis muscle over the top of the bones of the forearm.

The radial arm line starts at the crease of the wrist on the medial border of the tendon of the brachioradialis muscle and continues up the medial border of the muscle to the elbow crease. This line is manipulated using the thumb which moves the muscle medially in order to find the myofascial channel between the brachioradialis muscle and the flexor carpi radialis muscle.

On the posterior surface of the arm there is only one treatment line to consider (Fig. 12.6).

The posterior arm line starts at the centre of the wrist crease, between the heads of the ulna and radius bones. Moving up towards the elbow the line follows the border of the extensor digitorum muscle.

Working all the arm lines involves finding the natural movement of the associated muscles in order to soften and deepen the myofascial channels without pressing against the bones.

Myofascial back lines

In common with all the treatment lines used in Thai massage there are differences in opinion as to where the back lines run. Often they are compared with the bladder meridians used in Chinese acupuncture. Because the arrangement of muscles on the back is so complex and multi-layered it is difficult to say exactly which muscles these lines relate to. That said however, in practice the lines are easy to find and use.

There are two medial back lines, one on either side of the spinal column. To locate the lines the thumbs are positioned side by side on the spinous process of a vertebra. They will fall naturally into two channels either side of the spine. Although these channels can be worked from the pelvis to the seventh cervical vertebra it is more practical to stop at the lower edge of the scapulae. In general the channels follow the medial borders of the erector spinae muscles.

There are also two lateral lines on the back. These are located by moving the thumbs laterally from the medial back lines. The thumbs rise up over a ridge of muscle and fall down the other side. In general these lines follow the lateral borders of the erector spinae muscles from the pelvis to the shoulder blades.

These lines are manipulated by walking the palms up the muscle ridge from the pelvis to the lower edge of the scapulae, exchanging the pressure slowly from hand to hand, creating a slight torsion around each vertebra. Once at the scapulae the thumbs take over, following the medial back lines down the spine, vertebra by vertebra until the pelvis. At each vertebra the aim is to engage with the fascia and muscle and push the tissues upwards. It is not unusual to feel or hear a click of release at a vertebra with these movements but it is not specifically the aim of the process. Some people click easily and some do not.

We can also work the lateral back lines while kneeling to the side of our patient. In this case, we engage the lateral back line using the heel of

Deltoid muscle

Triceps muscle

Brachioradialis muscle

Extensor carpi radialis longus muscle

Anconeus muscle

Extensor digitorum muscle

Extensor carpi radialis brevis muscle

Extensor digiti minimi muscle

Abductor pollicis longus muscle

Extensor pollicis brevis muscle

Extensor pollicis longus muscle

Flexor carpi ulnaris muscle

Extensor carpi ulnaris muscle

Posterior arm line

Figure 12.6   Posterior view of the arm showing the path of the posterior arm line.

our hand and bend the erector spinae muscle towards the spinal column. Our other hand rests on the pelvis.

Thai massage as myofascial massage

Thai massage is mostly concerned with the manipulation of the sen. The unfolding of this process is really quite simple. It does not matter whether the line is worked from the extremity toward the torso or from the torso toward the extremity. The general technique is to work up and down each line, feeling for any tightness in the tissue. Where there is tightness, the area is worked a little more to soften the tissue and equalize the feel of the entire line. This process is often referred to as 'clearing energy blocks'. Unlike shiatsu or acupressure there is no method, apart from touch, with which to assess the lines and there is no method of balancing the energy between the sen. The guiding principle is to work to soften all the lines on the limbs and let nature take care of the rest.

There are various ways to work the sen. They are mostly worked with the thumbs or palms. Occasionally they are worked with the knees, elbows or the soles of the feet. Whichever tool is used, the most important thing is the sensitivity of the massage practitioner. The practitioner needs to feel what is happening. When the patient knows that they are being felt they relax, letting go of any fear that they might be hurt or broken.

Usually Thai massage practitioners press into the line to the point where the tissue tightens and resists. They then add a little more pressure. Working with attention on the myofascial pathway requires some modification to this approach. Simply pressing until the tissue resists leaves no room for movement or change in response to the massage practitioner's input. If the massage practitioner learns to feel the response in the tissue they will often find as they increase the pressure that the connective tissue shows a direction in which it prefers to go. The practitioner follows the direction of the patient's body.

This way of working requires a very alive attention with each and every move. There is no repetition of a technique. Every technique has to be rediscovered in the moment. This sounds like a slow process but it is not. Learning to work like this takes a little time but soon the sensation of the massage practitioner's body wakes up.

The massage practitioner feels for the softening of the tissue and connects with the elasticity and inherent movement of the fascia. It may draw their hands up towards the patient's head or down towards their feet. This natural movement is followed until the first barrier of resistance is met. The practitioner then allows the elasticity of the patient's body to push their thumbs back out, following the same path in which they came in. This basic movement is never the same. The connective tissue changes with each pass along a myofascial pathway. With each pass the massage practitioner can expect to work a little deeper. Even the direction of movement in the connective tissue may change with the work.

In Thai massage, rhythm is very important. That rhythm is a combination of the practitioner's action and the response of the patient's tissues to that action. The rhythm arises in the moment and helps the muscle to soften. Muscle tissue consists of cells and fibres, organized in a connective tissue web, suspended in fluid. Working like this encourages the muscle to change from a more solid to a more relaxed and liquid state. The muscle is expressing a quality called thixotrophy; which describes the way in which a colloidal combination of solid matter suspended in fluid changes state in response to the heat and the quality of the movement administered.

The muscle changes its quality in response to the heat of the practitioner's contact and the rhythm of their movement. The resulting softening of the ground substance improves the flow of nutrients to the cells and waste from the cells to the lymphatic system (Oschman 2000, p. 171). Rhythmic kneading of the muscle also encourages venous, lymphatic and tissue drainage (Chaitow 2003, p. 174). The softening and loosening of the myofascial pathways further enhances this process by easing and encouraging that flow between adjacent muscles. In addition, this combination can be expected to reduce pressure on the peripheral nerves effectively reducing 'noise' flowing through the nervous system.

Thai massage and neuromuscular technique

One of the techniques included under the general heading of Neuromuscular Technique is the 'c-bend'; recognized as one of the few ways of modifying connective tissue status and lengthening muscle through a process of 'tension loading'. The technique involves using the thumbs or the heel of the hand to introduce a 'c-bend' into the target muscle, until the first barrier of resistance is met. The barrier is engaged until the therapist feels a release in the tissue. This would typically occur between 5 and 30 seconds. Using this technique encourages muscle lengthening without the risk of initiating a stretch reflex. Although the c-bend can be applied as a series of rapid, snapping thrusts with the intention of breaking up rigid tissue, when its aim is to lengthen muscle the process is slower and smoother (Chaitow 2003, pp. 32–33).

The c-bend enlists the help of the muscle spindles and Golgi tendon receptors within the muscles. The muscle spindles detect and adjust the length of the muscle while the Golgi tendon receptors detect how hard the muscle is working (Chaitow 2003, p. 3). Applying a c-bend, signals to the nervous system that the muscle is under load and the nervous system lengthens the muscle to reduce the risk of overload and damage.

In Thai massage, rhythmic manipulation of the sen is a major part of the massage. Using a myofascial approach to the sen, the massage practitioner invariably follows the border of a muscle. As they push into the myofascial pathway they often find themselves applying a c-bend to the muscle. Although in Thai massage it is not usual to hold the c-bend for long, the rhythmic repetition of the movement along the length of the muscle still has the desired effect of lengthening and softening the muscle.

When I studied NMT with Leon Chaitow one of the first attempts we made at applying a c-bend was to the erector spinae muscle. The movement involved using the medial border of the muscle to c-bend it away from the spine. In Thai massage it is more practical to use the lateral border of the erector spinae muscle to apply a c-bend toward the spine. This is the lateral back line. It works just as well. The c-bend is repeated along the length of the spine from the edge of the pelvis to the lower edge of the scapula. One hand works while the other rests (Fig. 12.7).

When manipulating the 1st outside leg line on the upper leg the massage practitioner can use the myofascial pathway to apply a c-bend along the length of the rectus femoris muscle from the corner of the knee to the pelvis. In this case the work usually begins by applying a c-bend using the palm to warm up and soften the muscle before applying a stronger c-bend with both thumbs. The muscle is bent over the top of the femur (Fig. 12.8).

The c-bend can also be applied when working the 2nd outside leg line on the upper leg. This myofascial pathway follows the anterior border

Figure 12.7 Applying a 'c-bend' to the erector spinae muscle.

Figure 12.8 Applying a 'c-bend' to the rectus femoris muscle.

Figure 12.9   Applying a 'c-bend' to the iliotibial tract.

of the iliotibial tract. Here the c-bend is applied only using the thumbs. The aim of the movement is to bend the iliotibial tract down and under the femur. This c-bend encourages lengthening of the tensor fascia latae muscle (Fig. 12.9).

The c-bend can similarly be applied to the 3rd outside leg line as well and the 1st and 2nd inside leg lines.

The same technique can be applied to all four treatment lines on the forearm. Here the sen can be felt as myofascial pathways between the muscles of the forearm. For each line the massage practitioner uses the thumb to c-bend the target muscle across the bones of the forearm (Fig. 12.10).

The examples given here are just that; there are many more possibilities and variations. When the sen are felt for as myofascial planes rather than as 'energy lines' the entire massage unfolds as a

continuous and rhythmic application of c-bends. Although the application of the c-bend in Thai massage does not have the aim of breaking up fibrous tissue nor of holding the muscle for more than a second at its barrier, it does nevertheless have the desired effect of lengthening and softening the muscle. The Thai massage practitioner's aim is to gain just a little more length and softness muscle by muscle throughout the patient's body. The accumulated effect is quite profound; undoubtedly more than the sum of the parts.

Conclusion

One of the main sources of modern myofascial techniques is Rolfing. Ida Rolf started teaching her system in the 'therapeutic' scene that developed around Fritz Perls, Will Schutz and the Esalen Institute in the mid 1960s. This period at Esalen, in California, saw the birth of a confrontational style of group therapy called 'encounter'. The Institute also came to be regarded as the centre of the 'human potential' movement. Ida Rolf's system fitted this environment well. Early Rolfing was a fairly confrontational style of bodywork and the ten-session series became a fashionable adjunct to psychotherapy with the belief that it would reach the parts that the 'talking cure' could not.

Rolfing is based on the concept of an 'ideal body' which, for Ida Rolf, was a body better orientated to gravity. The aim of the Rolfing series was to bring the client closer to this ideal. In my experience of the work in the hands of one of Rolf's direct students there was little talk and the work was clearly a matter of the therapist 'knowing' what was right for my body; a knowing that now takes between six and seven hundred hours of training to acquire. Perhaps, because of this origin, myofascial techniques are generally taught and used within the context of a diagnosis and treatment approach to bodywork; the therapist becomes the expert on the patient's body.

In comparison, at between 60 and 100 hours, the Thai massage practitioner's training is quite meagre. And, in the absence of a system of diagnosis on which to base a treatment plan it would

Figure 12.10   Applying a 'c-bend' to the flexor carpi radialis muscle.

seem that the practitioner of Thai massage has little more to offer the patient than attention to the relationship, to the unfolding rhythm of the work and to relaxation. However, if we consider that the massage might actually be a myofascial workout from the feet to the top of the head, we begin to understand just why this humble massage technique is, in practice, fascinating and deeply effective. We may well be improving the flow of blood as it carries oxygen and nutrients to the cells. We may well be assisting the drainage of lymph as it carries toxins away from the cells. We may well be reducing the pressure of muscles and connective tissue bindings leaning against the nerves, thereby reducing the extraneous noise flowing through the nervous system.

Thai Massage Master, Pichet Boonthume, tells his students to work the lines until the limbs become like jelly and everything else will be fine. If those lines are myofascial pathways and, through the rhythmic application of c-bends, they can be used to lengthen the muscles, soften and smooth the connective tissue matrix and enhance the exchange of fluids and information from cell to cell throughout that matrix, we must marvel at the wisdom of the ancients. As modern technology permits us to peek into places where those ancients could only go with their senses we may well find the same thread of perennial wisdom running through NMT and Thai massage as well as a number of other medical systems of similar origin.

References

Brust H: *The Art of Traditional Thai Massage*, Bangkok, 1990, Editions Duang Kamol.

Brust H: *The Art of Traditional Thai Massage for Advanced Practitioners*, Bangkok, 1996, Editions Duang Kamol.

Chaitow L: *Modern Neuromuscular Techniques*, Edinburgh, 2003, Churchill Livingstone.

Feuerstein G: *Yoga, The Technology of Ecstacy*, Wellingborough, 1990, Crucible.

Gold R: *Thai Massage: A Traditional Medical Technique*, St Louis, MO, 2007, Mosby Elsevier.

Iyengar BKS: *Light on Yoga*, London, 1984, Unwin.

Juhan D: *Job's Body: A Handbook for Bodywork*, New York, 2003, Station Hill Press.

Kinder H, Hilgemann W: *Atlas of World History*, Middlesex, 1978, Penguin Books, p 43.

Langevin HM, Churchill DL, Cipolla J: The FASEB, *Journal* 15, 2001.

Larson D: The Role of Connective Tissue as the Physical Medium for the Conduction of Healing Energy in Acupuncture and Rolfing, *Am J Acupunct* 18(3), 1990.

Maciocia G: *The Foundations of Chinese Medicine*, Edinburgh, 1991, Churchill Livingstone, p 152.

Manaka Y: *Chasing the Dragon's Tail*, Brookline, MA, 1995, Paradigm Publications.

McPartland JM, Skinner E: The Biodynamic Model of Osteopathy in the Cranial Field, *EXPLORE* 1(1), 2005.

Mercati M: *Thai Massage*, London, 1998, Marshall Publishing, p 10.

Milne H: *The Heart of Listening*, Berkeley, CA, 1995, North Atlantic Books, p 48.

Motoyama H: *Theories of the Chakras*, New Delhi, 2003, New Age Books.

Oschman JL: *Energy Medicine*, Edinburgh, 2000, The Scientific Basis. Churchill Livingstone.

Rapgay L: *Tibetan Medicine, No 3*, Dharamsala, India, 1981, The Library of Tibetan Works and Archives, pp 11–14.

Rolf I: *Rolfing*, Rochester, VT, 1989, First Healing Arts Press.

Tortora GJ, Grabowski SR: *Principles of Anatomy and Physiology*, New York, 1996, Harper Collins.

Appendix

Nimmo, chiropractic and myofascial pain

Jeffrey Cohen, Russell W. Gibbons, Michael Schneider and Howard Vernon

Introduction

Raymond Nimmo was a pioneering research clinician and practitioner whose background in chiropractic offered him a sound understanding (at the time) of the way the nervous system operated in relation to musculoskeletal pain. Nimmo's work with trigger points paralleled that of Janet Travell, with whom he communicated. In this appendix there are three documents:

1. A short extract from a book from 2001 on Nimmo's work, compiled with two of his chiropractic colleagues and collaborators, Drs Michael Schneider DC and Jeffrey Cohen DC that sets out in summary form his ideas on technique.
2. An article by Jeffrey Cohen and Russell W. Gibbons (1998) that expands on these introductory notes and offers information on Nimmo's history.
3. An article by Howard Vernon and Michael Schneider (2009) that provides a context in chiropractic for treatment of myofascial pain, including reference to Nimmo.

These articles are published within the context of this text on *Modern Neuromuscular Techniques*, in order to increase awareness of the multiple strands that have contributed to current knowledge.

Nimmo notes on technique

Michael Schneider DC, Jeffrey Cohen DC

The application of the Receptor-Tonus Method consists of the following:

1. The detection and elimination of noxious points which generate nerve impulses. Such impulses coming from sources other than proper centres are physiologically unlawful. They set up devious routes in the nervous system and may produce trouble anywhere in the body. In the autonomics, they produce vasoconstriction of blood vessels, with consequent ischaemia, hypoxia, pain and cellular degeneration. They apparently invade any system of nerves, including the cranial nerves, or even brain centres.
2. The elimination of hyper- or hypotonia of muscles. Only when this is accomplished is it possible for osseous structures to assume normal relationships. Aberration of the tonus system is the cause of skeletal misalignment and curvature.
3. The normalizing of ligaments and tendons. When under tension from muscle or joint pull, these structures are affected. Being rich in nerve supply, especially sensory and proprioceptors, they become foci of irritation to the nervous system.

All work is specific to, and exclusive to, the **nervous system**. It does not make any difference where you begin the corrective treatment, however, it would be well to begin in the area of the patient's chief complaint of pain.

Hold manual pressure for about three to eight seconds. **Five seconds** is probably best. Nothing is gained by holding a long contact. These points do not leave while pressure is being applied, but later. Treatment starts the process. It is far better to hold a point several times at five seconds at a time, than it is to hold it for thirty or sixty seconds. Prolonged pressure produces a pressure anesthesia which will beguile the operator into thinking he has eliminated the trigger point. When this occurs, the point will more than likely return.

Some say that a rubbing, stroking, circular movement, or a vibrating contact should be used. This is merely complicating the process, and gaining nothing. Those who say this are trying to camouflage this work, and usually call it something else. What is being done here is inhibition. You are trying to **inhibit a facilitated process**. You are trying to achieve quiescence in these particular points. What is accomplished is a raising of the stimuli threshold so that the point will cease firing impulses into the nervous system.

When normal, muscles palpate as soft, homogenous, relaxed, and are not painful to properly applied pressure. This is true of all palpable muscles. Never treat a point that is not painful, for then the treatment itself may become the irritant. When no longer painful, the job is done. Leave it alone. If you over treat a muscle, all you can do is leave it alone. This rule applies to all trigger points, and all muscles.

Pressure is what clears the muscles of hypermyotonia. Gliding on the longer muscles, after lubrication, so one will not pull hair or skin, which is very painful, is merely distributing the pressure equally over the muscle. The effect on lymph is not important. You are not, so-called, 'milking' the muscle. You are merely applying pressure, just as in any other place. Pressure, used correctly, clears out all these conditions, which are trigger points, hypermyotonia, and hypomyotonia. Whenever a hypertonic muscle is released, normal tonus appears in its opposite according to the working of Davis' Law; likewise, if a stimulus is made in a hypotonic muscle, hypertonus is temporarily released in the antagonist. The so-called 'weak' muscle regains its strength instantly. This is an aberration of the tonus function, which has been set into operation by abnormal stimuli, acting in accordance with Davis' Law.

Raymond L. Nimmo and the evolution of trigger point therapy, 1929–1986

Jeffrey H, Cohen DC,[1] Russell W, Gibbons Litt D[2]

Dr. Raymond L. Nimmo (1904–86) was the definitive chiropractic pioneer in the now widely accepted field of soft tissue and trigger point therapy. This article explores how Nimmo was able to make the radical conceptual leap from moving bones to working with muscles that move the bones. Also discussed are the neurophysiological explanations that Nimmo evolved in the 1950s for the trigger point phenomenon, formulations that are still regarded as highly sophisticated half a century later. Finally, the article describes how Nimmo, with a basic chiropractic education absent of much of the background in the biological and physical sciences of today's preparation, was able to combine his clinical experiences and intellectual formulation to arrive at a theory that became widely accepted. (J Manipulative Physiol Ther 1998; 21:167–72).

Introduction

On November 20, 1980, William Bachop, Ph.D., chairman of the Department of Anatomy at National College of Chiropractic, wrote to Raymond L. Nimmo, D.C., of Granbury, Texas and posed the following question, a question suggesting the seemingly ever-present conflict between laboratory research and clinical practice outcomes in the 'technique' wars of chiropractic for most of this century:

> *The Nimmo technique is used in all parts of the chiropractic world, and I asked why should a chiropractor in private practice in a small town in Texas make a discovery that had seemingly eluded the chiropractors on the faculties of the colleges…with the time, funding and facilities to do research (Bachop 1980)?*

Nimmo's reply explored many of the issues involving research techniques within the profession in its formative years, but in some respects he did not address another central question that could be raised about Nimmo and the practitioners who have been credited with 'discoveries' of other techniques. That question should have some significance and interest in this postcentennial period of chiropractic, when the profession can correctly claim to having elevated its preclinical, professional and clinical studies to standards that have achieved parity in the health care community.

Nimmo was one of the many chiropractors trained in the second and third decades of this

[1]Private practice of chiropractic, Pittsburgh, PA.
[2]Editor Emeritus, *Chiropractic History*, Pittsburgh, PA.

century who had virtually no prechiropractic academic training in the basic sciences, and whose instruction in anatomy, physiology, neurology and the other fundamentals for treating the human body were under chiropractors (although some of these did have university training). Their own backgrounds did not suggest lives of research, writing and clinical instruction, yet they each became important in the lexicon of chiropractic technique after the initial debates between D. D. Palmer and his early associates, Willard Carver, S. M. Langworthy, Alva Gregory, Joy Loban and A. P. Davis (Gatterman & Lee 1995).

Discussion

Raymond L. Nimmo (1904–86) (Fig. 1) was a 1926 Palmer graduate who was to become the definitive pioneer in the now widely accepted area of soft tissue and trigger point therapy. His history and experience is similar to others who evolved specific technique research in this period. Among them were Joy Loban (1889–19?), who advocated an early nonforce technique (Gibbons 1991); Leo Spears (1894–1956), largely known for his hospital but an early formulator of 'painless' adjustments (Rehm 1991); Thomas Lake (1887–1950), who developed endonasal therapy (Gibbons & Thomas 1995); and Frederick W. Illi (1901–1984), developer of the sacroiliac physiology of spinal biomechanics (Gaucher-Peslherbe 1995).

Nimmo's background is known. His contemporaries shared with him an absence of a grounding in the basic sciences or even in academics (although the early lives of Loban and Lake have still to be fleshed out). They advocated specific technique instruction with a passionate fervour that gained thousands of followers during their lives. Unlike them, Nimmo's technique, termed Receptor-Tonus (RT), has survived its founder (Illi's work may correctly have evolved into conceptual chiropractic theory rather than a technique). Although other techniques have become either discarded or little-used, Nimmo's technique survived. Although developed in the limited chiropractic world of the 1950s, his concepts are compatible with contemporary medical thought in this area. Nimmo was born in Fort Worth in 1904, where he lived most of his life,

with the exception of his college and military experience. He attended Tarleton State University in Stephenville in 1923 and a year later entered the Palmer School of Chiropractic, receiving his D.C. in 1926. That decade the Palmer School graduated several individuals who introduced new chiropractic techniques—Spears, Gonstead, Gillet—although other schools would also produce contemporaries (Hugh and Vinton Logan and Illi at Universal; DeJarnette at the Nebraska College).

Although he travelled in the Navy, and briefly practised in Illinois, Oklahoma and Georgia, Nimmo practised for 30 years in Fort Worth. He moved to suburban Granbury in 1956. In his invited essay response to National College anatomist Bachop, Nimmo traced the evolution of his theoretical and clinical process to RT, much of which involved instruction by those who had originated other techniques:

In 1935 I took what Logan called Basic Technique, which he took from Dr. John Hurley's Aquarian Age Healing. Dr. Hugh and Dr. Vinton were in Hurley's first class. I subsequently taught BT for a while ... [I practiced] what was called Chromaffin Synapse Therapy ... which we thought was the sacral ganglia, but was actually releasing muscles ... [yet both] got results, sometimes spectacularly (Nimmo 1981).

A review of chiropractic techniques by Lee and Gatterman (Gatterman & Lee 1995) listed almost 100, with multiple developers in many instances, yet some explored by Nimmo were not included:

I took what was called Bio-Engineering ... D. C. McIntosh taught what he called the McIntosh system of Fascia Release ... we would palpate for tensed fascia, then release it. What it was, of course, was tensed musculature (Nimmo 1981).

Later Nimmo met Ida Rolf, Ph.D., the founder of the Rolfing school, and investigated her methods. Rolf's work led Nimmo to speculate:

[In Rolfing,] the theory was that muscles were bound down by connective tissue, and had to be freed ... [I determined] that certain muscles were

not affected. Rolf worked on all of them, even on the ribs where there were no muscles. When I found that muscles such as the latissimus and the hamstrings were not affected, I sought to discover why, and determined that these muscles are affected, just not as often. I eventually solved all of this. A piece in Scientific American *explained tonus, which has never been taught in the schools. It is hypermyotonia which causes the so-called subluxation and other distortions (Nimmo 1981, 1971).*

In his practice, Nimmo observed 'spots on the shoulders which when pressed on referred pain to various areas, and the results were spectacular in case after case' (Nimmo 1981). He called these 'Noxious Generative Points.' In 1952, he discovered the work of Janet Travell, M.D., perhaps the foremost physician to research myofascial pain and dysfunction, who became prominent in the 1960s as personal physician to President John F. Kennedy. Travell related her fascination with examining muscles in cadavers in the dissection laboratory.

Travell, who had on several occasions expressed to one of the authors (J.H.C.) her admiration for Nimmo's work (Travell J., personal communication), discussed trigger points in a Symposium on Connective Tissue. This apparently prompted Nimmo to search the literature further and to reach his thesis that became the foundation for the Receptor-Tonus therapy:

I realized what every patient can understand, but many chiropractors seemingly cannot, that no bone can move unless a muscle moves it, and no muscle moves a bone unless a nerve impulse reaches it. I decided the lumbar lordosis was due to tight sacrospinalis muscles. I would release them, but the patient would go back into the same position, with return of pain. I looked for muscles that pulled down the front of the pelvis, which were of course, the quadriceps ... (Travell J. Personal communications, 1991 Oct 20 and 1990 Apr 26) (Nimmo 1981).

Thus, a Texan with a year of college and 18 months of classroom and clinic experience during the Palmer School's classical period entered a decades-long quest to eliminate or at least control

pain. In his 1980 letter to Bachop, Nimmo said that he found it difficult to write, yet he came through with quotable expressions, such as '... there are certain essentials necessary in order for us to escape from the mossy-fingered grip of orthodoxy and improve when a superior method is evident' (Nimmo 1981).

Nimmo declared that

in Receptor-Tonus we strive to teach nothing that does not have a physiological basis. The discovery of certain laws gives validity and substance to this principle of practice. It is ensconced in physiology, and consequently can stand the white light of scientific scrutiny (Nimmo 1981).

His therapy was summarized from a chiropractic perspective by Gatterman and Lee (Fig. A.1):

Nimmo found noxious generative points in muscles that referred pain in characteristic patterns. Viewing these hypersensitive areas, the trigger points of Travell, as abnormal reflex arcs he developed a manual technique designed to reduce the irritable loci. He referred to the inter-relationship of muscle tonus and the central nervous system as 'reverberating circuits,' whereby the stimulus was self-perpetuating until the cycle was broken.... This procedure referred to by Travell as ischemic compression offers a noninvasive chiropractic technique instead of the common medical practice of injection of the painful trigger points (Gatterman & Lee 1995).

The following is a brief description of the neurophysiology on which RT is based, according to Nimmo in 1986, the year of his death:

Although it is generally called the Nimmo Technique, the correct designation is Receptor-Tonus Technique for the reason that it deals exclusively with muscle tonus and nerve receptors which initiate pain. The early development of the method was necessarily somewhat experimental and empirical. It was different from anything I had ever been taught but it was the most efficient method and permanent release from pain I had ever used or observed (Nimmo 1986).

To fully understand RT, one must have a basic understanding of the concept of tonus (Fig. A.2):

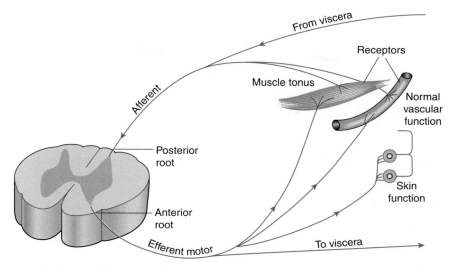

Figure A.1   The normal reflex arc (Nimmo 1971).

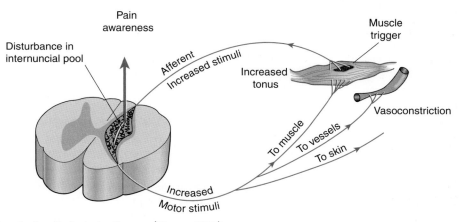

Figure A.2   The physiopathological reflex arc (Nimmo 1971).

Tonus is not an exclusive property of isolated muscle. It is an interaction between a muscle and the spinal cord by the sympathetics. Muscles project a continuous stream of impulses through the posterior root to the gray matter of the cord where the internuncial neurons increase the stimuli which are transmitted through the anterior root and upon reaching the muscle produce a slight pull. This is normal tonus. Tersely stated, the internuncial neurons in the cord are highly excitatory. In their reactive relationships with one another there is a self re-exiting process, which increases and prolongs the motor discharge induced by the incoming stimuli from sensory nerves. Livingston observed that when a volley of sensory stimuli entered the cord for two milliseconds, the discharge through the ventral root lasted 20 milliseconds—in this case ten times longer. Guyton called this the after discharge (Nimmo 1986).

The malfunction of this normal process results in a hypertonic muscle (Fig. A.3). Nimmo states,

Hypermyotonia may result from various insults such as accidents, exposure to cold drafts or from occupations requiring prolonged periods of postural strain such as typing or driving an automobile for many hours without rest (Nimmo 1986).

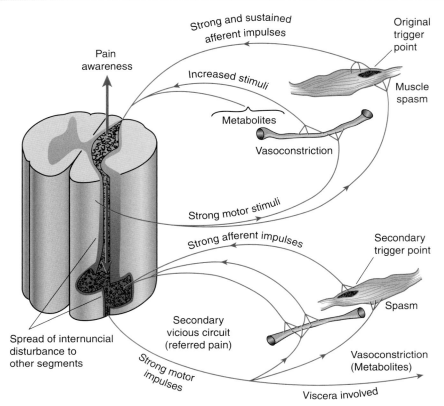

Figure A.3   Vicious physiopathological reflex circuit arising from peripheral structures with referred phenomena (Nimmo 1971).

Increased sensory input to the cord from such 'insults' results in an increased stream of efferent impulses to the muscles, causing a constant state of abnormal contraction.

This in turn causes additional increase in sensory impulses back to the cord, which are again amplified in the internuncial pool, causing even more efferent impulses to the muscle. The result is a vicious, self-perpetuating cycle, with the muscle getting tighter and tighter. This process, occurring in the sympathetic nerves, is beyond voluntary control. Reflex spillover in the sympathetic nerves also causes local vasoconstriction, trapping metabolites in the area (Nimmo 1986).

The focus of irritability within this area of abnormal muscle contraction and vasoconstriction becomes the trigger point. As this process continues, it spreads to other levels of the cord, causing secondary trigger points to develop in other muscles as well as the well known phenomenon of referred pain (Fig. A.4). It is fascinating to compare this diagram with Figure 5, which is from Travell and Simon's 1983 masterpiece *Myofascial Pain and Dysfunction—The Trigger Point Manual* (Travell & Simons 1983). The similarities are striking and suggest one concept developed concurrently by two outstanding independent researchers.

The difference between Nimmo's and Travell's treatment methods is significant. Travell advocated injections to the trigger point and later spray and stretch and 'ischemic compression' to relax the involved muscle. On the other hand, Nimmo states, '*I have found that a proper degree of pressure, sequentially applied, causes the nervous system to release a hypertonic muscle*' (italics are Nimmo's). Nimmo did not see the trigger point as an object to be injected, stretched, massaged or dissolved by ultrasound (Cohen & Schneider 1990; Nimmo 1981).

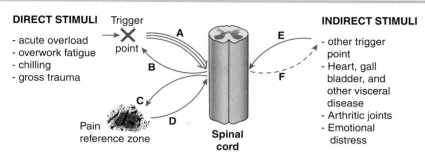

Direct and indirect stimuli. (Reprinted by permission from Travell JG, Simons DG. Myofascial pain and dysfunction: the trigger point manual. Vol. 1. Baltimore: Williams & Wilkins; 1983 p. 15.)

He saw the trigger point as the result of a neurological chain of events that must be approached through the nervous system. This puts RT squarely in the realm of chiropractic; it is not merely an adjunctive therapy, as is so often thought. Nimmo spent 30 years evolving and refining this approach empirically. Every time a patient presented with a new problem, he painstakingly figured out which muscles were involved, consulted his anatomy books, and developed a method of applying pressure to that muscle, as well as muscles seemingly remote from the primary problem that contained secondary trigger points. Nimmo determined that all primary and secondary trigger points must be eliminated to eliminate this vicious cycle. This requires precise application of proper pressure to all involved muscles in the appropriate sequence (Nimmo 1986, Cohen & Schneider 1990, Nimmo 1981).

In a videotape made in the early 1980s, Nimmo explored the philosophical and the scientific approach of his practice and research methodology, recalling that his philosophy classes departed from anatomical and physiological facts to make questionable deductions for the subluxation theory 'which was then upper cervical and later HIO.' Nimmo declared that 'understanding the principles upon which Receptor-Tonus is based has simplified many problems, and brought explanation to many others. We can now explain how D. D. Palmer restored hearing to Harvey Lillard by making a thrust to the fourth thoracic vertebra' (Nimmo 1984).

Nimmo circulated a paper published in 1957 by Arizona practitioner Stanley Hayes, in which Hayes proposed a 'new hypothesis for consideration' of the chiropractic subluxation concept.

Citing the Lillard case, Hayes said that the traditional chiropractic adjustment was:

> based on the idea that force should be used to remove nerve disturbance at any point in the spine where such disturbance appears to exist. Most clinical results are actually secured by releasing abnormal states of tension in the ligaments (and possibly muscles) closely associated with the spine (Hayes 1957).

Later in 1957, Nimmo would also author an article in the *Journal of the NCA* titled 'Receptors, effectors and tonus—a new approach' (Nimmo 1957), which he subsequently reprinted as the first number of an occasional RT newsletter called *The Receptor*. In this paper, Nimmo made this conclusion about his work:

> I believe that a full knowledge of this approach will give one the anatomical and physiological right to fully eighty percent of all illness. I have subscribed to many techniques, putting all to thorough test, and I have found almost all of them valuable. After much experience working with this principle I am convinced that it is anatomically and physiologically sound (Nimmo 1957).

Nimmo stressed the necessity of cooperation with the larger health care community even at a time when there was evidence of the overt and covert antichiropractic activity within many parts of mainline medicine. 'Chiropractic cannot be insular,' he declared many times in a lengthy videotape (Nimmo 1984). He cited not only Travell but Bonica, head of the Department of Anesthesiology at the University of Washington medical school, whom he quoted as saying that 'medicine does not know the basic principles of pain,' lamenting the absence of any teaching in medical schools and any widely-supported pain research (Travell & Simon 1983; Nimmo 1984, 1969).

Travell's work in *The American Practitioner* and her 1983 book *Myofascial Pain and Dysfunction: The Trigger Point Manual* were frequently referenced. Nimmo stressed dialogue with medicine and cited cases in which he had recommended surgery even after attending surgeons had not recommended that course. His departure from medical procedures for low back pain was essentially the trigger point injection, asserting that conservative manipulative procedures utilizing RT could effect the same results. Three medical researchers at George Washington University Medical Center conducted a 'randomized, double-blind evaluation of trigger point injection' in 1988, concluding that 'this study indicates that the critical factor in giving relief of pain is not the injected substance but rather, some type of mechanical stimulus to the trigger point' (Garvey et al. 1989).

Nimmo summarized the RT Method as being based on two main principles: a method that removes the origin of nerve impulses producing abnormal, painful and pathological processes in the body. In 1970, he wrote of RT that

> It clears trigger points, those described in the current literature, but many more not yet known, as well as inaccessible to the methods of other professions. It eliminates those factors which hold the body or parts thereof in a state of misalignment and distortion. The first frees the body from pain, the second further frees it of pain and straightens it up.

What may be exceptional about Nimmo's technique is the wide acceptance that it achieved through the series of classes which he conducted throughout the United States and Canada, starting in 1958. Nimmo declared that 'no other concept introduced to our profession has had so great an impact upon our professional thinking in a like period of time' (Nimmo 1963). In the same publication, Nimmo wrote that he had received a request from the Department of Health, Education and Welfare (which preceded the present Health & Human Services) for all copies of *The Receptor*, to 'be placed in the Department of New Medical Discoveries of the Library of Congress.'

A striking example of the advanced state of Nimmo's thought appeared recently in the journal *Advances in Physical Therapy* (Makous 1995). What is described as a 'unique intraoral approach' to treating temporomandibular joint disorder discusses a manual trigger point treatment for tensor veli palatini muscle. This technique, along with methods for treating all the muscles of mastication, was taught by Nimmo in his seminars throughout the 1960s and 70s and was published in *The Receptor* in 1980 (Nimmo 1981).

Conclusion

Several conclusions are offered about Raymond Nimmo and his technique, from the collaborative effort of both a practitioner of his teaching and a lay observer of the history of the profession (Fig. A.5).

Adjustive Techniques (percentage of use by DCs)	
Diversified	91.1
Gonstead	54.8
Cox/Flexion-Distraction	52.7
Activator	51.2
Thompson	43
SOT	41.3
NIMMO/Tonus Receptor	40.3
Applied Kinesiology	37.2
Logan Basic	30.6
Cranial	27.2
Palmer Upper Cervical/HIO	26
Meric	23.4
Pierce-Stillwagon	19.7
Other	15
Pettibon	6.3
Barge	4.1
Grostic	3.4
Toftness	3.3
Life Upper Cervical	2
NUCCA	1.5

From Table 9-11, Chiropractic Treatment Procedures. *Job Analysis of Chiropractic*, NBCE, Greeley, CO, 1993, p. 78.

Figure A.5   Adjustive techniques.

Adjustive Techniques (percentage of use by DCs)

Diversified	91.1
Gonstead	54.8
Cox/Flexion-Distraction	52.7
Activator	51.2
Thompson	43
SOT	41.3
NIMMO/Tonus Receptor	40.3
Applied Kinesiology	37.2
Logan Basic	30.6
Cranial	27.2
Palmer Upper Cervical/HIO	26
Meric	23.4
Pierce-Stillwagon	19.7
Other	15
Pettibon	6.3
Barge	4.1
Grostic	3.4
Toftness	3.3
Life Upper Cervical	2
NUCCA	1.5

From Table 9-11, Chiropractic Treatment Procedures. *Job Analysis of Chiropractic*, NBCE, Greeley, CO, 1993, p. 78.

1. Nimmo, although a pioneer graduate with but a rudimentary exposure to anatomy, physiology and neurology, evolved a sophisticated approach to technique in the alleviation of myofascial pain. This approach was a dramatic paradigm shift from the traditional chiropractic theories of the day, which emphasized the 'bone on nerve' concept.
2. As a chiropractor, he introduced basic concepts in trigger point therapy that were complementary to those being advanced by such recognized medical pioneers as Travell. He supported these concepts with extensive medical references and was completely up to date on current scientific literature (Travell J. Personal communications, 1991 Oct 20 and 1990 Apr 26) (Nimmo 1963).
3. The Nimmo technique, in competition with many contemporary adjustive procedures, has survived for almost half of the profession's history and is currently used by 40 percent of chiropractors according to a study conducted in 1993 by the National Board of Chiropractic Examiners (Job analysis of chiropractic 1993).

In time, the 'small town chiropractor from Texas' may obtain some posthumous recognition in the larger literature of the healing arts, for Raymond Nimmo was a legitimate pioneer in the identification and treatment of pain, which remains as a primary challenge to practitioners of all schools in these final years of the twentieth century.

Council on chiropractic guidelines and practice parameters

Chiropractic management of myofascial trigger points and myofascial pain syndrome: a systematic review of the literature

Howard Vernon, DC, PhD,[a] and Michael Schneider, DC[b]

Abstract

Objectives: Myofascial pain syndrome (MPS) and myofascial trigger points (MTrPs) are important aspects of musculoskeletal medicine, including chiropractic. The purpose of this study was to review the most commonly used treatment procedures in chiropractic for MPS and MTrPs.

Methods: The Scientific Commission of the Council on Chiropractic Guidelines and Practice Parameters (CCGPP) was charged with developing literature syntheses, organized by anatomical region, to evaluate and report on the evidence base for chiropractic care. This article is the outcome of this charge. As part of the CCGPP process, preliminary drafts of these articles were posted on the CCGPP website www.ccgpp.org (2006-8) to allow for an open process and the

[a]Canadian Memorial Chiropractic College, Toronto, Ontario, Canada.
[b]School of Health and Rehabilitation Sciences, University of Pittsburgh, Pittsburgh, Pa.
Submit requests for reprints to: Howard Vernon, DC, PhD, Canadian Memorial Chiropractic College, 6100 Leslie St, Toronto, Ontario, Canada M2H 3J1 (e-mail: *hvernon@cmcc.ca*).
Paper submitted April 29, 2008; in revised form May 14, 2008; accepted June 1, 2008.0161-4754/$34.00 Copyright © 2009 by National University of Health Sciences.doi: 10.1016/j.jmpt.2008.06.012

broadest possible mechanism for stakeholder input. PubMed, Excerpta Medica Database, Cumulative Index to Nursing and Allied Health Literature, and databases for systematic reviews and clinical guidelines were searched. Separate searches were conducted for (1) manual palpation and algometry, (2) chiropractic and other manual therapies, and (3) other conservative and complementary/alternative therapies. Studies were screened for relevance and rated using the Oxford Scale and Scottish Intercollegiate Guidelines Network rating system.

Results: A total of 112 articles were identified. Review of these articles resulted in the following recommendations regarding treatment: Moderately strong evidence supports manipulation and ischaemic pressure for immediate pain relief at MTrPs, but only limited evidence exists for long-term pain relief at MTrPs. Evidence supports laser therapy (strong), transcutaneous electrical nerve stimulation, acupuncture, and magnet therapy (all moderate) for MTrPs and MPS, although the duration of relief varies among therapies. Limited evidence supports electrical muscle stimulation, high-voltage galvanic stimulation, interferential current, and frequency modulated neural stimulation in the treatment of MTrPs and MPS. Evidence is weak for ultrasound therapy.

Conclusions: Manual-type therapies and some physiologic therapeutic modalities have acceptable evidentiary support in the treatment of MPS and TrPs (J Manipulative Physiol Ther 2009;32:14-24).

Key Indexing Terms: *Myofascial Pain Syndromes; Myofascial Trigger Points; Chiropractic; Musculoskeletal Manipulations.*

Ever since the seminal work of Travell and Rinzler (1952) in 1952, the role of myofascial trigger points (TrPs) in myofascial pain syndrome (MPS) has become an accepted part of musculoskeletal clinical practice. Along with Simons (Travell & Simons 1983), Travell first identified the importance of myofascial pain and its localization in what they termed *trigger points*, providing the first classification of diagnostic criteria for TrPs. They also provided detailed maps of the pain referral patterns from TrPs in all the muscles of the body. Myofascial pain syndrome is currently thought to be the leading diagnosis among pain management specialists (Harden et al. 2000)

and the leading diagnosis in pain patients reporting to general practitioners (Skootsky et al. 1989).

Interest in myofascial tenderness extends throughout the history of chiropractic. It might be said that local paraspinal tenderness, as part of the manifestations of the 'subluxation,' was a central feature of chiropractic thinking from its inception. Arguably, the work of Ray Nimmo (Nimmo 1962, 1984, 1992) represents the earliest and perhaps still most established thinking on this topic among chiropractors. Cohen and Gibbons (Cohen et al. 1998) describe his work as 'a conceptual leap from moving bones to working with muscles that move bones.' Schneider (1994, 2001) has provided a collection and review of all of Nimmo's works. Nimmo's explanations in the 1950s of the pathophysiology of TrPs are still regarded as accurate and highly sophisticated.

Other chiropractic authors who have written on this topic include Schneider (Schneider 1990, 1994, 1995, 2001), Perle (Perle 1989, 1995), Hains (Hains 2002, 2002), and Hammer (Hammer 2007) whose seminal textbook is now in its third printing. There are also numerous case reports and technical reports relating to various soft tissue techniques in chiropractic. In the field of MPS, chiropractic is generally regarded as one of the complementary and alternative medical (CAM) therapies. The CAM therapies are quite commonly used in the treatment of myofascial pain and TrPs (Harris & Clauw 2002), and there is considerable overlap between chiropractic approaches and CAM therapies in this field.

Methods

The search strategy for this review was constrained by the need to identify only those studies of chiropractic treatments (manual therapy and other conservative therapies) that were not directed at clinical complaints associated with any of the specific body regions that have been designated as other reviews in the Council on Chiropractic Guidelines and Practice Parameters (CCGPP) process. In other words, no study was selected of the effect of a chiropractic treatment specifically indicated for back pain, neck pain, upper limb pain (shoulder, elbow, wrist), and

A. The Oxford Rating Scale (Phillips et al. 2001; Sackett et al. 2000).
1a: Systematic review, with homogeneity of RCT's.
1b: Individual RCT with narrow confidence interval.
1c: All or none.
2a: Systematic review, with homogeneity of cohort studies.
2b: Individual cohort study (including low quality RCT; eg <80% follow-up).
2c: Outcomes Research; Ecological studies.
3a: Systematic review with homogeneity of case-control studies.
3b: Individual case-control study.
4: Case-series (and poor quality cohort and case-control studies).
5: Expert opinion without explicit critical appraisal, or based on physiology, bench research or 'first principles'.
B. The SIGN Checklist.
1. ++ = All or most methodological criteria have been fulfilled/bias has been maximally reduced.
2. + = Some of the criteria have been fulfilled/bias has been somewhat reduced.
3. − = Few or no criteria fulfilled/bias is clearly present.

Fig A.6   Rating scales for included studies.

lower limb pain (hip, knee, ankle, and foot) of any kind (i.e., for any category of diagnosis). Only studies of chiropractic treatments for MPS and TrPs were considered. Therefore, the inclusion criteria for this search were as follows: manual therapies, trigger points, myofascial pain syndrome (MeSH headings: musculoskeletal manipulations, myofascial pain syndrome [not exploded to temporomandibular joint]), conservative therapies, laser, acupuncture, ultrasound (US), electrotherapy, naturopathy; 1965 to 2007; English, German; human studies.

After the primary search was conducted, a number of secondary searches were conducted based upon 'related links,' especially emphasizing systematic or clinical reviews, randomized clinical trials, and conservative treatments (vs musculoskeletal manipulations only), as well as searches of additional works by the authors identified in the primary search. Finally, citation reviews were conducted manually to identify any additional suitable studies.

This search was conducted in the PubMed; Cumulative Index to Nursing and Allied Health Literature; Index to Chiropractic Literature (ICL); Manual, Alternative, and Natural Therapy System (MANTIS); Excerpta Medica Database; National Guidelines Clearinghouse; Database of Abstracts of Reviews of Effects; and Turning Research Into Practice databases. Selected publications were rated on the Oxford Rating Scale (Phillips et al. 2001, Sackett et al. 2000) as well as the Scottish Intercollegiate Guidelines Network (SIGN) Checklist (Fig. A.6).

This review accepted all levels of published evidence for narrative description: clinical guidelines, systematic reviews, clinical trials, cohort or case series, case studies, and clinical reviews. For evidence rating, recommendations were constructed and rated according to the Oxford Rating Scale (Phillips et al. 2001, Sackett et al. 2000) as follows:
Consistent level 1 studies
Consistent level 2 or 3 studies or extrapolations from level 1 studies
Level 4 studies or extrapolations from level 2 or 3 studies
Level 5 studies or troublingly inconsistent or inconclusive studies at any level.

Results

Manual Therapies

Systematic Reviews of Manual Therapies. Two completed systematic reviews were identified (Fernandez de las Penas et al. 2005, Rickards 2006). These reviews were rated (Oxford Scale) as 1a evidence with a 2+ quality rating on the SIGN Checklist.

Fernandez de las Penas et al. (2005) used the following selection criteria for acceptable studies:

clinical or randomized controlled trials in which some form of manual therapy (strain/counter-strain, ischemic compression, transverse friction massage, spray and stretch, muscle energy technique) was used to treat (myofascial trigger points) MTrPs (p. 29).

Mobilization and manipulation were apparently not explicitly included. It should be noted that the criterion applied to the 'clinical category' in this search was 'MTrPs,' although MPS was referenced later in their review. No additional, more specific criteria related to clinical complaints in any of the body regions (i.e., back pain, neck pain, limb pain, etc.) were used. It would appear that this search strategy is consistent with the one devised for this review, as other CCGPP reviews dealt with the chiropractic management of pain complaints specific to these body regions.

Fernandez de las Penas et al. (2005) identified 7 acceptable trials (SIGN = 2+/Oxford Scale ratings = 1b), 4 of which obtained a sufficiently high quality score (>5/10 on the Physiotherapy Evidence Database Scale).

- Gam et al. (1998) (Physiotherapy Evidence Database score = 6/10)
- Jaeger & Reeves (1986) (2/10)
- Hanten et al. (2000) (3/10)
- Hong et al. (1993) (6/10)
- Hou et al. (2002) (5/10)
- Hanten et al. (1997) (5/10)
- Dardzinski et al. (2000) (1/10)

The interventions used in these studies were as follows (number of studies in parentheses): spray and stretch (2), soft tissue massage (2), ischaemic compression (2), occipital release exercises (1), strain/counterstrain (SCS) (1), and myofascial release (1). An important finding was:

Only 2 studies ... test(ed) the specific efficacy (efficacy beyond placebo) of various manual therapies in the treatment of MPS (Gam et al., 1998 [massage] and Hanten et al., 2000 [occipital release]). These studies found no difference between interventions (p. 30) (Fernandez de las Penas et al. 2005).

Another important issue from this group of studies is the duration of treatment. Most of these studies (4) investigated only the immediate effects on pain and tenderness (Jaeger & Reeves 1986, Hong et al. 1993, Hou et al. 2002, Hanten et al. 1997). One study investigated the short-term treatment effects of ischaemic compression vs exercises over 5 treatments (Hanten et al. 2000), whereas 2 investigated longer-term effects (6 months) of a course of, in one case, massage added to US therapy (Gam et al. 1998) and, in the other case, SCS in addition to exercises (Dardzinski et al. 2000). In both of the latter studies of a course of therapy, the manual therapy used (massage or SCS) was included among other therapies, making it impossible to identify the distinct contribution of the manual therapy to the reported outcomes.

Fernandez de las Penas et al. (2005) conclude that there are very few randomized controlled studies (RCTs) of any type of manual therapy in the treatment of MTrP (MPS) and, as a result, 'the hypothesis that manual therapies have specific efficacy beyond placebo in the management of MPS caused by MTrPs is neither supported or refuted by the research to date' (p. 33). They do acknowledge that there is some evidence for improvement in some groups within these trials and that this warrants further research.

In Rickards' (2006) review, the inclusion criteria included RCTs of a conservative (in this section: manual only) therapy for active TrPs, not latent TrPs, in which a patient-related pain outcome was used and in which an explicit diagnosis of TrP was made including at least local tenderness and a taut muscle band. Studies were rated on a 20-point scale; however, no cutoff score was used for inclusion. Rickards included the following studies: Chatchawan et al. (2005), Fernandez de las Penas et al. (2006), Hanten et al. (1997), Hou et al. (2002), and Edwards & Knowles (2003).

For the purposes of the present review, the following comments apply to this group of studies: (1) The study of Chatchawan et al. (2005) of massage therapies clearly identified the target group as chronic low back pain and would be included in the CCGPP review on low back pain. (2) The study of Fernandez de las Penas et al. (2006) is included below. (3) The studies of Hanten et al and Hou et al are included in the review by Fernandez de las Penas et al above. (4) Edwards and Knowles' trial (2003) did not include a manual therapy (only active stretching and dry needling were investigated). Therefore, for manual therapies, Rickards' review does not add anything substantial to the present review.

A Cochrane Collaboration Protocol entitled 'Non-invasive physical treatments of myofascial pain' Kilkenny et al. (2007) was identified. This protocol currently contains no results. However, it was used as a source of additional references, particularly on published clinical trials and systematic reviews.

Practice Guidelines on Manual Therapy. The following practice guidelines were identified:
Institute for Clinical Systems Improvement (ICSI).
  Assessment and management of chronic pain. Bloomington (MN): Institute for Clinical Systems Improvement (ICSI); 2005 Nov. p. 77 No recommendation for physical (manual) therapies in the treatment of MPS or TrPs.
Work Loss Data Institute. *Pain (chronic).* Corpus Christi (TX): Work Loss Data Institute; 2006. 261 p. *Myofascial pain syndrome, physical therapy: 14-21 days.*

RCTs of Manual Therapy. In addition to Fernandez de las Penas et al (Gam et al. 1998), our search identified 3 RCTs (Oxford Scale rating = 1b or 2b) of the effect of spinal manipulation on local paraspinal muscular tenderness in the dorsal spine (Terrett & Vernon 1984 [2+/2b]), cervical spine (Vernon et al. 1990 [2+/2b]), and lumbopelvic area (Cote et al. 1994 [2+/2b]). All 3 studies investigated only the immediate effect of the interventions on local muscular pain thresholds (electrical stimulus in Terrett and Vernon (1984) and pressure stimulus in Vernon et al. (1990) and Cote et al. (1994). Immediate and statistically significant increases in pain thresholds were found for spinal manipulation as compared with mobilization in the cervical and dorsal paraspinal muscles, but not in the lumbopelvic soft tissues.

Vicenzino et al. (1996) (2+/1b) reported on the immediate effect of a cervical mobilization on pressure pain threshold (PPT) of tender points on the lateral epicondyle in patients with 'tennis elbow.' Only the mobilization (described as 'manipulation' in this study) resulted in statistically significant increases in lateral epicondyle PPTs vs placebo and control conditions.

Greene et al. (1990) (2+/1b) investigated the effect of 4 different treatments given 3 times over 3 days on skin resistance levels. Subjects with thoracic TrPs were randomized to receive osteopathic manipulative treatment (OMT), laser treatment, OMT plus laser, and sham laser. No significant differences in effects were noted between these groups.

Atienza Meseguer et al. (2006) (2+/1b) studied 54 subjects with trapezius TrP treated with classic SCS, modified SCS, and control. Both treatment groups showed immediate improvement in PPT vs controls, but not vs each other.

Fryer and Hodgson (2005) (2+/1b) compared manual pressure release to sham myofascial release in 37 subjects with upper trapezius myofascial TrPs. A statistically significant increase in PPT was obtained immediately after the intervention in the manual pressure group vs controls that was found to be due to a change in tissue sensitivity.

Fernandez de las Penas et al. (2006) (2+/1b) compared ischaemic compression to transverse friction massage in 40 subjects with myofascial TrPs in the upper trapezius muscle. Both groups obtained significant improvement in PPT within 2 minutes. No difference was found between the groups.

Conclusion: RCTs

A total of 14 RCTs were retrieved. Quality scores ranged widely for the 7 trials reviewed by Fernandez de las Penas et al. (2005). Ten of 14 trials we identified involved only immediate changes in TrP or tender point ratings. Two other trials reported outcomes for short courses of treatments over 3 to 5 days (Hanten et al. 2000, Greene et al. 1990), whereas 2 others reported outcomes at 6 months (Gam et al. 1998, Dardzinski et al. 2000). The outcomes of the 'immediate' trials can be summarized as demonstrating effectiveness in reducing tenderness for spinal manipulation (2 of 3 trials), spray and stretch (2 trials), ischaemic compression (3 trials), transverse friction massage (1 trial), and SCS (1 trial). One trial of mobilization failed to show any significant changes in tenderness scores vs controls. It would appear that there is moderately strong evidence to support the use of some manual therapies in the immediate relief of TrP tenderness.

The 2 trials of short-term effects (3–5 days) demonstrated the effectiveness of osteopathic manipulation and ischaemic compression, respectively, in reducing TrP tenderness. One long-term trial reported that SCS demonstrates clinically important changes in TrP tenderness and general pain over 6 months, whereas the other showed that massage produced limited effect. It would appear that there is only limited evidence to support the use of manual therapies over longer courses of treatments in the management of TrPs and MPS.

Case Reports of Manual Therapy Twenty-six case reports in the chiropractic literature were identified from ICL or MANTIS (Appendix A). These reports covered TrP treatments in patients with hand pain, low back pain due to a TrP in the quadratus lumborum muscle, wrist pain, fibromyalgia, upper quarter syndrome, MPS, and general TrPs.

Clinical Reviews of Manual Therapy Up-to-date clinical reviews (Hong 2004, Gerwin 2005, Alvarez & Rockwell 2002, Simons 2002, Harden 2007, Lavelle et al. 2007) by noted experts in the field of myofascial pain have endorsed the use of a variety of manual therapies in the treatment of TrPs and MPS. These are classed as level 5 (Oxford Rating) evidence.

Harden (2007) notes that the principal aims of therapy for MPS are relief of pain and inflammation, prevention of further injury, reducing spasm, correcting abnormal postures, and improving circulation. He endorses the following therapeutic modalities for accomplishing these aims:

- In the acute stage:
  o Ice
  o Iontophoresis
  o US
  o Splinting
- Postural and ergonomic education
- Massage
- Myofascial release
- Exercises and postural correction
- Laser therapy: efficacy undetermined
- Acupuncture: efficacy undetermined

Hong (2004) recommends that the first principle of treatment of MPS is the identification and treatment of the presumed primary lesion (section 1). Only after this has been done, and if there is persistence of pain from the active TrPs, should direct treatment to the TrPs be performed. Hong suggests that, at this point in the therapeutic process, release of muscle tightness is the first objective. He identifies 7 steps in the treatment process for the active TrPs themselves:

i. Pain recognition: treating the active TrPs and not the latent ones.

ii. Identify the key TrP: Among active TrPs, one will be the most painful and most provocative of referred pain.

iii. Conservative vs aggressive treatment: This principle applies to the treatment of the primary lesion as well as the key TrP. Treatment should begin with what he describes as 'non-invasive treatment including physiotherapy' and progress toward more invasive forms of therapy.

iv. Acute vs chronic TrPs: Distinguishing these helps guide therapy in the acute vs chronic stages of pain.

v. Superficial vs deep TrPs: Different therapeutic modalities are needed the more deeply located is the TrP.
  a. Superficial: deep pressure massage.
  b. Deep: stretch, US, laser, acupuncture, acupressure, or local injection.

vi. Individual preference: Each patient may have levels of comfort and familiarity with various forms of treatment that should then be tailored to this need.

vii. Other considerations: cost, time, etc.

Hong places considerable importance on manual therapies for TrPs. He indicates the following as important aspects of manual therapy (p. 40):

- Stretching of shortened muscles (or taut band)
- Improving local circulation
- Counterirritation
- Other reflex effects

Gerwin (2005) also endorses the treatment protocol that separately addresses therapies for the local TrP vs therapies for the perpetuating factors. In the former category, he specifically endorses manual TrP compression for focal TrP release, followed by myofascial release techniques for local stretching and then 'therapeutic stretch' for the longer-range elongation of the body segments. In the case of perpetuating factors, he includes correction of postural faults as well as joint dysfunction. This should be followed by an active programme of physical conditioning, stretching, and endurance, including preventative strategies. Unfortunately, no studies were provided as evidence for this approach.

Simons (2002) reviews the mechanisms of TrP formation and perpetuation to guide the appropriate treatment approach. The therapies endorsed in his review are as follows:

- Postisometric relaxation and release
- Trigger point (manual) pressure release
- Combinations of the above 2 therapies
- Trigger point massage

Only the work of Lewit (1986) is cited as support for this approach. Other noninvasive therapies that Simons merely mentions as additional to the approach described above include facilitatory techniques, acupuncture, SCS, microcurrent, US, and laser.

Alvarez and Rockwell's (2002) review only provides a list of noninvasive treatment modalities that include acupuncture, osteopathic manual medicine techniques [sic], massage, acupressure, US, heat, ice, diathermy, transcutaneous electrical nerve stimulation (TENS), and 'spray and stretch' techniques. For these modalities, no clinical trial evidence was provided. The only support was a reference to the authoritative work described in Travell and Simons' (1983) manual.

Lavelle et al. (2007) endorse the following treatments as efficacious: spray and stretch, TENS, physical therapy, and massage.

Critique of Clinical Reviews

Manual Therapies. All 6 reviews from within the last 5 years endorsed manual therapies for TrP treatment in MPS. None of these reviews provided a single reference to a clinical trial to support this position. None of the 11 trials reviewed above was cited in any of these reviews. As such, there is discordance, even at the level of

renowned experts' reviews, between the apparent consensus on the use and types of manual therapies in treating TrPs vs the evidence from the published literature.

Other therapies. Only Harden (2007) cites the clinical trial of Esenyel et al. (2000) (US + stretching vs dry needling + stretching vs stretching alone) and the case series of Simunovic et al. (1998) (laser therapy) as clinical studies of these sorts of therapies as well as the review of laser therapy by Gam et al. (1998). The other reviews provide no support in the form of any clinical study for their recommendation on noninvasive therapies for TrPs.

Evidence Synthesis of Manual Therapies. Tables A.1 and A.2 summarize the literature retrieved in this review.

Clinical Practice Recommendations of Manual Therapies.

1. There is moderately strong evidence to support the use of some manual therapies in providing immediate pain relief at TrPs. The evidence level is B.
2. There is only limited evidence to support the use of manual therapies over longer courses of treatment in the management of TrPs and MPS. The evidence level is C.

Other Conservative Therapies

Systematic Reviews of Other Conservative Therapies. Two published reviews were identified for treatment methods other than manual therapies

Table A.1   Literature review: all studies

Study type	Oxford level	Number
Systematic reviews	1a	2
Systematic review protocols		1
Practice guidelines	1a	2
RCTs	1b	11
RCTs	2b	3
Case series	4	3 (Grobli; Anderson; Crawford)
Case reports	5	17
Clinical reviews (selected: 2000–2005)	5	6

Table A.2   Literature review: randomized clinical trials of manual therapy for MPS or TrPs (all rated as Oxford 1b, unless otherwise noted as 2b)

RCT	Time	Manual therapy	Outcome
Terret & Vernon 1986 (2b)	Immediate	Spinal manipulation	Spinal manipulation > mobilization
Jaeger & Reeves 1986	Immediate	Spray and stretch	Significant intragroup effects
Greene et al 1990	3 d	Osteopathic manipulative therapy	No difference between OMT with or without laser and vs control
Vernon et al 1992 (2b)	Immediate	Spinal manipulation	SMT > control
Hong et al 1993	Immediate	Spray and stretch, deep manual pressure	Deep pressure massage was more effective than comparison modalities.
Cote et al 1994 (2b)	Immediate	Spinal manipulation	Spinal manipulation = control
Hanten et al 1997	Immediate	Manual mobilization	No significant differences between mobilization, exercise, and control
Gam et al 1998	6 mo	Massage	No significant differences between massage with real or sham US or control
Hanten et al 2000	5 d	Ischaemic compression	Ischaemic compression > exercise for pain and tenderness
Dardzinski et al 2000	6 mo	SCS	Clinically important intragroup changes
Hou et al 2002	Immediate	Ischaemic compression	Ischaemic compression > control
Fryer & Hodgson 2005	Immediate	Manual pressure release vs sham control	Manual pressure release > control
Fernandez–de–las Penas et al 2006	Immediate	Ischaemic compression and transverse friction massage	Ischaemic compression = transverse friction massage
Atienza Meseguer et al 2006	Immediate	SCS	SCS > control

SMT, Spinal manipulation therapy.

(Rickards 2006, Cummings & White 2001). In Rickards' (2006) review, the inclusion criteria included RCTs of a conservative therapy for active TrPs, not latent TrPs, in which a patient-related pain outcome was used and in which an explicit diagnosis of TrP was made including at least local tenderness and a taut muscle band. Studies were rated on a 20-point scale; however, no cutoff score was used for inclusion. It should be noted that no trials for acupuncture were included in this review (below). A total of 18 trials were included in this review (Tables A.3-A.6). Rickards' (2006) conclusions were based on the following schema:

- Significant evidence: consistent findings in multiple high-quality RCTs
- Moderate evidence: consistent findings in multiple lower-quality evidence and/or a single high-quality RCT
- Limited evidence: a single low-quality RCT

- Unclear evidence: inconsistent or conflicting results from multiple RCTs
- No evidence: no evidence identified
- Evidence of adverse effect: RCTs with lasting negative changes

Rickards' conclusions for each therapy were as follows:

Laser: Significant evidence that laser may be effective in the short term. Type, dose, and frequency of treatments require additional research.

TENS: Evidence (unqualified?) that TENS may be effective in providing immediate relief at TrPs.

Other electrotherapies: Limited evidence for the effectiveness of frequency modulated neural stimulation (FREMS), high-voltage galvanic stimulation (HVGS), electrical muscle stimulation (EMS), and interferential current (IFC).

Table A.3   Studies of laser therapy from Rickards (2006) (n = 6 studies)

Study	Treatments	Outcomes
Gur et al. (2004)	Laser vs placebo	Laser > placebo
Snyder–Mackler et al. (1989)	Laser vs placebo	Laser > placebo
Ceccherelli et al. (1989)	Laser vs placebo	Laser > placebo
Hakguder et al. (2003)	Laser and stretching vs placebo and stretching	Laser > placebo
Ilbuldu et al. (2003)	Laser vs dry needling vs placebo	Laser > dry needling Laser > placebo
Altan et al. (2003)	Laser + exercise + stretching vs placebo + exercise + stretching	Laser = placebo (other treatments thought to contribute to improvement)

Table A.4   Studies of electrotherapy from Rickards (2006) (n = 5 studies)

Study	Treatments	Outcomes
Graff–Radford et al. (1986)	A: TENS mode A B: TENS mode B C: TENS mode C D: TENS mode D E: Placebo TENS	B > C, D > A, E (B = 100 Hz)
Farina et al. (2004)	FREMS vs TENS	FREMS = TENS
Hsueh et al. (1997)	A : Placebo electrotherapy B : TENS C : EMS	TENS > EMS, placebo
Ardic et al. (2002)	A: TENS + stretching B: EMS + stretching C: Stretching	A = B > C
Tanrikut et al. (2003)	A: HVGS + exercise B: Placebo HVGS + exercise C: Exercise	A > B, C

Table A.5   Studies of magnet therapy from Rickards (2006) (n = 3 studies)

Study	Treatments	Outcomes
Brown et al. (2002)	Magnets vs placebo	Magnets > placebo
Smania et al. (2005)	A: RMS B: TENS C: Placebo US	A > B > C
Smania et al. (2003)	A: RMS B: Placebo RMS	A > B

RMS, Repetitive magnetic stimulation.

Table A.6   Studies of US therapy from Rickards (2006) (n = 4 studies)

Study	Treatments	Outcomes
Gam et al. (1998)	A: US + massage + exercise B: Placebo US + massage + exercise C: Control	A = B = C
Maljesi & Unalan (2004)	A: High–power US B: Conventional US	A > B
Lee et al. (1997)	A: Placebo US B: US C: Electrotherapy D: US + electrotherapy	C > A
Esenyel et al. (2000)	A: US + stretching B: TrP injection + stretching C: Stretching	A, B > C

US: Moderate evidence that US is no more effective than placebo.

Magnets: Preliminary evidence that magnets may be effective.

It was noted that most trials involved either immediate or short-term effects and that much more research, especially on the longer-term effects, was needed.

Table A.7   Studies of acupuncture therapy from Cummings and White (2001) (n = 3)

Study	Treatments	Outcomes
Birch & Jamison (1998) (neck pain)	A: Superficial acupuncture + heat B: Wrong point superficial acupuncture C: NSAID	At 3 mo: A > B, C
Johannson et al. (1991) (facial pain or headache)	A: Acupuncture B: Occlusal splint C: No treatment control	At 3 mo: A = B > C
Kisiel & Lindh (1996) (neck pain)	A: Manual acupuncture B: Physiotherapy	At 6 mo: A = B

IP,;NSAID, nonsteroidal anti-inflammatory drug.

Cummings and White (2001) reviewed all trials up to 2000 of 'Needling Therapies' for myofascial pain. Three of these trials involved what could be described as 'standard' acupuncture typical of the type used by some chiropractors. This is distinguished from deep dry needling and any injection-type therapies that would not be standard chiropractic treatment approaches. For the present review, any trials that specifically identified one of the regional complaint areas in the CCGPP (i.e., low back pain, neck pain) without specifying the treatment of TrPs were excluded (Table A.7). Cummings and White (2001) concluded that marked improvements were demonstrated in most treatment groups. However, dry needling techniques alone did not appear to be superior to other treatments in the treatment of myofascial TrPs. As well, they could not find evidence for a specific efficacy of these techniques beyond placebo. They called for more placebo-controlled trials.

A Cochrane Collaboration Protocol entitled 'Non-invasive physical treatments of myofascial pain' (Kilkenny et al. 2007) was identified. This protocol currently contains no results. However, it was used as a source of additional references, particularly on published clinical trials and systematic reviews.

RCTs of Other Conservative Therapies. Both Rickards (Rickards 2006) and Cummings and White (Cummings & White 2001) used specific inclusion and exclusion criteria that resulted in the exclusion of numerous studies, either because they were not RCTs or for various methodologic reasons. These excluded trials will not be listed or reviewed here, as that would both duplicate and undermine the methods and conclusions of these reviews. Several trials have been identified in the present search that either have been published since these reviews or were not identified at all in these reviews (probably because of the inclusion of MANTIS and ICL databases in the present search) in the following areas:

Acupuncture. There is some additional evidence that a course of deep acupuncture to TrPs is effective in the treatment of myofascial pain for up to 3 months (Table A.8).

Laser. The study of Greene et al. (1990) of laser vs osteopathic manipulation (OMT) alone vs OMT + laser vs sham laser to thoracic paraspinal muscle TrPs over 3 days involved measuring only local skin resistance. No measures of pain or tenderness response were made. This study would not have qualified for Rickards' review and does not, as well, for the present review.

Olavi et al. (1989) compared infrared laser to placebo laser over various active TrPs located throughout the body. Pressure pain thresholds were measured immediately after and then 15 minutes after treatment. A statistically significant difference favouring the laser group was found, especially at 15 minutes.

Electrotherapy. No additional studies were retrieved.

Exercise. No additional studies not already included in Rickards (2006) under 'physical therapies' were retrieved.

Table A.8   Additional acupuncture trials

Study	Treatments	Outcomes
Ceccherelli et al. (2006) (neck pain)	A: Somatic acupuncture B: Somatic acupuncture + auricular acupuncture	At 1 and 3 mo: A = B (both = positive effect on pain)
Itoh et al. (2004) (low back pain)	A: Acupuncture at traditional points B: Superficial acupuncture at TrPs C: Deep acupuncture at TrPs	At 3 mo: A > B, C (not statistically significant)
Ceccherelli et al. (2002) (low back pain)	A: Superficial acupuncture to TrP B: Deep acupuncture to TrP	At 3 mo: B > A
Goddard et al. (2002) (jaw pain)	A: Acupuncture B: Sham acupuncture	Immediately: A = B
Ceccherelli et al. (2001) (shoulder)	A: Superficial acupuncture to TrP B: Deep acupuncture to TrP	At 1 and 3 mo: B > D

Spray and stretch.   The study of Hou et al. (2002) was included in section 3 and was included in the reviews of both Fernandez de las Penas et al. (2005) and Rickards (Kilkenny et al. 2007) under the category of manual therapy. This is because most treatment groups received ischaemic compression with or without a variety of other physiologic therapies. One of these therapies was spray and stretch, making Hou et al. (2002) the only published clinical trial to investigate this therapy. Hou et al found that the addition of spray and stretch to ischaemic compression provided immediate benefit in reducing TrP sensitivity. There are no other published clinical trials of spray and stretch therapy for management of pain from TrPs. Notwithstanding this, it is often cited by clinical experts as a valuable treatment of TrPs.

Ultrasound.   Srbely and Dickey (2005, 2007) applied therapeutic-intensity vs low-intensity US to trapezius TrPs in 44 subjects. Pressure pain thresholds over trapezius TrPs increased 44% (14.2%) in the first group, whereas no increase was obtained in the second group.

   Evidence Synthesis of Other Conservative Therapies. Table A.9 summarizes the evidence retrieved in this review.

   Clinical Practice Recommendations.

1. *Laser*: There is substantial evidence that laser therapy is effective in the treatment of TrPs and MPS. The evidence level is A.

Table A.9   Literature review: all studies of other conservative therapies

Study type	Oxford level	Number
Systematic reviews	1a	2
Systematic review protocols		1
Practice guidelines	1a	2
RCTs	1b	29

2. *TENS*: There is moderately strong evidence that TENS may be effective in providing immediate relief at TrPs. The evidence level is B.
3. There is limited evidence for the effectiveness of other forms of electrotherapy: FREMS, HVGS, EMS, and IFC. The evidence level is C.
4. *US*: There is conflicting evidence as to whether US is no more effective than placebo or is somewhat more effective than other therapies in the treatment of TrPs and MPS. The evidence level is C.
5. *Magnets*: There is some evidence that magnets may be effective in the treatment of TrPs and MPS. The evidence level is B.
6. *Acupuncture*: There is some evidence that a course of deep acupuncture to TrPs is effective in the treatment of myofascial pain for up to 3 months. The evidence level is B.

Table A.10 Summary of recommendations

Topic	Conclusion and strength of evidence rating
Manipulation/ mobilization	Rating B: short-term relief There is moderately strong evidence to support the use of some manual therapies (manipulation, ischaemic pressure) in providing immediate relief of pain at MTrPs. Rating C: long-term relief There is limited evidence to support the use of some manual therapies in providing long-term relief of pain at MTrPs.
Conservative nonmanipulation	Rating A: laser therapies There is strong evidence that laser therapy (various types of lasers) is effective in the treatment of MTrPs and MPS. Rating B: TENS, magnets, and acupuncture There is moderately strong evidence that TENS is effective in the short-term relief of pain at MTrPs. There is moderately strong evidence that magnet therapy is effective in the relief of pain at MTrP and in MPS. There is moderately strong evidence that a course of deep acupuncture to MTrPs is effective in the treatment of MTrPs and MPS for up to 3 mo. Rating C: electrotherapies, US There is limited evidence for the effectiveness of EMS, HVGS, IFC, and FREMS in the treatment of MTrPs and MPS. There is conflicting evidence that US is no more effective than placebo or is somewhat more effective than other therapies in the treatment of MTrPs and MPS.

Conclusion

The published evidence for the treatment of MPS and TrPs by common chiropractic treatments has been reviewed. Although publications ranging from systematic reviews and clinical trials to clinical reviews were included in the review, the evidence ratings were developed only on the basis of the clinical trial evidence. Manual-type therapies and some physiologic therapeutic modalities have acceptable evidentiary support in the treatment of MPS and TrPs (Table A.10).

> **Practical Applications**
>
> - There is evidence that manual therapies are useful in short-term relief of TrP pain.
> - There is evidence that laser and acupuncture are useful in the short- and long-term relief of MPS.

References

Altan L, Bingol U, Aydae M, Yurtkuran M: Investigation of the effect of GA AS laser therapy on cervical myofascial pain syndrome, *Rheumatol Int* 25:23–27, 2003.

Alvarez DJ, Rockwell PG: Trigger points: diagnosis and management, *Am Fam Physician* 65:653–660, 2002.

Ardic F, Sarhus M, Topuz O: Comparison of two different techniques of electrotherapy on myofascial pain, *J Back Musculoskelet Rehabil* 16:11–16, 2002.

Atienza Meseguer A, Fernandez de las Penas C, Navarro-Poza JL, Rodriguez-Blanco C, Bosca Gandia JJ: Immediate effects of the strain/counterstrain technique in local pain evoked by tender points in the upper trapezius muscle, *Clin Chiropr* 9:112–118, 2006.

Bachop W: Letter to Raymond Nimmo, Nov 20, 1980.

Birch S, Jamison RN: Controlled trial of Japanese acupuncture for chronic myofascial neck pain: assessment of specific and nonspecific effects of treatment, *Clin J Pain* 14:248–255, 1998.

Brown CS, Ling FW, Wan JY, et al: Efficacy of static magnetic field therapy in chronic pelvic pain: a double-blind pilot study, *Am J Obstet Gynecol* 187:1581–1587, 2002.

Ceccherelli F, Altafini L, Lo Castro G, et al: Diode laser in cervical myofascial pain: a double-blind study versus placebo, *Clin J Pain* 5:301–304, 1989.

Ceccherelli F, Bordin M, Gagliardi G, et al: Comparison between superficial and deep acupuncture in the treatment of shoulder myofascial pain: a randomized and controlled study, *Acupunct Electrother Res* 26:229–238, 2001.

Ceccherelli F, Rigoni MT, et al: Comparison of superficial and deep acupuncture in the treatment of lumbar myofascial pain: a double-blind randomized controlled study, *Clin J Pain* 18:149–153, 2002.

Ceccherelli F, Tortora P, Nassimbeni C, et al: The therapeutic efficacy of somatic acupuncture is not increased by auriculotherapy: a randomised, blind control study in cervical myofascial pain, *Complement Ther Med* 14:47–52, 2006.

Chatchawan U, Thinkhamrop B, Kharmawan S, et al: Effectiveness of traditional Thai massage versus Swedish massage among patients with back pain associated with myofascial trigger points, *J Bodywork Mov Ther* 9:298–309, 2005.

Cohen J, Gibbons R, Raymond L: Nimmo and the Evolution of Trigger Point Therapy, 1929-1986, *J Manipulative Physiol Ther*, 21(3), 1998.

Cohen JH, Schneider M: Receptor-tonus technique: an overview, *Chiropr Technique* 2:13–16, 1990.

Cote P, Mior SA, Vernon H: The short-term effect of a spinal manipulation on pain/pressure threshold in patients with chronic mechanical low back pain, *J Manipulative Physiol Ther* 17:364–368, 1994.

Cummings TM, White AR: Needling therapies in the management of myofascial trigger point pain: a systematic review, *Arch Phys Med Rehabil* 82:986–992, 2001.

Dardzinski JA, Ostrov BE, Hamann LS: Myofascial pain unresponsive to standard treatment. Successful use of strain and counterstrain technique in physical therapy, *J Clin Rheum* 6:169–174, 2000.

Edwards J, Knowles N: Superficial dry needling and active stretching in the treatment of myofascial pain—a randomised controlled trial, *Acupunct Med* 21:80–86, 2003.

Esenyel M, Caglar N, Aldemir T: Treatment of myofascial pain, *Am J Phys Med Rehabil* 79:48–52, 2000.

Farina S, Casarotto M, Bennelle M, et al: A randomised controlled study on the effect of two different treatments (FREMS and TENS) in myofascial pain syndrome, *Eura Medicophys* 40:293–301, 2004.

Fernandez de las Penas C, Alonso-Blanco C, Fernandez-Camero J, et al: The immediate effect of ischemic compression technique and transverse friction massage on tenderness of active and latent myofascial trigger points: a pilot study, *J Bodywork Mov Ther* 10:3–9, 2006.

Fernandez de las Penas C, Sohrbeck Campo M, Fernandez Carnero J, et al: Manual therapies in myofascial trigger point treatment: a systematic review, *J Bodywork Mov Ther* 9:27–34, 2005.

Fryer G, Hodgson L: The effect of manual pressure release on myofascial trigger points in the upper trapezius muscle, *J Bodywork Mov Ther* 9:248–255, 2005.

Gam AN, Warming S, Larsen LH: Treatment of myofascial trigger points with ultrasound combined with massage and exercise: a randomized controlled trial, *Pain* 77:73–79, 1998.

Garvey TA, Marks MR, Wiesel SW: A prospective randomized, double-blind evaluation of trigger-point injection therapy for low-back pain, *Spine* 14:962–964, 1989.

Gatterman M, Lee HK: Chiropractic adjusting techniques. In: Peterson D, Weise G, editors. *Chiropractic: an illustrated history*, Chicago, 1995, Mosby, pp 240–261.

Gaucher-Peslherbe PL: *Fred Illi and sacroiliac dynamics*, Lombard, IL, 1995, Lecture at the National College of Chiropractic.

Gerwin RD: A review of myofascial pain and fibromyalgia—factors that promote their persistence, *Acupunct Med* 23:121–134, 2005.

Gibbons RW: Joy Loban and Andrew P Davis: itinerant healers and schoolmen, *Chiropr History* 11(1):23, 1991.

Gibbons RW, Thomas T: *Lake and endo-nasal therapy*, Lombard, IL, 1995, Paper delivered at National College of Chiropractic.

Goddard G, Karibe H, McNeill C, et al: Acupuncture and sham acupuncture reduce muscle pain in myofascial pain patients, *J Orofac Pain* 16:71–76, 2002.

Graff-Radford SB, Reeves JL, Jaeger B: Management of head and neck pain: the effectiveness of altering perpetuating factors in myofascial pain, *Headache* 27:186–190, 1986.

Greene C, Debias D, Helig D, et al: The effect of helium-neon laser and osteopathic manipulation on soft-tissue trigger points, *J Am Osteopath Assoc* 90:638–639, 1990.

Gur A, Sarac AJ, Cevik R, et al: Efficacy of 904 nm gallium arsenide low level laser therapy in the management of chronic myofascial pain in the neck: a double-blind and randomized controlled trial, *Lasers Surg Med* 35:229–235, 2004.

Hains G: Chiropractic management of shoulder pain and dysfunction of myofascial origin using ischemic compression techniques, *J Can Chiropr Assoc* 46:192–200, 2002.

Hains G: Locating and treating low back pain of myofascial origin by ischemic compression, *J Can Chiropr Assoc* 46:257–264, 2002.

Hakguder A, Birtane M, Gurcan S, et al: Efficacy of low level laser therapy in myofascial pain syndrome: an algometric and thermographic evaluation, *Lasers Surg Med* 33:339–343, 2003.

Hammer W: *Functional soft tissue examination & treatment by manual methods*, ed 3, Sudbury (Mass), 2007, Jones & Bartlett.

Hanten W, Olson S, Butts N, et al: Effectiveness of a home program of ischemic pressure followed by sustained stretch for treatment of myofascial trigger points, *Phys Ther* 80:997–1003, 2000.

Hanten WP, Barret M, Gillespie-Plesko M, et al: Effects of active head retraction with retraction/extension and occipital release on the pressure pain threshold of cervical and scapular trigger points, *Physiother Theory Pract* 13:285–291, 1997.

Harden RN: Muscle pain syndromes, *Am J Phys Med Rehabil* 86(Suppl):S47–S58, 2007.

Harden RN, Bruehl SP, Gass S, et al: Signs and symptoms of the myofascial pain syndrome: a national survey of pain management providers, *Clin J Pain* 16:64–72, 2000.

Harris RE, Clauw DJ: The use of complementary medical therapies in the management of myofascial pain disorders, *Curr Pain Headache Rep* 6:370–374, 2002.

Hayes S: A new hypothesis for consideration on the subluxation, *J Natl Chiropr Assoc* 27(7):9–11, 68–69, 1957.

Hong CZ: Myofascial pain therapy, *J Musculoskelet Pain* 12:37–43, 2004.

Hong CZ, Chen YC, Pon CH, et al: Immediate effects of various physical medicine modalities on pain threshold of an active myofascial trigger point, *J Musculoskelet Pain* 1:37–53, 1993.

Hou CR, Tsai LC, Cheng KF, et al: Immediate effects of various physical therapy modalities on cervical myofascial pain and trigger point sensitivity, *Arch Phys Med Rehabil* 83:1406–1414, 2002.

Hsueh TC, Cheng PT, Kuan TS, et al: The immediate effectiveness of electrical nerve stimulation and electrical muscle stimulation on myofascial trigger points, *Am J Phys Med Rehabil* 76:471–476, 1997.

Ilbuldu E, Cakmak A, Disci R, et al: Comparison of laser, dry needling and placebo laser treatments in myofascial pain syndrome, *Rheumatol Int* 25:23–27, 2003.

Itoh K, Katsumi Y, Kitakoji H: Trigger point acupuncture treatment of chronic low back pain in elderly patients—a blinded RCT, *Acupunct Med* 22:170–177, 2004.

Jaeger B, Reeves JL: Quantification of changes in myofascial trigger point sensitivity with the pressure algometer following passive stretch, *Pain* 27:203–210, 1986.

Job analysis of chiropractic, Greeley (CO), 1993, National Board of Chiropractic Examiners, p 78.

Johannson A, Wenneberg B, Wagersten C, et al: Acupuncture in treatment of facial muscular pain, *Acta Odontol Scand* 49:153–158, 1991.

Kilkenny MB, Deane K, Smith KA, et al: Non-invasive physical treatments of myofascial pain (protocol), *Cochrane Library*, 2007.

Kisiel C, Lindh C: Smartlindring med fysikalsk terapi och manuell akupnktur vid myofasciella nackoch skuldersmartor, *Sjukgymnasten* 12(Suppl):24–31, 1996.

Lavelle ED, Lavelle W, Smith HS: Myofascial trigger points, *Med Clin North Am* 91:229–239, 2007.

Lee JC, Dt Lin, Hong C: The effectiveness of simultaneous thermotherapy with ultrasound and electrotherapy with combined AC and DC current on the immediate pain relief of myofascial trigger points, *J Musculoskelet Pain* 5:81–90, 1997.

Lewit K: Post-isometric relaxation in combination with other methods of muscular facilitation and inhibition, *Man Med* 2:101–104, 1986.

Makous E: Treating temporomandibular joint disorder with unique intraoral approach, *Adv Phys Ther* 6:6–7, 1995.

Maljesi J, Unalan H: High power pain threshold ultrasound technique in the treatment of active myofascial trigger points: a randomized, double-blind case-control study, *Arch Phys Med Rehabil* 85:833–836, 2004.

Nimmo RL: A technique for the correction of muscular imbalance of the temporomandibular joints, *Granbury (TX): The Receptor* 2(2):1–8, 1981.

Nimmo RL: An open letter to the chiropractic profession, *Dig Chiropr Econ* 1:51, 1969.

Nimmo RL: *Development of chiropractic (video cassette)*, Pasadena (TX), 1984, Texas College of Chiropractic.

Nimmo RL: Receptors, effectors, and tonus: a new approach, *J Natl Chiropr Assoc* 27(11):21, 1957.

Nimmo RL: *Some remarks on the development of receptor-tonus technique. Privately circulated response to Bachop*, Granbury (TX), 1981, R. L. Nimmo.

Nimmo RL: Specificity and the law of facilitation in the nervous system, *Granbury (TX): The Receptor* 2(1):1–8, 1971.

Nimmo RL: Technique for the immediate release of headache and neck pain, *Granbury (TX): The Receptor* 2(3):1–15, 1986.

Nimmo RL: *The development of chiropractic through the perspective of Dr. Raymond Nimmo [videorecording]*, Pasadena (Tex), 1984, Texas Chiropractic College.

Nimmo RL: *The receptor-tonus method course of instruction. Distributed at seminars*, Included in letter to Dr. Stanley Hayes, Tucson (AZ).

Nimmo RL: *The receptor-tonus method*, Pasedena (Tex), 1992, Texas Chiropractic College.

Nimmo RL: *The receptor-tonus method: directory*, 1962, Self-published.

Olavi A, Pekka G, Pertti K, et al: Effects of infrared laser therapy at treated and non-treated trigger points, *Acupunct Electrother Res* 14:9–14, 1989.

Perle SM: Myofascial trigger points, *Chiropr Sports Med* 9:106–108, 1995.

Perle SM: Understanding trigger points: key to relieving myotogenous pain, *Chiropr J* 3:17, 1989.

Phillips B, Ball C, Sackett D, et al: *Levels of evidence*, Oxford, UK, 2001, Oxford Centre for Evidence-based Medicine.

Rehm WS: Price of dissension: the private wars of Leo L. Spears, *Chiropr History* 15(1):33, 1991.

Rickards LD: The effectiveness of non-invasive treatments for active myofascial trigger point pain: a systematic review of the literature, *Int J Osteopath Med* 9:120–136, 2006.

Sackett DL, Straus SE, Richardson, et al: *Evidence-based medicine: how to practice and teach EBM*, Edinburgh, Scotland, 2000, Churchill Livingstone.

Schneider M: Receptor-tonus technique assessment, *Chiropr Tech* 6:156–159, 1994.

Schneider M: Tender points/fibromyalgia vs trigger points/myofascial pain syndrome: a need for clarity in terminology and differential diagnosis, *J Manipulative Physiol Ther* 18:398–406, 1995.

Schneider M, Cohen J: The Collected Writings of Nimmo & Vannerson, *J Manipulative Physiol Ther* 32(1):14–24, 2001.

Schneider MJ: Snapping hip syndrome in a marathon runner: treatment by manual trigger point therapy—a case study, *Chiropr Sports Med* 4:54–58, 1990.

Simons DG: Understanding effective treatments of myofascial trigger points, *J Bodywork Mov Ther* 6:81–88, 2002.

Simunovic Z, Trobonjaca T, Trobonjaca Z: Treatment of medial and lateral epicondylitis—tennis and golfer's elbow—with low level laser therapy: a multicentre double-blind, placebo-controlled clinical study on 324 patients, *J Clin Laser Med Surg* 16:145–151, 1998.

Skootsky SA, Jaeger B, Oye RK: Prevalence of myofascial pain in general internal medicine, *West J Med* 151:157–160, 1989.

Smania N, Corato E, Fiaschi A, et al: Repetitive magnetic stimulation: a novel approach for myofascial pain syndrome, *J Neurol* 252:307–314, 2005.

Smania N, Corato E, Fiaschi A, et al: Therapeutic effects of peripheral repetitive magnetic stimulation on myofascial pain syndrome, *Clin Neurophysiol* 114:350–358, 2003.

Snyder-Mackler L, Barry AJ, Perkins AI, et al: The effects of helium-neon laser irradiation on skin resistance and pain in patients with trigger points in the neck or back, *Phys Ther* 69:336–341, 1989.

Srbely J, Dickey JP: Randomized controlled study of the antinociceptive effect of ultrasound on trigger point sensitivity: novel applications in myofascial therapy, *Clin Rehabil* 21:411–417, 2007.

Srbely J, Dickey JP: Stimulation of myofascial trigger points causes systemic physiologic effects [abstract], *J Can Chiropr Assoc* 49:75, 2005.

Tanrikut A, Ozaras N, Ali Kaptan H, et al: High voltage galvanic stimulation in myofascial pain syndrome, *J Musculoskelet Pain* 11:11–15, 2003.

Terrett AC, Vernon H: Manipulation and pain tolerance. A controlled study of the effect of spinal manipulation on paraspinal cutaneous pain tolerance levels, *Am J Phys Med* 63:217–225, 1984.

Travell JG, Simons DG: *Myofascial pain and dysfunction: the trigger point manual*, Baltimore, 1983, Williams & Wilkins.

Travell J, Rinzler S: The myofascial genesis of pain, *Postgrad Med* 11:425–434, 1952.

Travell J, Simons DG: *Myofascial pain and dysfunction: the trigger point manual*, Baltimore Md, 1983, Williams and Wilkens.

Vernon HT, Aker P, Burns S, et al: Pressure pain threshold evaluation of the effect of spinal manipulation in the treatment of chronic neck pain: a pilot study, *J Manipulative Physiol Ther* 13:13–16, 1990.

Vicenzino B, Collins D, Wright A: The initial effects of a cervical spine manipulative physiotherapy treatment on the pain and dysfunction of lateral epicondylalgia, *Pain* 68:69–74, 1996.

Further Reading

Anderson RU, Wise D, Sawyer T, et al: Integration of myofascial trigger point release and paradoxical relaxation training treatment of chronic pelvic pain in men, *J Urol* 174(1):155–160, 2005.

Brewer G, Kampschroeder F, Moore L: Trigger point and transverse frictional massage: a case report, *Chiropr* 6:40–42, 1990.

Cohen JH, Gibbons RW, Raymond L: Nimmo and the evolution of trigger point therapy, 1929–1986, *J Manipulative Physiol Ther* 21:167–172, 1998.

Crawford JS, Simpson J, Crawford P: Myofascial release provides symptomatic relief from chest wall tenderness occasionally seen following lumpectomy and radiation in breast cancer patients, *Int J Radiat Oncol Biol Phys* 34(5):1188–1189, 1996.

Daniells E, Wood T: Chiropractic care protocol versus stretching in the treatment of active trigger point in the extensor muscles of the hand and fingers. In *Proceedings of the World Federation of Chiropractic, 7th Biennial Congress*, Toronto, ON, 2003, pp 311–312.

Davies C: Trigger point therapy for carpal tunnel syndrome: self-applied massage of the forearms and scalenes, *J Am Chiropr Assoc* 39:18–23, 2002.

De Franca G, Levine L: Quadratus lumborum and low back pain, *J Manipulative Physiol Therap* 14:142–149, 1991.

Grobli C, Dejung B: Non-medical therapy of myofascial pain, *Schmerz* 17:475–480, 2003.

Han SC, Harrison P: Myofascial pain syndrome and trigger point management, *Reg Anaesth* 22:89–101, 1997.

Hong C: Specific sequential myofascial trigger point therapy in the treatment of a patient with myofascial pain syndrome associated with reflex sympathetic dystrophy, *Australas Chiropr Osteopath* 9:7–11, 2000.

Howitt SD, Wong J, Zabukovec S: The conservative treatment of trigger thumb using Graston Technique and Active Release Techniques®, *J Can Chiropr Assoc* 50:249–254, 2006.

Hsieh H, Hong C: Effect of chiropractic manipulation on the pain threshold of myofascial trigger point: a pilot study. In *Proceedings of: International Conference on Spinal Manipulation*, 1990, pp 359–363.

Hunter G: Specific soft tissue mobilization in the management of soft tissue dysfunction, *Man Ther* 3:2–11, 1998.

Hyde T: Graston technique: a soft tissue treatment for athletic injuries, *DC Tracts* Fall, 2003.

Kasunich NJ: Changes in low back pain in a long distance runner after stretching the iliotibial band, *J Chiropr Med* 2:37–40, 2003.

Kaye MJ: Evaluation and treatment of a patient with upper quarter myofascial pain syndrome, *J Sports Chiropr Rehabil* 15:26–33, 2001.

Leahy P: Improved treatments for carpal tunnel and related syndromes, *Chiropr Sports Med* 9(1):6–9, 1995.

Leahy PM: *Active release techniques: soft tissue management system for the upper extremity*. Colorado Springs, CO, 1996, Self-published.

Leahy PM, Mock LE: Myofascial release technique and mechanical compromise of peripheral nerves of the upper extremity, *Chiropr Sports Med* 6:139–150, 1992.

Melham TJ, Sevier TL, Malnofski MJ, et al: Chronic ankle pain and fibrosis successfully treated with a new noninvasive augmented soft tissue mobilization technique (ASTM): a case report, *Med Sci Sports Exerc* 30(6):801–804, 1998.

Mock LE: Myofascial release treatment of specific muscles of the upper extremity. Part 1, *Clin Bull Myofasc Ther* 2(1):5–23, 1997.

Mock LE: Myofascial release treatment of specific muscles of the upper extremity. Part 2, *Clin Bull Myofasc Ther* 2(2/3):5–22, 1997.

Mock LE: Myofascial release treatment of specific muscles of the upper extremity. Part 3, *Clin Bull Myofasc Ther* 2(4):51–69, 1997.

Mock LE: Myofascial release treatment of specific muscles of the upper extremity. Part 4, *Clin Bull Myofasc Ther* 3(1):71–93, 1998.

Mulcahy R, Johnson J, Witt R: Treatment of myofascial pain utilizing an activator instrument on trigger points, *Chiropractic* 9:45–46, 1994.

Schneider M: *The collected writings of Nimmo and Vannerson: pioneers of chiropractic trigger point therapy*, Pittsburgh (Pa), 2001, Michael Schneider.

Such GW: Manual care of the hyoid complex, *Top Clin Chirop* 9:54–62, 2002. c/r.

Vernon H, Schneider M: The Collected Writings of Nimmo & Vannerson, *J Manipulative Physiol Ther* 32(1):14–24, 2009.

Walsh MJ, Wise P: Chiropractic treatment of fibromyalgia: two case studies, *Chiropr J Aust* 31:42–46, 2001.

Index

Note: Page numbers followed by *b* indicate boxes, *f* indicate figures and *t* indicate tables.

A

abdominal reflex areas, 143–148
  Mackenzie's, 104, 104*f*, 106*f*
abdominal release techniques, specific,
  153, 189–192, 214
  technique A, 190–192, 190*f*
  technique B, 190*f*, 192
abdominal symptoms, differential,
  149*b*
abdominal tissues, pain variables, 146
abdominal (and pelvic) treatment,
  general, 141–154, 189
  applications, 214
  assessing origin of pain, 145–146
  chronic pelvic pain, 153–154
  junctional tissues, 142–143
  mesenteric attachment stress,
    146–148, 147*f*, 148*f*
  objectives, 141–142
  organ dysfunction, 143
  technique, 148–154, 148*b*, 149*b*, 149*f*
abnormal neural movement, 8–9
accommodation, 268–269
acetylcholine (ACh), 60
active release technique® (ART), 155
acupressure, 173, 254
  mechanisms of pain relief, 81
  pain thresholds and, 79
  points (*tsubo*), 132–133, 136
acupuncture
  applied kinesiology and, 79–82
  mechanisms of pain relief, 81
  meridians (channels), 278, 279–280,
    281–282
  model of pain genesis, 14–15
  needling, 79, 211
  periosteal, 93, 94*t*

trigger point therapy, 308, 308*t*,
  309, 309*t*
acupuncture points, 75–76, 78–86
  active, 78
  Ah shi, 44, 82, 90
  Akabane, 82, 83–84, 84*t*, 85*f*
  Alarm, 82, 83*f*, 83*t*
  Associated, 82, 83, 84*f*, 84*t*
  Lief's basic spinal NMT, 132–133,
    136–137
  morphology, 78–79
  treatment, 80–81
  vs other points, 211
  vs trigger points, 78–86, 78*f*
adaptation, soft tissue, 211
adenosine triphosphate (ATP), 15, 16,
  60, 204
adhesion breaking techniques, 161,
  189–192, 190*f*
adrenocortical hormones, 39–40
2-AG, 170
agonist contract–relax (ACR), 166
Ah shi acupuncture points, 44, 82, 90
Akabane acupuncture points, 83–84,
  85*f*
Akabane points, acupuncture, 82, 84*t*
Alarm acupuncture points, 82, 83*f*, 83*t*
aldosterone, 87
Alexander technique, 215
algometrics, 66*b*
alpha-motor neurons (α-efferents), 178*f*
  pain–spasm–pain cycle, 16
  PINS technique, 269, 270
American neuromuscular therapy
  (NMT), 9*b*, 123, 221–246
  aims, 9
  application, 224–225, 226*f*
  basic techniques, 226–230

  categories of influences on health,
    222–223, 222*t*
  history, 40–41, 221–222
  original six factors, 223–224
  platform, 222–224
  sequencing, 225
  soft tissue manipulation (STM),
    171–184
  specific methods, 230–244
  vs Lief's European NMT, 244–246
anandamide (AEA), 170
angina pectoris, 62, 149
annulospiral receptors, 4, 178*f*, 252, 269
anxiety
  hyperventilation and, 69, 204–205
  motor unit involvement, 10*b*
  see also stress
aortic aneurysms, 148*b*, 149
appendicitis, 75–76, 82, 89
applications of NMT, 213–215
applied kinesiology
  acupuncture and, 79–82
  Bennett's neurovascular reflex
    points, 86, 117
  proprioceptive adjustment, 177
armouring, Reich's defensive, 12–13
arms
  circulation of, 102*f*, 103*b*
  Thai massage, 284–285, 284*f*, 285*f*
arterial disease of legs, 102*f*, 103*b*
Asokananda, 277
assessment, 36–37, 97–98, 205–207
  American NMT, 225
  digital, 97, 98*f*
  facilitated spinal tissues, 54–55, 55*f*
  lifting skin folds, 105–106, 107*f*
  PINS, 255, 256
  skin distraction, 109

assessment (*Continued*)
stretching superficial tissue,
106–109, 107*f*, 108*f*
visual, 102*b*
see also palpation
Associated acupuncture points, 82, 83,
84*f*, 84*t*
associated techniques, 36, 155–202
asymmetry, 255
ATP *see* adenosine triphosphate
Atreya, 276
autonomic activity, 249–250
autonomic effects, trigger points, 61
axon transport, 6
Ayur-veda, 275, 276
nadis, 278–279, 282

B

back
muscles, 20
Thai massage, 285–286
see also spinal treatment, Lief's basic
back pain
abdominal disorders causing, 149*b*
see also low back pain
Baldry, P
abdominal reflex areas, 145
fibromyalgia and myofascial pain
syndrome, 71
trigger points, 14–15, 80
Beal, Myron, 53–55
behavioural factors, soft tissue
dysfunction, 13
bending loading, 186
Bennett's neurovascular (NV) reflexes,
84–86, 117, 118*f*, 119*b*
abdominal region, 145
Bigelow, N, 49–50
Bimbisara, King, 276
biochemical influences, 222–223, 222*t*
biomechanical influences, 222–223,
222*t*
biomechanical terms, 24*b*
bladder dysfunction, 102*f*, 103*b*, 143
blood pressure, 87
bloodless surgery, 161, 189–192, 190*f*
Boas' point, 82
bones, 258
brachial plexus, 235
Bradley, Dinah, 67–68
bradykinin, 14, 16
breathing function
compound stress influences, 69
trigger point monitoring, 67–68
see also hyperventilation
breathing retraining, 206, 209, 215

Brewer's point, 82
British College of Osteopathic
Medicine, 38
Buddhism, 276, 277
Butler, D, 6, 8–9

C

C bend technique, 187, 187*f*, 287–288
Thai massage, 287–288, 287*f*, 288*f*
calcium ions, 14–15, 60, 64
cardiovascular disease, 52
carotid artery, 238
carpal tunnel syndrome, 62
case records, 128–129
case reports of manual therapy,
304, 305*t*
central nervous system (CNS)
contradictory reporting to, 5
reporting stations, 3–4, 3*b*
central sensitization, 17, 50–51
cerebral birth injury, 174
cerebrospinal fluid, 280
cervical lamina supine, NMT American
version™, 234–236, 237*f*
chain fibres, 4, 252, 269
Chaitow, Boris, 36, 275
abdominal release techniques, 189,
191–192
Chapman's reflexes, 86, 110
INIT hypothesis, 216–217
NMT development, 37–38, 40
NMT methods, 125
positional release techniques, 194
skin rolling method, 184–185
spinal treatment, 139
trigger points, 67
Chaitow, Leon, 253, 275–276
c-bend technique, 287
NMT American version™,
222–224
Champneys, 35–36
Chapman's neurolymphatic reflexes,
86–89
abdomino-pelvic NMT, 144, 144*f*
acupuncture points and, 80
characteristics, 86
clinical value, 86–87, 89
diagnosis and treatment, 110–117
explaining results of NMT, 87
groupings, 116–117
Lief's basic spinal NMT, 132, 137,
139, 139*b*
location, 111*t*, 114*f*, 115*f*, 116*f*
mechanisms, 87
Nimmo's dismissal of, 88–89
palpation, 89

research evidence, 87–88
treatment, 89, 253–254
chill-and-stretch techniques, 64, 67,
157–160, 159*f*, 209
Chinese medicine, traditional
see traditional Chinese medicine
chiropractic
Nimmo's work and, 41–42,
292–299, 298*f*, 298*t*
positional release techniques, 194
trigger point and myofascial pain
syndrome management,
299–300, 301*f*
chronic pelvic pain (CPP), 153–154,
207–208
clasp-knife reflex, 270
clinical practice, 203–219
evidence-based recommendations,
305, 309–310, 310*t*
guidelines on manual therapy, 303,
305*t*
indications for NMT, 213–215
clinical reviews of manual therapy,
304–305, 305*t*
Cohen, Jeffrey, 291–299
collagen, 39, 280
colonic dysfunction, 143
compartment syndrome, 47
complementary and alternative
medical (CAM) therapies, 300
compression
American NMT, 227
flat, 227, 228*f*
ischaemic (static) *see* ischaemic
compression
loading, 186
with manipulation, 227
pincer, 227, 228*f*
trigger points, 64, 65*b*, 66*b*, 66*f*
see also pressure
connective tissue, 280, 281
chemical structure, 39
as communication system, 77
deformation characteristics, 28–29
function of circulation, 39–40
involvement in NMT, 38–40
network, 22–30
responses to stress, 10–11, 12
connective tissue massage/
manipulation (CTM), 89–93, 103
assessment methods, 105–109, 107*f*,
108*f*
chronic pelvic pain, 154
method and mechanism, 90
connective tissue zones (of
dysfunction), 101–103, 102*f*, 103*b*
Lief's basic spinal NMT, 135, 137,
139*b*

constipation, 87, 102f, 103b
contextual thinking, 203–205
contract–relax (CR), 166
contract–relax agonist–contract
    (CRAC), 166
contractures, localized, 99
corkscrew technique, 236–238, 238f
Council on Chiropractic Guidelines
    and Practice Parameters
    (CCGPP), 299, 301f
craniosacral therapy, 27–28, 194
cranium, posterior, NMT American
    version™, 234, 236f
creep, 24, 27
Crohn's disease, 149
cross-fibre friction, 164
cross-talk, neural, 5
crystalline properties, living systems,
    27, 28f
Cyriax, James, 22, 254
cystitis, interstitial (IC), 142b, 153

D

de qi, 282
deep tissue release, 160–161, 161f
deformation characteristics, connective
    tissue, 28–29
DeLany, Judith
    NMT American version™, 40–41,
        221–246
    trigger points, 67
dermatomes, 104, 105f
diagnostic methods, 97–122
    see also assessment; palpation
diastasis recti, 153
digestive disorders, 143
disuse muscular atrophy, low back
    pain, 20
Dittrich, R.J., referred phenomena, 46
Dowling, Denis, 36, 50, 124, 247–274
Dvorak & Dvorak, referred
    symptomatology, 44
dynamic neutral, 194
dyspareunia, 153

E

ease, position of, 193–194, 193f,
    251–252
effleurage, 164, 226, 226f, 227
elastin, 39
elbow technique, 156–157, 157f
electroacupuncture according to Voll
    (EAV), 82
electrotherapy, 306, 307t, 308, 309

emotional factors
    NMT American version™, 223–224
    sensitization, 52
    soft tissue dysfunction, 12
    treatment approaches and, 206–207
emotional release, 207, 215
end points, PINS technique, 256, 257t,
    258
endocannabinoids, 77–78, 169, 170
endomysium, 23, 281
endorphins, 79, 81, 169
energy concepts, 25–26, 27b
enkephalins, 79, 81
enthesopathy/enthesitis, 60
epicondylitis, 62
epimysium, 281
erector spinae, 20
    c-bend technique, 287, 287f
    NMT American version™, 242–244,
        243f
European (Lief's) neuromuscular
    technique, 9b, 123
    abdominal release methods,
        189–192
    aims, 9
    basic spinal treatment, 129–140
    Chapman's reflexes and, 87
    history, 37–38
    vs American NMT, 244–246
    see also Lief, Stanley
evaluation before treatment, 205–207
    see also assessment
Evans, Howard, 124, 275–290
Evans, J., reflex pain, 46
exercise therapy, 308
extracellular matrix, 39
extrafusal fibres, 178f, 252, 269–270
eye
    assessing dominant, 102b
    symptoms, 46–48

F

facilitated positional release (FPR),
    252–253
facilitating methods, 194
facilitation, 17, 50, 51–56
    causes of local, 55–56
    Korr's research, 52, 53f
    palpatory assessment, 54–55, 55f
    segmental (spinal), 51
    tension headache, 52–53
    trigger points as areas of local,
        51–56, 208
fascia, 280, 281
    biomechanical terms, 24b
    as communication system, 77

energy and changes in, 25–26
    functional continuities, 24–25
    layers, 281
    network, 22–30
    PINS technique, 257
    stress responses, 26–30
    stretching methods, 188–189
fascial planes, Rolfing, 279–280
fatigue, back muscles, 20
fetal position, influences of, 17–19
fibromyalgia, 15
    connective tissue massage, 89
    diagnostic criteria, 70
    mechanisms of pain, 17, 48–49, 52
    pathophysiology, 69–71
    sites of tender points, 70–71, 70f
    terminology, 22
    vs myofascial pain syndrome, 71,
        72t
fibrosis, 22
    interneural, 8
    palpatory diagnosis, 100–101
    subfascial tissue, 46
fibrositis, 22, 48
    pathophysiology, 69–71
    see also fibromyalgia
fibrotic change, 211
    mechanisms, 11, 15
    therapeutic approaches, 15, 22, 211
finger technique, NMT, 127–128, 127f
flexor carpi radialis, c-bend technique,
    288f
flight or fight response, 249–250
flower spray receptors, 4, 178f, 252, 269
forearm technique, 156
friction
    American NMT, 227
    transverse or cross-fibre, 164
    vibration and, 164
frozen shoulder, 62
functional genomics, 7
functional pathology of locomotor
    system, 165, 211
functional positional release
    approaches, 36
functional technique, 194, 253

G

gall bladder dysfunction, 102f, 143, 149
gamma-motor neurons (γ-efferents), 4,
    178f, 252–253
    massage, 164
    PINS technique, 269
gastric ulcer, 82
gastrointestinal dysfunction, 48
gender differences, pain sensitivity, 14

gene expression, neural influences, 6–8, 7b
general adaptation syndrome (GAS), 10–11, 40
genomics, functional, 7
Gibbons, Russell W, 291, 292–299
gliding techniques, American NMT, 226, 226f, 227
global factors, 222–223
Goetz, Eduard, 251
Golgi end-organs, 3
Golgi tendon receptors (organs), 3–4, 178f
    massage therapy, 165
    muscle energy technique, 167, 168f
    PINS technique, 270
    proprioceptive adjustment, 177, 177f
Goodheart, George, 79, 133, 137
greater occipital nerve, 265, 265f
ground substance, 39
Gutstein, R, 46–49, 143
gynaecological dysfunction, 143

H

habituation, 268–269
hamstring problems, 212–213
hand, practitioner's non-treating, 129
Hatha Yoga, 278–279
head, connective tissue zones, 102f, 103b
headache
    connective tissue zones, 102f
    hyperalgesic skin zones, 185
    migraine, 261–266, 263f, 264f, 266f
    muscle tension/contraction component, 263–264
    PINS, 248–249
    tension, 52–53, 61
Head's zones, 81
heart disease, 102f, 103b
hiatus hernia, 149
high-velocity, low-amplitude (HVLA) mobilization, 267–268
hip pain, 266–268, 267f, 268f
histiocytes, 24
history taking, 121
Ho, Mae-Wan, 27
hormones, 39–40
5-hydroxytryptophan, 47
hyperalgesic skin zones (HSZ), 185
    assessment, 104–109, 109f
    treating overlying tissues, 185–186, 186f, 189
hypermobility, 13–14
hypertonicity, muscle, 11, 248

inhibition therapy, 249
    Nimmo's views, 295–296
    PINS technique, 258, 270
hyperventilation, 69, 204–205
hysteresis, 24
hysteria, 49–50

I

ice-chilling, 158–160
ileitis, 143
iliolumbar ligament, NMT American version™, 241–242, 242f
iliotibial band (ITB)
    c-bend technique, 287–288, 288f
    case study, 267–268, 267f
    friction syndrome, 196
    Ober's test, 196
    studies, 197f, 198, 198f
    techniques, 187, 196–198, 196f
Illi, Frederick W, 293
increased tolerance to stretch, 169
indications for NMT, 213–215
induration, 99
    technique, 161–162, 162f
inflammation, 16, 29–30, 47
inflammatory soup, 14
Ingber, Donald, 23
inhibition, 164, 249–251
    Nimmo's receptor-tonus method, 291–292
    possible mechanism of action, 268–271
    see also progressive inhibition of neuromuscular structures; reciprocal inhibition
INIT see integrated neuromuscular inhibitor technique
insertions, muscle, 133, 257
integrated neuromuscular inhibitor technique (INIT), 67, 162, 216–217
    methods, 216–217, 216f, 217f
integrins, 7, 280
intercostal muscles
    European NMT, 135, 148–150, 149f
    NMT American version™, 240–241, 241f
interosseous ligaments, 257
interspinales, 20
interstitial cystitis (IC), 142b, 153
intertransversari, 20
intrafusal fibres, 4, 178f, 252
irritable bowel syndrome (IBS), 87
irritation, 210
ischaemia
    localized, 15, 16

NMT American version™, 223–224
PINS technique, 269
within trigger points, 60, 64
ischaemic compression (trigger point release), 42, 162–163, 227
    pressure considerations, 66b, 229
    research evidence, 302
    technique, 65b, 66f, 229–230
isolytic contraction, 170
    iliotibial band, 197–198
    INIT methods, 217
isometric contractions, 166
    iliotibial band, 197
    INIT methods, 216–217, 216f, 217f
    pulsed, 170
    trigger point treatment, 209
isotonic contraction, concentric, 170
isotonic eccentric contraction
    rapid, 170
    slow, 170
isotonic eccentric stretch, 170

J

Jivaka Kumar Bhaccha, 276, 277
joints, 258
    mobility tests, 121
    as sources of muscular pain, 14, 15
    stability, 30
    treatment approaches, 206
    trigger point-related restriction, 62, 62t
Jones' tender points, 44, 90–93, 91f, 92f, 93f
    abdominal region, 145, 151, 152b
    spinal region, 137
    strain/counterstrain approach, 194, 248, 251–252
jump sign, 56, 59, 63

K

Kellgren, J.H, 45
kidney dysfunction, 143
kneading, 164
knee problems, 212–213
Korr, Irwin
    facilitation, 52, 53f
    somatic dysfunction, 4–5, 6–7, 7b, 8

L

Lake, Thomas, 293
Langevin, Helene, 77, 281–282
laser therapy, 306, 307t, 308, 309

lateral rectus sheath, 151
latissimus dorsi syndrome, 46
leg, Thai massage, 283–284, 283*f*, 284*f*
legs
    arterial disease, 102*f*, 103*b*
    venous lymphatic disturbance,
        102*f*, 103*b*
levator scapulae, NMT American
    version™, 231–232, 232*f*
Lewit, K
    C and S bends, 187
    functional pathology of the
        locomotor system, 165, 211
    hyperalgesic skin zones, 105, 185
    skin distraction method, 109, 109*f*
Lief, Peter, 38
    general vs specific approach, 209–210
    palpation, 100
Lief, Stanley, 38
    abdominal release techniques,
        189–192
    general vs specific approach, 209–210
    NMT development, 35–36, 37–38,
        40, 275
    NMT methods, 125
    skin rolling method, 184–185
    see also European (Lief's)
        neuromuscular technique
ligamentous attachments, 258
ligaments, 30
linea alba, treatment, 153
Littlejohn, J. Martin, 251
liver dysfunction, 102*f*, 103*b*, 143
liver pump technique, 182*f*, 183–184
load, 24
Loban, Joy, 293
local adaptation syndrome (LAS),
    10–11, 40
locally dysfunctional states, 222–223
long-term potentiation, 51
low back pain
    abdominal disorders, 149*b*
    Chapman's reflexes and, 87
    role of muscles, 19–20
    therapeutic choices, 20–21
    trigger points, 62
lubrication, skin, 128–129, 225
lymphatic pump techniques, 181–184,
    182*f*
lymphatic stasis, 61
lymphatic system, physiology, 88

M

McBurney's point, 75–76, 82, 89
McConnell, Carl, 2
McKenzie exercises, 194

Mackenzie's abdominal reflex areas,
    104, 104*f*, 106*f*
magnet therapy, 307, 307*t*, 309
Maitland, G, 8–9
Manaka, Yoshio, 281
Mann, Felix, 75–76, 93
massage, 163–166
    research evidence, 302
    see also Thai massage
mechanical interface (MI), 8, 9
mechanotransduction, 77
medical acupuncture model, 14–15
Mennell, J., trigger points, 67
menopausal symptoms, 48
Mense and Simons, causes of muscle
    pain, 16, 17, 47*b*
mesentery, attachment stress, 146–148,
    147*f*, 148*f*
MET *see* muscle energy technique
mid-lumbar syndrome, 46
mid-sacral syndrome, 46
mid-thorax, posterior, NMT American
    version™, 232–234, 233*f*
migraine headache, 261–266, 263*f*, 264*f*,
    266*f*
mobility tests, 121
mobilization, before rehabilitation, 13
mobilizers, 18
monoarticular muscles, 19
motor units, selective involvement, 10*b*
Moule, Terry, 36, 211–213
Moule, Tom, 36, 211–212
multifidus, 20
multijoint muscles, 19
muscle(s)
    categorization, 18*b*
    multijoint or monoarticular, 19
    origins and insertions, 133, 257
    stabilizers and mobilizers, 18
    see also phasic muscles; postural
        muscles
muscle energy technique (MET), 36,
    123, 166–171
    alternative versions, 170–171, 171*f*
    definition, 166
    iliotibial band, 197–198
    integrated use *see* integrated
        neuromuscular inhibitor
        technique
    joint problems, 206
    low back problems, 20–21
    mechanisms, 166–170, 168*f*
    origins, 166, 166*f*
    sequencing of therapy, 172
    stretching time, 171
    trigger point treatment, 67, 209
muscle fibre types, 18, 20
muscle spasm

mechanisms, 16, 17
    paraspinal, 20
muscle spindles, 4, 178*f*
    damage, 6
    facilitated positional release, 252–253
    massage, 164, 165
    PINS technique, 269–270
    proprioceptive adjustment, 177,
        177*f*, 178*f*
    strain/counterstrain, 252
    trigger points, 64
muscle tone, 30
    see also hypertonicity, muscle
muscle tonus, 294–295, 295*f*
muscular pain
    causes, 47*b*
    local, 47
    mechanisms, 14–17
    medical acupuncture model, 14–15
    neuropathic, 47
    subgroups, 15–16
    see also somatic dysfunction
muscular tension, pain from, 48
musculoskeletal system, 2
Myers, T, 24–25, 25*f*, 26*f*
myodysneuria, 46–49
    pathophysiology, 69–71
    see also fibromyalgia
myofascia, 281
myofascial massage, Thai massage as,
    286
myofascial meridians, 24–25
myofascial pain, 15
myofascial pain syndrome (MPS)
    chiropractic management, 299–300,
        301*f*
    clinical practice recommendations,
        305, 309–310, 310*t*
    fibromyalgia and, 71, 72*t*
myofascial pathways, 279–282
myofascial release (MFR), 188–189
    cautions, 189
    methodology, 188–189, 188*f*
    research evidence, 302
    S and C bends, 186–188, 187*f*
    stages or levels, 188
myofascial trigger points *see* trigger
    points
myopia, 46
myotendinotic changes, 270
myotherapy, Bonnie Prudden, 254
myotomes, reflex, 104, 104*f*

N

nadis, Ayur-vedic, 278–279, 282
naprapathy, American, 161

naturopathy, 35–36
needling, 79, 211, 308
nerve(s)
    connecting primary and end points, 256
    deformations, 8
    influences on gene expression, 6–8, 7b
    irritation, 14
    lesions/dysfunction, causing muscle pain, 47
    transport, 6
nerve growth factors (NGFs), 6
nerve root syndromes, 43–44
neural cross-talk, 5
neural entrapments/compressions, 223–224
neural movement, abnormal, 8–9
neural reporting stations, 3–4, 3b, 178f
neural tension, adverse, 8–9
neurolymphatic reflexes, Chapman's
    see Chapman's neurolymphatic reflexes
neuromuscular lesion, 38, 100
neuromuscular technique (NMT), 9, 9b, 35–42, 247–248
    aims, 9, 124b
    associated approaches, 36, 155–202
    basic, 123–140, 141–154
    clinical use, 203–219
    commonly used approaches, 125
    defining, 123–124
    finger technique, 127–128, 127f
    general vs specific, 209–210
    historical overview, 35–38
    low back problems, 20–21
    sequencing of therapy, 172
    site of application, 38–39
    thumb technique, 125–127, 126f
    tissues involved, 38–42
    unique aspects, 124–125
    use of lubricant, use of, 128–129
    see also American neuromuscular therapy; European (Lief's) neuromuscular technique
neuromuscular therapy (NMT), American version™
    see American neuromuscular therapy
neuropeptides, 16
neurotrophic function, 6, 7, 8
neurovascular (NV) reflexes see Bennett's neurovascular reflexes
Nimmo, Raymond L, 36, 124–125, 291, 300
    on Chapman's reflexes, 88–89
    chiropractic perspectives, 41–42, 292–299, 298f, 298t

evolution of trigger point therapy, 292–299, 296f, 297f
    influence on American NMT, 40–41, 221–222
    receptor-tonus (RT) method, 40, 291–292, 293, 294–296, 297–299
NMT see neuromuscular technique
NMT American version™ see American neuromuscular therapy
nociception, positional release therapy and, 195
nociceptors
    causes of irritation, 14
    sensitization, 15, 16–17, 47
norepinephrine (NE), 185
Northup, George, 75
noxious generative points (NGPs), 40–41, 294
    see also trigger points
nuclear bag fibres, 4, 252, 269
nuclear chain fibres, 4, 252, 269
nutritional factors, 223–224

O

Ober's test, 196
occipital release exercises, 302
occipitalis muscle, 234
oedema, 16, 99
ophthalmic division, trigeminal nerve, 265, 265f
organ dysfunction
    basic abdomino-pelvic NMT, 143
    connective tissue zones, 101–103, 102f, 103b
    Mackenzie's abdominal reflex areas, 104, 106f
    segmental associations, 54
origins, muscle, 133, 257
Oschman, J., energy concepts, 26, 27b
osteopathic lesion, 51
osteopathy, 248
    facilitation, 50, 51–56
    fascial changes, 26
    history, 250–251
    inhibition, 249
    muscular pain, 15
    point and/or pressure techniques, 251–254
    STAR or TART, 59–60
ovarian dysfunction, 143

P

Pacinian corpuscles, 3–4, 30
pain
    assessment, 256

identifying sources, 2
    mechanisms, 47b
    patterns, 43–51
    radicular, 43–44
    receptors see nociceptors
    reduction, static compression, 229
    referred see referred pain and symptoms
    static compression, 229
    see also muscular pain
pain–spasm–pain cycle, 16, 17
pain threshold
    acupressure and, 79
    individual variations, 14
pain zones
    essential, 59
    spill-over, 59
palpation, 98–104
    Chapman's neurolymphatic points, 89
    deeper, 100
    diagnostic, 98f, 99–103
    facilitated spinal tissues, 54–55, 55f
    skin assessment, 99
    trigger points, 62–63
parasympathetic activity, 250
Parkinson's disease (PD), 266
patient positioning, 54–55, 129
    abdomino-pelvic NMT, 147, 148
    NMT American version™, 231, 233b, 234
    PINS technique, 259
patterns
    pain, 43–51
    somatic dysfunction, 3
    of use, functional, 12
pectoralis minor release, 179–181, 181f
pedal lymphatic pump technique, 182f, 184
pelvic disease, 142b
pelvic pain, chronic (CPP), 153–154, 207–208
percussion techniques, 172–175
    soft tissue treatment, 172–173
    traditional Chinese medicine (TCM), 173–174, 173f
    Western, 174–175, 174f
perimysium, 23, 281
periosteal acupuncture, 93, 94t
periosteal pain points, 14, 93, 94t, 133
petrissage, 164
phasic muscles, 6, 18
    fetal position, 19
    list of major, 21–22
    responses to stress, 17, 18

physical therapy, positional release techniques, 194
physiological factors, soft tissue dysfunction, 12
PINS *see* progressive inhibition of neuromuscular structures
piriformis muscle syndrome, 175
piriformis muscle technique, 157, 175–177, 176*f*
piston thrust method, iliotibial band, 196*f*, 197
point and/or pressure techniques
    non-osteopathic, 254
    osteopathic, 251–254
portal circulatory dysfunction, 143
positional release techniques (PRT), 193–195
    abdominal muscles, 151, 152*b*
    hyperalgesic skin zones, 185–186, 186*f*
    methodology, 174–177, 193–194
    proposed mechanisms, 195
    safety, 194–195
positioning, patient *see* patient positioning
post-isometric relaxation (PIR), 60, 167, 168*f*
posterior cranium, NMT American version™, 234, 236*f*
posterior mid-thorax, NMT American version™, 232–234, 233*f*
postural/biomechanical dysfunctions, 223–224
postural muscles, 6, 18
    fetal position, 17–19
    list of major, 21, 21*f*, 22
    responses to stress, 17, 18
postural re-education, 206, 209, 215
posture
    balanced and imbalanced, 29*f*
    practitioner's, 126, 129–130, 130*f*
practice guidelines on manual therapy, 303, 305*t*
practitioners
    non-treating hand, 129
    posture, 126, 129–130, 130*f*
pranatherapy, 275
pressure
    acupuncture points, 82, 83
    algometrics, 66*b*
    American NMT, 229
    application variables, 186–187
    Bennett's neurovascular points, 85
    Chapman's neurolymphatic reflexes, 110–116
    digital assessment, 97, 98*f*
    forms of direct therapeutic, 186
    Lief's basic NMT, 126

mechanisms of action, 269
Nimmo's receptor-tonus method, 291, 292
PINS technique, 258, 259, 269–270
proprioceptive adjustment, 177
threshold, 66
variable, 125, 128, 131–132
see also compression; point and/or pressure techniques
pressure bars, 225, 226*f*, 228*f*, 230
prevertebral muscles, 20
primary points, PINS, 256, 257*t*, 258
progressive inhibition of neuromuscular structures (PINS), 36, 124, 247–274
    application, 261–268
    background, 248–249
    contraindications, 271
    method, 254–268
    possible mechanism of action, 268–271
    procedure, 255–261
    side-effects, 271
proprioception
    mechanisms altering, 5–6
    muscle spindle function, 4
    positional release therapy and, 195
proprioceptive adjustment, 177, 177*f*
proprioceptive neuromuscular facilitation (PNF), 60, 123, 166
prostaglandins, 14, 16
prostatic dysfunction, 143
Prudden, Bonnie, myotherapy, 254
pseudoradicular syndromes, 44
psoas techniques, 178–179, 180*f*
psychological factors, pain perception, 17
psychosocial influences, 222–223, 222*t*
pudendal nerve, 175–176
pulsations, abdominal, 148*b*
pulsed isometric contractions, 170
pump techniques, 181–184

Q

quadratus lumborum, NMT American version™, 244, 245*f*
quantum theory, 27

R

Rabagliatti, Dr, 37, 38–39
radicular pain, 43–44
randomized controlled trials (RCTs)
    manual therapies, 295*f*, 302, 303–305, 305*t*

other conservative therapies, 308
receptor-tonus (RT) method (Nimmo), 40, 291–292, 293, 294–296, 297–299
reciprocal inhibition (RI), 60, 167, 168*f*
recommendations, evidence-based, 305, 309–310, 310*t*
records, case, 128–129
rectal sheath, treatment, 148–150
rectus capitis posterior, precautions, 234
rectus femoris muscle, c-bend technique, 287, 287*f*
referred pain and symptoms, 43–51
    as cause of muscle pain, 47–48
    difference to radicular pain, 43–44
    five variations, 44
    non-radicular patterns, 44–46, 45*f*
reflex arc
    normal, 295*f*
    physiopathological, 294–295, 295*f*, 296*f*
reflex patterns and areas, 75–78
reflex phenomena, 43–74, 248
    historical perspectives, 44–46
    models of generation, 44–50, 45*f*, 49*f*
reflex points, variety of, 75–96
reflexology, 254
rehabilitation, mobilization before, 13
Reich's armouring, 12–13
reporting stations, neural, 3–4, 3*b*, 178*f*
respiratory function, Chapman's reflexes and, 87
restriction of motion, 255
reticulin, 39
Rolf, Ida and Rolfing, 26, 254
    fascia, 279–280, 281
    Nimmo and, 293–294
    Thai massage and, 275–276, 288–289
rotation loading, 186
rotatores, 20
roulement, 164
Ruffini end-organs, 3

S

S bend technique, 187–188, 187*f*
sacroiliac dysfunction, assessment, 205
sacroiliac ligament, NMT American version™, 241–242, 242*f*
sacrospinalis, elbow technique, 156, 157*f*
SAID acronym, 13
scar tissue, 23, 109
    treatment, 143
    see also fibrosis

Schneider, Michael, 291–292, 299–300
SCS *see* strain/counterstrain
sebaceous dysfunction, 48
segmental associations, organ
    dysfunction, 54
segmental facilitation, 51
Selye, Hans, 10, 68–69, 81, 210–211
sen (treatment lines), 277–278, 282–283,
    282*f*
    acupressure points and, 136
    arm, 284–285, 284*f*, 285*f*
    Ayur-vedic nadis and, 278–279
    back, 285–286
    Chinese meridians and, 278
    leg, 283–284, 283*f*, 284*f*
    methods of working, 286
    myofascial pathways and, 279–282
sensitivity, 255
sensitization, 15, 16–17, 47
    central, 17, 50–51
    factors affecting susceptibility, 52
    mechanisms, 50*f*, 51–52
    tension headache and, 52–53
sensory receptors, muscles and joints,
    3–4, 3*b*
septa, 257
serratus posterior superior, NMT
    American version™, 232, 233,
    233*f*, 234*f*
shearing loading, 186
shiatsu, 254.
shoulder
    elbow technique, 156–157, 157*f*
    frozen, 62
    pain, 255
    trigger point-related restriction, 62,
    62*t*
side-lying position, NMT American
    version™, 233*b*, 234*f*
Simons, David, 40–41
    fibromyalgia vs myofascial pain
        syndrome, 71, 72*t*
    trigger points, 56, 59, 60*b*, 61–63, 64,
    76
    see also Mense and Simons
skin
    changes, 99
    characteristics, trigger points, 63
    distraction, 109, 109*f*
    folds, lifting, 105–106, 107*f*
    hyperalgesic zones *see* hyperalgesic
        skin zones
    lubrication, 128–129, 225
    palpatory assessment, 99
    reflex effects, 104–109
    rolling, 105, 184–186, 184*f*, 226
    techniques, 184–198
    trophic changes, 54

small intestinal dysfunction, 143
soft tissue
    adaptation, 211
    lengthening, myofascial release,
        186–188
soft tissue approaches
    additional, 155–171, 156*b*
    joint problems, 206
soft tissue distress, 1–34
    causes, 12–22
    energy and fascial considerations,
        25–26
soft tissue manipulation (STM),
    171–184
sol–gel properties, 26, 226
Solomonow, M, 30
somatic dysfunction, 2–12, 38, 247–248
    aetiological pathways, 50*f*
    defined, 2
    evolution over time, 10–11, 12
    identifying sources of pain, 2
    influences on evolution, 3–5, 6–9
    sequence of therapy, 172
somatovisceral reflexes, 142, 145
Spears, Leo, 293
Speransky, A.D., 44–45, 117, 210–211
spinal lamina groove, NMT American
    version™, 239–240, 240*f*
spinal treatment, Lief's basic, 129–140
    applications, 214
    completion, 139–140
    deactivating trigger points, 131–132
    duration, 133
    lateral thigh and gluteal structures,
        139
    left hip position, 137–139, 138*f*
    left-side trunk, 135, 136*f*
    lower thoracic/upper lumbar area,
        135–137, 137*f*
    mechanics/economy of effort,
        130–131
    neck region, 130–131, 131*f*, 132–135,
        133*f*
    origins and insertions, 133
    posterior reflex centres, 132–133
    practitioner's posture, 129–130, 130*f*
    right hip position, 138*f*, 139
    right-side trunk, 135–137, 136*f*
    trapezius and sternomastoid,
        134–135
    variable pressure, 131–132
spleen dysfunction, 143
spleen pump technique, 182*f*, 183–184
splenii tendons, NMT American
    version™, 236–238, 238*f*
spondylogenic reflexes, 44
spondylotherapy, 174–175, 174*f*
sports injuries, 211–213

spray-and-stretch technique, 157–158,
    159*f*
    research evidence, 302, 309
St John, Paul, 40–41, 221–222
stabilizers, 18
STAR mnemonic, 59–60, 255
static compression *see* ischaemic
    compression
sternocleidomastoid, NMT American
    version™, 238–239, 239*f*
sternomastoid muscle, European
    NMT, 132, 134–135
Still, Andrew Taylor, 250–251, 281
Still technique, 253
Stoddard, A, 15
stomach dysfunction, 102*f*, 103*b*, 143
strain (biomechanical), 24
strain/counterstrain (SCS), 90,
    193–195, 248, 251–252
    integrated use *see* integrated
        neuromuscular inhibitor
        technique
    mechanism of effect, 195
    research evidence, 302
stress
    biomechanical, 24
    connective tissue responses, 10–11,
        12
    fascial responses, 26–30
    flight or fight response, 249–250
    helpful role, 210–211
    hyperventilation, 69
    muscle responses to psychological,
        10*b*
    postural and phasic muscle
        responses, 17, 18
    reducing effects of massage,
        164–165
    trigger point production, 62, 68–69
stressor stimulus, 40
stretching, 28–29
    Bennett's neurovascular points, 85
    hyperalgesic skin zones, 109, 109*f*,
        185
    iliotibial band, 198–199, 198*f*
    increased tolerance to, 169
    myofascial release, 188–189, 188*f*
    PINS technique, 269–270
    proprioceptive adjustment, 177
    superficial tissue, assessment,
        106–109, 107*f*, 108*f*
    time in MET, 171
    trigger points, 60, 64–67
structural factors, soft tissue
    dysfunction, 13
suboccipital triangle, 235, 236*f*
substance P, 16
sudomotor changes, 48, 54

superficial back line, Myers', 24–25, 25f
superficial front line, Myers', 24–25, 26f
sweating, abnormal, 48
sympathetic nervous system, 87, 105, 146, 249–250
sympathetically mediated pain (SMP), 185
symphysis pubis, treatment, 151
synchronicity, 203–205
systematic reviews
    manual therapies, 301, 302–303, 305t
    other conservative therapies, 305–306, 307t, 308t, 309t

T

Tantrism, 278–279
tapotement, 164
TART acronym, 59–60
Tasker, Dain L, 251
taut bands, 16, 59, 60
temperature
    assessment, 97, 98f
    changes, 99
tender points
    fibromyalgia, 70–71, 70f
    Jones' see Jones' tender points
    strain/counterstrain approach, 193f, 194
    as trigger points, 76
tenderness, 99
tendomyosis, 44
tendon reflex, 4
tension headache, 52–53, 61
    see also headache
tension loading, 186
tensor fascia lata (TFL)
    shortening, 14
    techniques, 139, 196–198
    see also iliotibial band
Thai massage, 36, 124, 275–290
    acupressure points and, 136
    history and current status, 276–277
    as myofascial massage, 286
    NMT and, 287–288
    techniques, 283–286
    treatment lines see sen
Thai medicine, traditional, 277
Theravada Buddhism, 277
thermodynamics, soft tissue changes, 25–26
thermography, trigger points, 63b
thixotropy, 24, 25–26, 226
thoracic outlet, 134–135
thumb
    American NMT, 226f, 227

hypermobile, 127
Lief's basic spinal treatment, 129
technique, NMT, 125–127, 126f
tissue lifting techniques, 226
tissue texture changes, 255
tone, muscle, 30
    see also hypertonicity, muscle
tonus, muscle, 294–295
Torque unwinding, 253
traditional Chinese medicine (TCM)
    percussion methods, 173–174, 173f
    sen of Thai massage and, 278
    skin rolling method, 185
transcutaneous electrical nerve stimulation (TENS), 306, 307t, 309
transverse friction, 164
trapezius muscle
    European NMT, 134–135
    NMT American version™, 228f, 231
Travell, Janet
    central and attachment trigger points, 60b
    clinical signs of trigger points, 56, 62–63
    essential pain zone, 59
    features of trigger points, 64, 300
    influence on American NMT, 221–222
    mechanisms of pain genesis, 49–50
    Nimmo and, 40–42, 294, 297–298
    referred pain patterns, 56
    trigger point production, 62, 296, 297f
    trigger point therapy, 254, 296
trigeminal nerve, 265, 265f
trigger band technique, 253
trigger point release see ischaemic compression
trigger point therapy, 64–68, 208–209, 214
    alternatives to, 67–68, 68f
    attachment trigger points, 61
    basic abdomino-pelvic NMT, 142–143
    central trigger points, 60–61
    chill-and-stretch see chill-and-stretch techniques
    clinical practice, 214
    INIT methods, 162, 216–217, 216f, 217f
    ischaemic (static) compression see ischaemic compression
    Lief's basic spinal treatment, 131–132
    Nimmo's influence, 292–299, 296f, 297f
    percussion therapy, 172–175
    pressure considerations, 66b, 229
    recommendations, 305, 309–310, 310t

research evidence, 299–300, 301f, 305t, 306t, 307t, 308t, 309t
Travell's methods, 254, 296
vs acupuncture points, 78–86, 78f
vs other points, 211
trigger points (TrPs), 44, 56–69, 59f, 207–211
    abdominal region, 145
    active, 56, 59b
    as alarm signals, 204–205
    central and attachment, 59, 60b
    common sites, 57f, 59
    diagnosis, 62–63, 63b, 101
    distinguishing features, 76
    facilitation concepts, 51–56, 208
    features, 63–64
    fibromyalgia and, 71
    historical insights, 40–42, 44–50, 45f, 49f
    latent, 56, 59b
    mechanisms of pain genesis, 14–15, 16–17, 16f, 45f
    as monitors of function, 67–68
    neurotrophic flow effects, 8
    NMT American version™, 223–224
    non-pain symptoms, 61–62
    pain patterns, 43–51
    pelvic floor, 153, 154
    pelvic pain and, 207–208
    physiological role, 67, 204–205
    piriformis, 176, 176f
    production, 62, 62f, 296, 296f, 297f
    as repositioners, 204
    spinal region, 131–132, 134, 135, 139b
    stress burden and, 68–69
    tender points as, 76
trochanter, iliotibial band treatment over, 197
trophic changes, skin, 54
trophic neural influences, 6, 7, 8
tryptophan, 47
tsubo, 132–133, 136
twig snap method, iliotibial band, 196–197, 196f
Typaldos, Steven, 253

U

ultrasonography, iliotibial band, 197f, 198
ultrasound (US) therapy, 307, 307t, 309
umbilicus, treatment, 152–153
upper thoracic mobilization, pectoralis minor release, 179–181
ureteric dysfunction, 143
urgency–frequency syndrome, 142b

V

vapocoolant sprays, 157–158, 159*f*
Varma, Dewanchand, 37–38, 275
vasomotor changes, 48, 54
venous congestion, 16
venous lymphatic disturbance of legs, 102*f*, 103*b*
Vernon, Howard, 291, 299–300
vertebral artery, precautions, 234, 235*b*, 236*f*
vertebral veins, varicose, 149
vibration and friction, 164
visceroptosis effects, 146–148
viscerosomatic reflexes, 53–54, 55, 101
viscoelasticity, 24

viscoplasticity, 24
visual diagnosis, 102*b*
vulvar vestibulitis syndrome, 153

W

Wallace, Elaine, 253
Wat Pho, Bangkok, 276, 277
wind-up, 52
Wolff's law, 13, 22–23

X

X-signal system, 281

Y

Yoga, Hatha, 278–279
Youngs, Brian
  general vs specific approach, 209–210
  palpatory diagnosis, 100–101
  tissues involved in NMT, 38–40

Z

zones of dysfunction, connective tissue
  see connective tissue zones